ADVANCES IN Surgery

Editor-in-Chief
John L. Cameron

ELSEVIER

PHILADELPHIA LONDON TORONTO MONTREAL SYDNEY TOKYO

VOLUMES 1 THROUGH 57 (OUT OF PRINT)

VOLUME 59

VOLUME 58

Editor: Megan Ashdown (m.ashdown@elsevier.com)
Developmental Editor: Anirban Mukherjee

Reprints: For copies of 100 or more of articles in this publication, please contact the Commercial Reprints Department, Elsevier Inc., 360 Park Avenue South, New York, NY 10010-1710. Tel: (212) 633-3812; Fax: (212) 462-1935; E-mail: reprints@elsevier.com.

Publishing Office:
Elsevier Inc.
1818 Market Street,
Suite 3323
Philadelphia, PA 19103
United States

International Standard Serial Number: 0065-3411
International Standard Book Number: 978-0-443-47226-8

ADVANCES IN
Surgery

CONTRIBUTORS

EVAN T. ALICUBEN, MD, Assistant Professor of Cardiothoracic Surgery, Director for Thoracic Surgery Clinical Research, Director for Quality and Outcomes, Division of Thoracic and Foregut Surgery, University of Pittsburgh Medical Center, Pittsburgh, Pennsylvania, USA

ANDREA V. BARRIO, MD, FACS, Attending Surgeon, Breast Service, Department of Surgery, Memorial Sloan Kettering Cancer Center, New York, New York, USA

MATTHEW BARTEK, MD, MPH, General Surgeon, Critical Care Physician, and Palliative Care Physician, Division of Palliative Care and Geriatrics, Division of Trauma, Emergency Surgery, and Surgical Critical Care, Department of Surgery, Massachusetts General Hospital, Harvard Medical School, Boston, Massachusetts, USA

GEORGIA M. BEASLEY, MD, MHS, Associate Professor of Surgery with Tenure, Department of Surgery, Duke University Medical Center, Durham, North Carolina, USA

KAELA E. BLAKE, MD, FACS, Assistant Professor of Surgery, The University of Tennessee Health Sciences College of Medicine, Knoxville, Tennessee, USA

TYLER BOGACZYK, MD, Fellow, Division of Colon and Rectal Surgery, Department of Surgery, Lankenau Medical Center, Wynnewood, Pennsylvania, USA

ADOM BONDZI-SIMPSON, MD, MSc, Chief Resident, Department of Surgery, University of Toronto, Toronto, Ontario, Canada

CARLOS FERNANDEZ-DEL CASTILLO, MD, Professor of Surgery, Harvard Medical School, Jorge and Darlene Pérez Endowed Chair in Surgery, Director Emeritus, Pancreas and Biliary Surgery Program, Division of Surgical Oncology, Department of General Surgery, Massachusetts General Hospital, Boston, USA

MING-HUEI CHENG, MD, MBA, FACS, Professor and Chairman, A+ Surgery Clinic, Taipei, Taiwan

MIN-JEONG CHO, MD, Assistant Professor, Department of Plastic and Reconstructive Surgery, The Ohio State University, Columbus, Ohio, USA

IAN G. CHRISTIE, MD, Resident Physician, Division of Thoracic and Foregut Surgery, Department of Cardiothoracic Surgery, University of Pittsburgh, Pittsburgh, Pennsylvania, USA

KEVIN C. CHUNG, MD, MS, William C. Grabb Distinguished University Professor of Surgery, Charles B. G. De Nancrede Professor of Surgery, Plastic Surgery and Orthopaedic Surgery, Section of Plastic Surgery, University of Michigan Medical School, Ann Arbor, Michigan, USA

COURTNEY E. COLLINS, MD, FACS, Associate Professor of Surgery, Center for Abdominal Core Health, The Ohio State University College of Medicine, Columbus, Ohio, USA

ISABEL DeLAURA, MD, Resident, Department of Surgery, Duke University, Durham, North Carolina, USA

SAMEH HANY EMILE, MBBCh, MSc, MD, FACS, Professor, Department of Colorectal Surgery, Project Scientist, Ellen Leifer Shulman and Steven Shulman Digestive Disease Center, Cleveland Clinic Florida, Weston, Florida, USA

DINA M. FILIBERTO, MD, FACS, Associate Professor, Division of Trauma and Surgical Critical Care, Department of Surgery, University of Tennessee Health Science Center, Memphis, Tennessee, USA

DENISE W. GEE, MD, Associate Professor, Division of GI Surgery, Department of Surgery, Massachusetts General Brigham, Boston, Massachusetts, USA

JULIE HALLET, MD, MSc, Associate Professor, Division of General Surgery, Department of Surgery, University of Toronto, Research Chair in Patient-Centred and Quality Cancer Surgery, Toronto, Ontario, Canada

MOHAMMED HAMOUDA, MD, Postdoctoral Fellow, Division of Vascular and Endovascular Surgery, Department of Surgery, UC San Diego, La Jolla, California, USA

JON M. HARRISON, MD, Member of the Faculty, Section of Hepatobiliary and Pancreatic Surgery, Division of Surgical Oncology, Department of General Surgery, Massachusetts General Hospital, Boston, Massachusetts, USA

DANIEL I. HOFFMAN, MD, General Surgery Resident and Post-Doctoral Research Fellow, Center for Surgery and Public Health, Department of Surgery, Brigham and Women's Hospital, Boston, Massachusetts, USA

ANDREW J. KERWIN, MD, FACS, Professor of Surgery, Division Chief, Division of Trauma and Surgical Critical Care, University of Tennessee Health Science Center, Memphis, Tennessee, USA

SHOSHANA T. LEVI, MD, Fellow, Department of Surgical Oncology, The University of Texas MD Anderson Cancer Center, Houston, Texas, USA

HEATHER A. LILLEMOE, MD, FACS, Assistant Professor, Department of Surgical Oncology, Assistant Professor, Department of Breast Surgical Oncology, The University of Texas MD Anderson Cancer Center, Houston, Texas, USA

ELIZABETH J. LILLEY, MD, MPH, Assistant Professor of Surgery, Harvard Medical School, Affiliate Faculty, Surgical Oncologist and Palliative Care Physician, Department of Supportive Oncology, Center for Surgery and Public Health, Dana Farber Cancer Institute, Associate Surgeon, Division of Surgical Oncology, Department of Surgery, Brigham and Women's Hospital, Boston, Massachusetts, USA

JAMES D. LUKETICH, MD, Henry T. Bahnson Professor, Division of Thoracic and Foregut Surgery, Department of Cardiothoracic Surgery, University of Pittsburgh, Pittsburgh, Pennsylvania, USA

SAMUEL LUKETICH, Undergraduate Student, Department of Biology, University of Pittsburgh, Pittsburgh, Pennsylvania, USA

MAHMOUD B. MALAS, MD, MHS, RPVI, FACS, Professor and Chief, Joan Klein Jacobs Endowed Chair in Surgery, Director of Center for Learning and Excellence in Vascular and Endovascular Research (CLEVER), Division of Vascular and Endovascular Surgery, Department of Surgery, UC San Diego, La Jolla, California, USA

ELIZABETH A. MANNINO, MD, Surgical Critical Care Fellow, Division of Trauma and Surgical Critical Care, Department of Surgery, University of Tennessee Health Science Center, Memphis, Tennessee, USA

JOHN MARKS, MD, FACS, FASCRS, Professor, Division of Colon and Rectal Surgery, Department of Surgery, Lankenau Medical Center, Wynnewood, Pennsylvania, USA

JOHN MIGALY, MD, FASCRS, FACS, Mark M Ravitch Endowed Professor, Chair of the Division of Colon and Rectal Surgery, The Johns Hopkins Hospital, Baltimore, Maryland, USA

AVIHAI MOSCOVICI, MD, Fellow, Division of Colon and Rectal Surgery, Department of Surgery, Lankenau Medical Center, Wynnewood, Pennsylvania, USA

MARGARET H. O'CONNOR, MD, PhD, General Surgery Resident, Department of Surgery, Duke University Medical Center, Durham, North Carolina, USA

MARCO PAPPALARDO, MD, MSc, PhD, Associate Professor of Plastic Surgery, Division of Plastic and Reconstructive Surgery, Department of Medical and Surgical Sciences, University of Modena and Reggio Emilia, Italy

KATE R. PAWLOSKI, MD, MPH, Assistant Attending Surgeon, Breast Service, Department of Surgery, Memorial Sloan Kettering Cancer Center, New York, New York, USA

ARJUN PENNATHUR, MD, Professor of Cardiothoracic Surgery, Sampson Family Endowed Chair in Thoracic Surgical Oncology, Division of Thoracic and Foregut Surgery, University of Pittsburgh Medical Center, Pittsburgh, Pennsylvania, USA

BENJAMIN K. POULOSE, MD, MPH, FACS, Professor of Surgery and Robert M. Zollinger Lecrone-Baxter Chair, Chief of Division of General and Gastrointestinal Surgery, Center for Abdominal Core Health, The Ohio State University College of Medicine, Columbus, Ohio, USA

UZMA RAHMAN, MD, Fellow, Division of Cardiothoracic Surgery, The Johns Hopkins Hospital, Baltimore, Maryland, USA

AMANDA DOOLEY ROMERO, MD, Surgical Critical Care Fellow, Division of Trauma and Surgical Critical Care, Department of Surgery, University of Tennessee Health Science Center, Memphis, Tennessee, USA

CLAIRE B. ROSEN, MD, MSME, Fellow, Division of GI Surgery, Department of Surgery, Massachusetts General Brigham, Boston, Massachusetts, USA

ANTHONY T. SAXTON, MD, General Surgery Resident, Department of Surgery, Duke University, Durham, North Carolina, USA

RANDALL P. SCHERI, MD, Professor of Surgery, Duke University, Durham, North Carolina, USA

BRYAN SZEGLIN, MD, Halsted General Surgery Resident, Department of Surgery, The Johns Hopkins Hospital, Baltimore, Maryland, USA

BRANDON VU, MD, Fellow, Division of Colon and Rectal Surgery, Department of Surgery, Lankenau Medical Center, Wynnewood, Pennsylvania, USA

STEVEN D. WEXNER, MD, PhD (Hon), Professor and Vice Chair for Professional Development for the Department of Colorectal Surgery, Physician Executive Director and System Chair for Colorectal Surgery, Medstar Georgetown University Hospital, Washington, DC, USA

STEPHEN C. YANG, MD, FACS, MAMSE, Professor of Surgery and Oncology, The Arthur B. and Patricia B. Modell Endowed Chair of Thoracic Surgery, Vice Chair of Thoracic Surgery, Vice Chair of Professional Development, The Johns Hopkins Medical Institutions, Baltimore, Maryland, USA

KEVIN YEI, MD, Vascular Surgery Resident, Division of Vascular and Endovascular Surgery, Department of Surgery, UC San Diego, La Jolla, California, USA

ADVANCES IN
Surgery

CONTENTS

VOLUME 60 • 2026

limiting inflammation to severe peritonitis. A paradigm shift in the treatment of uncomplicated diverticulitis has been noted, with cumulating evidence challenging the routine use of antibiotics. High-quality evidence suggests that antibiotics may be safely omitted in healthy patients with mild AD. Nonetheless, surgery remains the mainstay treatment of patients with generalized peritonitis or recurrent, debilitating disease. In summary, current guidelines recommend an individualized approach to AD, balancing disease severity, comorbidities, quality of life, and patient preference in decision-making.

Chronic limb-threatening ischemia is the most advanced stage of peripheral arterial disease and typically requires revascularization to prevent limb-loss. The choice of open surgical bypass versus endovascular therapy should be individualized based on patients' anatomy, operative risk, and conduit availability. Patients who are suitable candidates for both bypass and endovascular intervention and have an adequate single-segment great saphenous vein should undergo open surgical bypass based on level 1 evidence.

Landmark trials have demonstrated that residual microscopic disease in the undissected axilla does not translate to a higher risk of nodal recurrence, which laid the groundwork for trials examining the omission of axillary surgery. The SOUND and INSEMA randomized trials demonstrated no difference in disease-free survival in patients with small, cN0 breast cancer treated with or without sentinel lymph node biopsy (SLNB). Postmenopausal patients with luminal breast cancer undergoing lumpectomy with a normal preoperative axillary ultrasound are ideally suited for omission of SLNB, as systemic therapy decisions are increasingly based on genomic assays rather than pathologic nodal status.

The advent of potent immune checkpoint inhibitor and other targeted therapies has transformed neoadjuvant therapy into a potentially more efficacious treatment strategy overall. Administering immunotherapy before surgery can enhance the immune system's ability to target melanoma cells, utilize neoantigens, and treat clinically occult and metastatic disease. Furthermore, it provides an opportunity for assessment of treatment response based on pathologic assessment and ultimately leads to better survival rates, lower recurrence, and minimizes overuse of adjuvant treatments. Continued clinical trials will further elucidate best practices with respect to treatment duration, choice, and treatment strategies.

Lymphedema is one of the most difficult surgical conditions to treat because of the destruction of tenuous lymphatic system. Historically, nonsurgical management and debulking procedures were performed to reduce volume without correcting the underlying lymphatic physiology. With the recent advances in technologies, microsurgical treatments to re-establish the lymphatic system are becoming increasingly popular. Studies have reported the efficacy of these procedures in the treatment and prevention of lymphedema. This article strives to deliver an understanding of the current landscape on lymphedema surgery to increase access, promote early surgical intervention, and to offer guidance to patients beyond myths regarding lymphatic surgery.

The dramatic rise in thyroid cancer incidence in recent decades is driven primarily by the detection of small, biologically indolent papillary microcarcinomas rather than a true increase in clinically significant disease. Robust long-term data now show that active surveillance is a safe and effective initial strategy for appropriately selected low-risk patients, with very low rates of progression and oncologic outcomes comparable to immediate surgery. Reflecting this evidence, contemporary guidelines endorse active surveillance as an alternative to upfront resection, emphasizing shared decision-making, structured ultrasound monitoring, and clearly defined triggers for intervention, shifting modern thyroid cancer care toward individualized care minimizing overtreatment.

Sarcoma of the Breast: A Rare and Heterogeneous Entity 127

Shoshana T. Levi and Heather A. Lillemoe

Breast sarcomas are a rare and pathologically diverse group of malignancies. They can arise de novo or in a previously irradiated field and tend to have poor prognostic outcomes. Given their rarity and the tendency to combine the various histologies in single analyses, data related to management and prognostic outcomes are somewhat limited. Surgical resection remains the mainstay of treatment with the intention for wide-margin resection, except in the case of radiation-associated angiosarcoma, where radical resection is associated with improved local control. Multidisciplinary treatment is common and is ideally undertaken at a high-volume sarcoma center to optimize outcomes.

interrupted for procedures, or never initiated due to concern for bleeding from injury sites. Current evidence supports initiation of pharmacologic prophylaxis within 24 hours of admission to reduce the risk of venous thromboembolism. Initiation within 24 hours of admission appears to be safe with low risk of bleeding from injuries, including progression of intracranial hemorrhage.

Esophagectomy remains the standard therapy for localized esophageal cancer, but postoperative function depends heavily on effective gastric conduit emptying. The aperistaltic conduit located in the negative pressure thoracic cavity is at risk of delayed gastric emptying leading to aspiration and pulmonary complications. This article summarizes historical and contemporary evidence evaluating pyloroplasty and alternative pyloric drainage strategies during esophagectomy. While earlier trials produced mixed results, recent level I evidence supports pyloroplasty as a safe adjunct that reduces gastric outlet obstruction and postoperative interventions. Meticulous conduit construction and vigilant postoperative assessment remain essential. There continues to be controversy, and an ongoing randomized trial, The PYNI-GAREREO Phase III Trial of Pyloroplasty Vs. No Pyloroplasty will be completed in the near future. (Trials.2023 Jun 19;24:412) and will add further level 1 evidence to this controversy.

Despite signing a consent form, many surgical patients subsequently report gaps in understanding an operation, its alternatives, and its impact on everyday life. Observational studies, patient surveys, and audio-recordings of preoperative interactions suggest that surgeons reliably meet legal requirements for informed consent but less often achieve informed, preference-concordant decisions–especially for older adults facing high-risk procedures. Emerging tools such as structured decision aids, scenario-based frameworks, risk visualization, and patient-reported outcome measures can improve knowledge, expectations, and satisfaction. This article reviews the state of the science, highlights practical communication frameworks, and outlines persistent gaps and future directions.

Serous cystadenomas (SCA) are benign, and resection is generally reserved for symptomatic patients. Variations in radiographic appearance are common and can obscure the diagnostic picture. As such, many SCA are misdiagnosed and either observed or resected under the presumption of a mucinous cyst or another cystic pancreatic etiology. Improved diagnostics are needed as these will limit the number of unwarranted resections to a few true indications.

Anastomotic leaks (ALs) are a significant source of morbidity and mortality. Every step should be implemented to prevent AL, including careful patient selection, optimizing patient's clinical and nutritional status, and ensuring proper technique. The appropriate management of an AL depends on several factors, such as patient's clinical status, the type of surgery, location of the AL, induction therapies, and the resources available. Surgeons should be familiar with the armamentarium of treatment modalities available to manage AL and use a patient-tailored approach when selecting the most appropriate treatment.

Watch and Wait in Patients with Clinical Complete Response After Neoadjuvant Therapy with Rectal Cancer: Is it Safe? **271**

Bryan Szeglin and John Migaly

The treatment of locally advanced rectal cancer has been transformed over the last century with nearly 40% of patients achieving complete eradication of their tumor with total neoadjuvant therapy alone. Nonoperative management with a watch-and-wait approach has now allowed a subset of patients the chance to avoid surgery altogether with 50% of watch-and-wait patients achieving long-term organ preservation. However, the other half of patients develop either local regrowth, which requires expeditious surgical intervention, or distant recurrence. Watch-and-wait is a reasonable option for select patients in a protocolized environment that can successfully deliver the recommended surveillance protocol, which ensures its safety.

Surgery on Patients Taking Glucagon-Like Peptide-1 Receptor Agonists **285**

Claire B. Rosen and Denise W. Gee

This article begins by providing historical insight into the discovery, development, and use of glucagon-like peptide-1 receptor (GLP-1R) agonist medications in the treatment of type 2 diabetes and obesity. Next, the mechanism of action and impacts of GLP-1R agonists are discussed, along with an overview of the Food and Drug Administration–approved GLP-1R agonists currently on the market. Comparison in effects on weight loss of the available GLP-1R agonists is briefly discussed, along with its use in the context of bariatric surgery. Finally, perioperative considerations for surgical patients using GLP-1R agonists are reviewed along with suggested recommendations.

The treatment of locally advanced rectal cancer has been transformed over the last century. While initially treated with surgery alone, adjuvant therapy with chemotherapy and radiation became common for locally advanced disease to prevent local and distant recurrence. Several trials subsequently showed benefit to moving this therapy into the neoadjuvant setting which led to improved oncologic outcomes, greater compliance, and similar surgical morbidity. In this article, we will explore this historical transition to a total neoadjuvant approach that can lead to cure in select patients and brings into question the role of surgery altogether.

Advances in Surgery 60 (2026) 1–14

ADVANCES IN SURGERY

Robotic versus Laparoscopic Colectomy for Cancer

Avihai Moscovici, MD*, Tyler Bogaczyk, MD, Brandon Vu, MD, John Marks, MD, FASCRS

Division of Colon and Rectal Surgery, Department of Surgery, Lankenau Medical Center, 100 East Lancaster Avenue, Medical Science Building, Suite 375, Wynnewood, PA 19096, USA

Keywords

- Robotic colectomy • Laparoscopic colectomy • Colorectal cancer
- Minimally invasive surgery • Technology adoption

Key points

- Minimally invasive surgery (MIS) for colorectal cancer provides equivalent oncologic outcomes to open surgery, with reduced perioperative morbidity and faster recovery.
- Laparoscopic colectomy is widely used yet remains challenging due to technical constraints and a steep learning curve, particularly with complex anatomy or high-body mass index patients.
- Robotic platforms overcome many limitations of laparoscopy, facilitates intracorporeal anastomosis, lowers conversion rates, and may improve functional outcomes without compromising safety.
- Adoption of robotic surgery is expanding but remains limited by cost, setup time, and need for structured training.
- Emerging technologies, including single port, artificial intelligence–assisted guidance and flexible robotic platforms, are expected to further advance MIS and precision in colorectal surgery.

INTRODUCTION

The evolution of colorectal minimally invasive surgery (MIS) can trace its roots back to the origin of laparoscopic surgery. In the 1980s, laparoscopic surgery was initially used to manage and treat gallbladder disease [1]. Compared to a

*Corresponding author. *E-mail addresses:* mosko85@gmail.com; moscovicia@mlhs.org

https://doi.org/10.1016/j.yasu.2026.03.001
0065-3411/26/

Abbreviations

AI	artificial intelligence
CME	complete mesocolic excision
CRM	circumferential resection margin
MIS	minimally invasive surgery
SILS	single-incision laparoscopic surgery
SP	single-port
TME	total mesorectal excision

traditional cholecystectomy, patients who underwent laparoscopic cholecystectomy were found to have less postoperative pain, faster return of diet, decreased hospital length of stay, and earlier return to normal activity [2,3]. With these promising outcomes, there was hope that laparoscopy could be used for colorectal pathology as well and usher in a new era of colorectal surgery.

The first series of laparoscopic colon resections were reported by Fowler [4] and Jacobs [5] in 1991 who described the technique for laparoscopic sigmoid resection and showed successful disease management with this approach. Subsequent studies highlighted the benefits of laparoscopic colorectal surgery, which included shorter operative times, faster return of diet, and reduced hospital length of stay [6,7]. However, despite the perceived benefits, the utilization of laparoscopic colorectal surgery was initially limited due to a steep learning curve, absence of randomized controlled trials, and concerns about oncological outcomes [8,9]. The safety and efficacy was further evaluated in the literature and showed acceptable morbidity (24%) and mortality (0%), adequate lymph node retrieval, and reduced length of stay compared to converted or open cases [10].

The early excitement surrounding laparoscopic colorectal surgery eventually became overshadowed by reports of tumor implantation at trocar and extraction sites. These implantations were thought to be different from the wound implantations seen in cancer patients who underwent open colectomy. In light of these reports, trepidation regarding oncologic adequacy emerged, and some even called for abandoning laparoscopic colectomy in the treatment of colorectal cancer [11–13]. Concerns arose around the oncologic suitability of laparoscopic colectomy and led to much debate regarding dissection approaches (medial to lateral vs lateral to medial) and extraction techniques [14–16].

LAPAROSCOPIC COLECTOMY FOR COLON CANCER

These significant questions demanded an answer and set the stage for the COST trial (2004), which marked a pivotal point in the debate over laparoscopic colectomy for colon cancer. The multicenter COST study disproved many of the early concerns regarding the laparoscopic approach, showing comparable 3-year recurrence rates between laparoscopic and open colectomy (16% vs 18%) and demonstrating that laparoscopic colectomy achieves equivalent oncologic endpoints, which were not inferior to open surgery in curable colon cancer [17]. Beyond oncologic safety, laparoscopic colectomy conferred several short-term clinical advantages compared with open surgery. Randomized trials and meta-analyses have since demonstrated reduced intraoperative blood loss, lower postoperative pain scores, shorter ileus duration, and earlier return of bowel function. Laparoscopy also improved postoperative pulmonary function and reduced both total and surgical morbidity rates, confirming the physiologic benefit of a laparoscopic approach in perioperative recovery [18,19].

Long-term follow-up studies further reinforced the oncologic equivalence of MIS colectomy. The Barcelona trial revealed that the laparoscopic approach was more effective than open surgery for treatment of colon cancer in terms of morbidity, hospital stay, recurrence, and cancer-related survival [20]. A subsequent project, based on the COST study group, presented a prospective randomized trial with a median follow-up of 7 years. Five-year disease-free survival (open 68.4% vs laparoscopic 69.2%) and overall survival (74.6% vs 76.4%) were similar, with no significant differences in recurrence rates (21.8% vs 19.4%) [21].

Further validation came from the COLOR trial, which in 2017 reported comparable 10-year outcomes for laparoscopic and open colectomy in patients with nonmetastatic colon cancer [22]. Disease-free survival (open 43.2% vs laparoscopic 45.2), overall survival (46.7% vs 48.4%), and recurrence rates (28.2% vs 29.4%) remained equivalent at decade-long follow-up. These findings established MIS colectomy for curable colon cancer as noninferior to open surgery regarding long-term oncologic outcomes and provided the foundation for widespread adoption of laparoscopic colectomy as the standard of care (Table 1).

Given that surgery alone represents definitive therapy for stage I and II disease and is a central component to stage III colon cancer treatment, these

Table 1
Comparison of laparoscopic versus open colectomy outcomes over time

Study	Lap Disease Free Survival (DFS) (%)	Open DFS (%)	*P* value
Barcelona Trial [20] (2002)	90.6	79.4	.03
COST Trial [17] (2004)	72.9	72.7	.70
COST Follow Up [21] (2007)	69.2	68.4	.94
COLOR Trial [22] (2017)	45.2	43.2	.96
	Lap overall survival (%)	Open overall survival (%)	*P* value
Barcelona Trial [20] (2002)	82.1	73.5	.14
COST Trial [17] (2004)	86	85	.51
COST Follow Up [21] (2007)	76.4	74.6	.93
COLOR Trial [22] (2017)	48.4	46.7	.83
	Lap recurrence (%)	Open recurrence (%)	*P* value
Barcelona Trial [20] (2002)	17	27	.07
COST Trial [17] (2004)	16	18	.32
COST Follow Up [21] (2007)	19.4	21.8	.25
COLOR Trial [22] (2017)	29.4	28.2	.73

studies establishing laparoscopic colon cancer surgery as a standard of care are among the most important research performed in colon cancer therapy in the past generation [23].

With laparoscopic colectomy established for colon cancer, attention naturally turned to whether similar benefits existed in rectal surgery, where technical demands are greater given the constraints of the pelvis and neoadjuvant radiotherapy. In developed countries, rectal cancer accounts for approximately 28% to 35% of all colorectal cancer cases [24]. The introduction of total mesorectal excision (TME), as a standardized surgical dissection technique, was a crucial development that significantly reduced rates of local recurrence [25]. A positive circumferential resection margin (CRM) is a strong predictor of local recurrence and distant metastases. Proper TME and a macroscopic completely intact mesorectal envelope more accurately reflects adequacy of lymphadenectomy, and grading TME completeness serves as a reliable predictor of local recurrence [24].

Over time, the management of rectal cancer has undergone a considerable paradigm shift. Multimodal treatment plans and strategies incorporating neoadjuvant chemotherapy and/or radiotherapy followed by radical resection have become the standard of care for locally advanced rectal cancer [25]. The adoption of TME with neoadjuvant chemoradiotherapy has reduced locoregional recurrence rates to under 10% and increased cancer-free survival rates to over 70% [26]. As discussed previously over the last 3 decades, technological innovations have revolutionized surgical practice. The advancement of minimally invasive platforms capable of achieving cancer control comparable to open surgery through less invasive means have been demonstrated [25]. Laparoscopic rectal resection has been shown to promote faster recovery and reduce hospital stays without compromising oncologic outcomes [24]. However, laparoscopic pelvic dissection remains technically demanding, leading to increased postoperative sexual dysfunction and higher conversion rates compared to open surgery. Initial concerns regarding the feasibility of MIS for rectal cancer stemmed from the 34% conversion rate to open surgery seen in the CLASICC trial [27].

The ALaCaRT Randomized clinical trial (2015) was unable to demonstrate noninferiority of laparoscopic surgery compared with open surgery based on composite oncologic endpoints, such as negative CRM, negative distal margin, and complete TME [28]. Nevertheless, subsequent long-term results did not reveal any significant differences in survival outcomes. These preliminary findings raised concerns among surgeons regarding the adequacy of laparoscopic surgery and questioned its routine use for rectal cancer surgery [25].

However, the more recent ACOSOG Z6051 trial supported the equivalent long-term outcomes and demonstrated that laparoscopic resection for rectal cancer was not inferior to open surgery with respect to disease-free survival (lap 75.2% vs open 73.2%) and rates of local (lap 2.1%, open 1.8%) or distant (lap 14.6%, open) 16.7% recurrence (Table 2) [29].

Table 2
Comparison of outcomes between ALaCaRT [28] and ACOSOG [29] trials

Outcomes	ALaCaRT (n = 462)			ACOSOG (n = 473)		
	Lap Rectal Resection	Open Rectal Resection	*P* value	Lap Rectal Resection	Open Rectal resection	*P* value
Successful resection (%)	82	89	.38	81.7	86.9	.41
Distal margin negative (%)	99	99	.67	98.3	98.2	.91
CRM >1 mm (%)	93	97	.06	87.9	92.3	.11
Complete or nearly complete TME (%)	97	99	.06	92.1	95.1	.20

Despite the encouraging oncologic and short-term outcomes, the technical constraints of conventional laparoscopy: 2-dimensional vision, limited instrument articulation, and suboptimal ergonomics, continued to challenge precision and contribute to surgeon strain, particularly in complex cases. These limitations hampered MIS adoption for colorectal surgery and provided the impetus for robotic-assisted colorectal surgery, designed to enhance dexterity, visualization, overall operative control, and lower the barriers for widespread MIS adoption.

In 2009, inspired by Heald's TME principle for rectal cancer: removal of the tumor together with its intact mesentery and primary lymphatic drainage, Hohenberger introduced the concept of complete mesocolic excision (CME) for colon cancer. This technique emphasized sharp dissection along the embryologic planes to separate the mesocolon from the parietal fascia, combined with central vascular ligation of the supplying arteries and draining veins at their origins, thereby aiming to improve lymph node harvest and reduce local recurrence rates [30].

However, long-term systematic reviews and meta-analyses demonstrated that CME only provided superior 3-year overall survival in patients with Stage III colon cancer. The technique was associated with increased risk of vascular injury and longer operative time compared with conventional D2 laparoscopic colectomy [31–33].

ROBOTIC COLECTOMY FOR COLON CANCER

The development of robotic-assisted colectomy emerged in response to overcome the aforementioned obstacles. Robotic systems provide 3-dimensional magnified vision, aiding in accurate identification of critical anatomy [24]. Tremor filtration and articulated wristed instruments also have the potential to enhance dissection precision and control, which is particularly helpful in narrow spaces or in patients with high body mass index. In addition, the robotic console reduces surgeon strain and fatigue by minimizing the postural demands inherent to laparoscopy [34]. When comparing the learning curve between conventional laparoscopic and robotic approaches for right colectomy, the robotic technique was found to have a shorter learning curve, with a reduction in operative time observed after approximately 16 cases compared to 25 cases for laparoscopy [35].

In aggregate, these advances have served to promote the adoption of MIS approaches for a larger group of surgeons. In particular, the robotic platform has facilitated an intracorporeal anastomosis by simplifying this step compared with conventional laparoscopy, as intracorporeal sewing is far easier robotically. In a laparoscopic right colectomy, the intracorporeal stapled ileocolic anastomosis, compared with the extracorporeal approach, has been associated with fewer short-term complications, particularly surgical site infections, shorter hospital stay, and earlier return of bowel function. An intracorporal anastomosis results in a smaller extraction wound in the abdominal wall, as the anastomosis is not performed through it. This approach also enables a right colon resection with less mobilization and mesenteric traction, potentially decreasing the risk of mesenteric twisting and shortening the time of an ileus. However, disadvantages of the intracorporeal technique include a steeper learning curve, the need for advanced laparoscopic/robotic suturing skills, and a risk of intraabdominal fecal spillage [36]. Robotic intracorporeal ileocolic anastomosis has been shown to be safe, notably faster, and easier than the laparoscopic technique (robotic 31.6 minutes vs laparoscopic 43.0 minutes) [37].

The major drawbacks of the robotic system include longer operative times, primarily due to operating room setup rather than the procedure itself, higher costs, further decrease of haptic feedback, as well as the physical separation of the surgeon from the patient [38].

In 2001, Weber and colleagues [39] performed the first robotic colectomies, marking the next step in the evolution of MIS. Following confirmation of its safety and feasibility, the technique was increasingly adopted by colorectal surgeons for the treatment of both benign and malignant conditions [40,41]. After the robotic approach provided encouraging outcomes with adequate oncological results, low morbidity, decreased blood loss, less postoperative pain, and fewer conversion rates, the natural subsequent move was to compare it to the conventional laparoscopic technique [42–44].

COMPARATIVE STUDIES: ROBOTIC VERSUS LAPAROSCOPIC COLECTOMY

In a 2022 systematic review and meta-analysis of 52,589 patients for robotic (n = 13,506) versus laparoscopic (n = 39,083) left colectomy, the overall complications, anastomotic leaks, and superficial wound infections were shown to be less common after robotic left colectomy. There were no significant differences in mortality or oncologic outcomes between the 2 approaches [45]. For right colectomy, a nationwide study in Denmark demonstrated that the robotic approach was associated with a higher lymph node yield (32.5 vs 28.4) and similar postoperative morbidity compared to the laparoscopic approach. Intracorporeal anastomosis was more commonly performed with the robotic approach (23.7% vs 4.5%) [46].

The ROLARR trial, together with subsequent follow-up studies, compared robotic and laparoscopic techniques for rectal cancer and revealed that robotic total mesorectal excision is both feasible and oncologically safe. However, it did not show a clear superiority over the laparoscopic technique in most perioperative outcomes, aside from earlier return of bowel function, a lower conversion rate, and shorter hospital stay [47,48]. Conversely, the REAL trial published in 2025 revealed better oncologic outcomes with the robotic system rather than with laparoscopic surgery, including decreased locoregional recurrence (robotic 1.6% vs lap 4%) and increased 3-year disease-free survival (87.2% vs 83.4%) among patients with mid- to low-rectal cancers. Furthermore, patients in the robotic group were noted to have superior postoperative sexual, urinary, and defecatory function after surgery [49].

A recent comprehensive analysis using the American College of Surgeons National Surgical Quality Improvement Program colectomy database between 2014 and 2020 included 229,862 colectomies to evaluate national trends in open, laparoscopic, and robotic approaches [50]. Overall, 54.2% were performed laparoscopically, 34.8% via open surgery, and 11.1% robotically. During this period, laparoscopic colectomy rates declined from 57.4% to 50.8%, and open surgery decreased from 38.4% to 34.4%, while robotic colectomy increased more than threefold (4.2% to 14.8%). Subgroup analysis showed that open surgery remained the predominant approach among patients with BMI less than 18.5 kg/m^2, high risk (American Society of Anesthesiologists [ASA] class 4–5), and for emergency cases; whereas robotic surgery rates were negligible in these high-risk groups [50]. These findings demonstrate a slow but clear national shift toward minimally invasive colectomy, with robotic surgery showing rapid expansion among selected patient populations (Table 3).

GLIMPSE OF THE FUTURE

The future of minimally invasive oncologic colorectal surgery continues to be shaped by the progressive adoption of new techniques and the rapid evolution of technology. As discussed in the previous section, open oncologic colorectal surgery will undoubtedly remain indispensable for urgent presentations, hemodynamically unstable patients, fragile patients, and in the hands of surgeons uncomfortable in their MIS skills. However, MIS is projected to continue expanding its share of elective colorectal cancer procedures. Current practice patterns and adoption trajectories suggest that robotic colectomy will increasingly supplant conventional laparoscopy. As robotic platforms become more widely available and their learning curves more favorable, their utilization is expected to increase substantially, further shifting the balance of MIS toward robotic surgery in the upcoming future [50,51].

Despite these trends, substantial variability in MIS colectomy utilization persists across institutions and geographic regions, shaped by differences in surgeon training, access to technology, and institutional resources [52]. Continued efforts to implement standardized training pathways, structured mentorship programs, and competency-based curricula will be essential to broaden MIS adoption and reduce disparities in care delivery [53].

Within this context, an important consideration for surgical training programs is the appropriate prioritization of laparoscopic versus robotic

Table 3
Trends for MIS colectomy approaches over time [50]

Approach	2014	2016	2018	2020
Open colectomy no. (%)	38.4	36.0	33.1	34.4
Laparoscopic colectomy (%)	57.4	55.0	54.8	50.8
Robotic colectomy (%)	4.2	9.0	12.1	14.8

approaches for MIS colectomy, as achieving proficiency in both modalities during residency remains a considerable challenge.

Robotic platforms have played an increasingly larger role in expanding MIS to more complex procedures, including obese patients, reoperative fields, and anatomically narrow confines such as the deep pelvis [54]. Looking ahead, next-generation robotic systems are expected to further influence the field by enhancing accessibility and expanding indications for surgery. Several systems have already been designed to facilitate complex procedures with minimal invasiveness, including the single-port (SP) robot, which can accommodate 1 camera and 3 instruments through an SP in the abdominal wall or transanally. The SP robot integrates the precision and control of robotic surgery with the cosmetic and recovery benefits of single-incision laparoscopic surgery (SILS) [55]. Initially implemented in transanal MIS and transanal total mesorectal excision, the SP robotic platform reflects a natural progression of concepts introduced by natural orifice transluminal endoscopic surgery (NOTES), namely the performance of advanced surgical interventions through a single natural orifice or access point. Leveraging these principles, the SP system will predictably be applied more widely to major oncologic colorectal resections. Comparative studies between the SP robotic and SILS techniques have shown similar operative times, complication rates, and pathologic outcomes, confirming the safety and efficacy of this approach [56]. Additional studies comparing multiport and SP platforms have reported comparable complication and conversion rates [57]. The anticipated development and integration of dedicated stapling and advanced energy devices, currently absent from the platform, are likely to address key technical limitations and thereby promote broader adoption of the system in the future.

Other developing frontiers in minimally invasive technology include the introduction of robotic flexible endoscopy platforms. These systems integrate articulating, wristed instruments through flexible endoscopes, enabling improved tissue manipulation and true triangulation. By combining flexibility with robotic precision, these platforms aim to extend the principles of MIS into both endoluminal and intracorporeal interventions, potentially bridging the gap between advanced endoscopy, natural orifice surgery, and robotic surgery. While there is promise, this field remains in an early stage of development and faces several barriers to broader clinical adoption. Current challenges that need to be overcome include the engineering complexity of constructing fully articulated, miniaturized robotic systems capable of operating safely in confined environments, substantial manufacturing and acquisition costs, and the need for dedicated training pathways for surgeons and operating room staff. Additional hurdles include the integration of reliable safety mechanisms to prevent device malfunction during critical steps and the optimization of device durability and stability [58].

Developments in data science and intraoperative informatics are also anticipated to reshape surgical practice for both the laparoscopic and robotic colectomy. Artificial intelligence (AI)–assisted error detection, identification of anatomic structures, procedural mapping, and real time digitalized instructions could potentially enhance performance and improve outcomes. It also has the possibility to enable objective skill assessment and personalized feedback, thereby shortening learning curves and promoting higher technical quality across the specialty [59]. In the long term, integration of robotic platforms with preoperative imaging and intraoperative decision-support systems may move colorectal surgery toward increasingly personalized, anatomy-guided, and precision-based operative strategies [60]. These AI adjuncts at this time are better suited to robotic systems than laparoscopic ones and will likely further hasten the migration of operations from the open or laparoscopic realm to robotics.

Lastly the promise of teleremote robotic surgery is becoming a reality, providing the possibility to offer expert robotic oncologic surgery to remote locations as well as training to inexperienced surgeons.

SUMMARY

Minimally invasive surgical approaches have provided significant short-term and long-term benefits to patients with colorectal cancer without any negative impact on oncologic outcomes. First performed in the early 1990s, the adoption of laparoscopic and then robotic surgical approaches have been slow but steady. Yet roughly one-third of cancer resections are still performed open. Laparoscopy allowed for the widespread visualization and analysis of operative technique, and unintentionally served to emphasize the primacy of surgical technique in the care of the colorectal cancer patient. Robotics have helped to improve adoption of MIS approaches for colorectal cancer. Robotic capabilities have also increased performance of more complex techniques such as intracorporeal anastomoses, natural orifice surgery, and the expansion of ever shortening postoperative stays. Additionally, the robot seems ideally poised to take advantage of expanding AI into the operating room to help with identification of anatomy and potential danger areas. At this time, there seems to be an equivalence to frequency of laparoscopic and robotic approaches for colon cancer. Robotic surgery is the clearly favored approach for rectal cancer surgery due to the technical challenges of the deep pelvis.

The pace of adoption and extent of research performed highlights the technical challenges of applying new surgical approaches in a high-stakes field, such as cancer surgery, where a technical shortcoming can result in decreased survival. It therefore should be emphasized that all of these techniques: scalpel, laparoscope and robot, are tools for surgeons to use to provide optimal cancer care to the patients in their own hands. Clearly these MIS approaches can benefit our cancer patients, but it remains the responsibility of us as surgeons to learn and master these new approaches to our patient for the best possible outcomes.

While economic pressures exist to provide optimal cancer care while controlling costs, it seems clear that these improved surgical tools and exciting further developments will continue to improve the care of our patients and merit further study.

CLINICS CARE POINTS

- The most important takeaway is that MIS, either laparoscopic or robotic, can be performed safely with patient benefits in patients with colorectal cancer.
- The dominant driver for the operation should be an optimal oncologic resection; the surgeon needs to adjust their approach according to their experience and expertise, but this can be achieved in an MIS fashion, robotically or laparoscopically.
- Robotic surgery offers its greatest benefits in TME dissection for distal rectal cancer and in intracorporeal anastomosis.
- Laparoscopic approaches are more versatile in complex reoperative situations.

Disclosures

J. Marks, MD,is a consultant and is on the speakers' bureau for Stryker, Intuitive, and Medtronic. He has received educational grant support from Medtronic. He also serves as a consultant to Virtual Incision, Arthrex, and Vascular Technologies, and as a Scientific Advisory Board member for Surg 270. The other authors have no disclosures.

References

[1] Mühe E. Laparoscopic cholecystectomy–late results. Langenbecks Arch Chir Suppl Kongressbd; 1991. p. 416–23.
[2] Bailey RW, Zucker KA, Flowers JL, et al. Laparoscopic cholecystectomy. Ann Surg 1991;(214):531.
[3] Club SS. A prospective analysis of 1518 laparoscopic cholecystectomies. N Engl J Med 1991;16(324):1073–8.
[4] Fowler D, White S. Laparoscopy-assisted sigmoid resection. Surg Laparosc Endosc Percutan Tech 1991;1(3):183–8.
[5] Jacobs M, Verdeja J, Goldstein H. Minimally invasive colon resection (laparoscopic colectomy). Laparoscopy Endoscopy & Percutaneous Techniques 1991;1(3):144–50.
[6] Schoetz DJ, Bockler M, Rosenblatt MS, et al. "Ideal" length of stay after colectomy: whose ideal? Dis Colon Rectum 1997;40(7):806–10.
[7] Phillips EH, Franklin M, Carroll BJ, et al. Laparoscopic colectomy. Ann Surg 1992;216(6):703–7.
[8] Joo JS, Amarnath L, Wexner SD. Is laparoscopic resection of colorectal polyps beneficial? Surg Endosc 1998;12(11):1341–4.
[9] Jansen A. Laparoscopic gastrointestinal and gallbladder surgery: will the promise be fulfilled? Scand J Gastroenterol 1992;27(S194):41–6.
[10] Falk PM, Beart RW, Wexner SD, et al. Laparoscopic colectomy: a critical appraisal. Dis Colon Rectum 1993;36(1):28–34.
[11] Cirocco W, Schwartzman A, Golub RW. Abdominal wall recurrence after laparoscopic colectomy for colon cancer. Surgery 1994;116(5):842–6.
[12] Fusco MA, Paluzzi MW. Abdominal wall recurrence after laparoscopic-assisted colectomy for adenocarcinoma of the colon - Report of a case. Dis Colon Rectum 1993;36(9):858–61.
[13] Fodera M, Pello MJ, Atabek U, et al. Trocar site tumor recurrence after laparoscopic-assisted colectomy. J Laparoendosc Surg 1995;5(4):259–62.
[14] Darzi A, Hill AD, Henry MM, et al. Laparoscopic assisted surgery of the colon. Operative technique. Endosc Surg Allied Technol 1993;1(1):13–5.

[15] Croce E, Azzola M, Russo R, et al. Laparoscopic colectomy: the absolute need for a standard operative technique. J Soc Laparoendosc Surg 1997;1(3):217.
[16] Roe AM, Harper R, Eltringham WK, et al. Intracorporeal laparoscopic resections for colorectal cancer: report of cases of abdominoperineal rectal excision and right hemicolectomy with 2 year follow-up. J R Soc Med 1994;87(9):519–21.
[17] Nelson H, Sargent DJ, Wieand HS, et al, Group TCO of STS. A comparison of laparoscopically assisted and open colectomy for colon cancer. N Engl J Med 2004;350(20): 2050–9.
[18] Schwenk W, Haase O, Neudecker J, et al. Short term benefits for laparoscopic colorectal resection. Cochrane database of systemic reviews 2005;2:1–59.
[19] Color Study Group, Hazebroek EJ. COLOR: a randomized clinical trial comparing laparoscopic and open resection for colon cancer. Surgical Endoscopy And Other Interventional Techniques 2002;16(6):949–53.
[20] Lacy AM, García-Valdecasas JC, Delgado S, et al. Laparoscopy-assisted colectomy versus open colectomy for treatment of non-metastatic colon cancer: a randomised trial. Lancet 2002;359(9325):2224–9.
[21] Fleshman J, Sargent DJ, Green E, et al. Laparoscopic colectomy for cancer is not inferior to open surgery based on 5-year data from the COST study group trial. Ann Surg 2007;246 (4):655–62.
[22] Deijen CL, Vasmel JE, de Lange-de Klerk ESM, et al. Ten-year outcomes of a randomised trial of laparoscopic versus open surgery for colon cancer. Surg Endosc 2017;31(6): 2607–15.
[23] van den Berg I, Coebergh van den Braak, Robert RJ, et al. Actual survival after resection of primary colorectal cancer: results from a prospective multicenter study. World J Surg Oncol 2021;19(1):96.
[24] Prete FP, Pezzolla A, Prete F, et al. Robotic versus laparoscopic minimally invasive surgery for rectal cancer: a systematic review and meta-analysis of randomized controlled trials. Ann Surg 2018;267(6):1034–46.
[25] Melstrom KA, Kaiser AM. Role of minimally invasive surgery for rectal cancer. World J Gastroenterol 2020;26(30):4394.
[26] Bonjer HJ, Deijen CL, Abis GA, et al. A randomized trial of laparoscopic versus open surgery for rectal cancer. N Engl J Med 2015;372(14):1324–32.
[27] Guillou PJ, Quirke P, Thorpe H, et al. Short-term endpoints of conventional versus laparoscopic-assisted surgery in patients with colorectal cancer (MRC CLASICC trial): Multicentre, randomised controlled trial. Lancet 2005;365(9472):1718–26.
[28] Stevenson ARL, Solomon MJ, Lumley JW, et al. Effect of laparoscopic-assisted resection vs open resection on pathological outcomes in rectal cancer: the ALaCaRT randomized clinical trial. JAMA 2015;314(13):1356–63.
[29] Fleshman J, Branda ME, Sargent DJ, et al. Disease-free survival and local recurrence for laparoscopic resection compared with open resection of stage II to III rectal cancer: follow-up results of the ACOSOG Z6051 randomized controlled trial. Ann Surg 2019;269(4):589–95.
[30] Hohenberger W, Weber K, Matzel K, et al. Standardized surgery for colonic cancer: complete mesocolic excision and central ligation–technical notes and outcome. Colorectal Dis 2009;11(4):354–64.
[31] Porter DJ. Complete mesocolic excision in colon cancer: a systematic review and meta analysis. World Journal of Surgery and Surgical Research 2019;2:1149.
[32] Li K, Li H, Wu A, et al, RELARC Study Group. Long-term survival on extent of lymphadenectomy for right-sided colon cancer: five-year follow-up results of a randomized controlled trial (RELARC Trial). Ann Surg 2025; https://doi.org/10.1097/SLA.0000000000006941.
[33] Hayashi K, Passera R, Meroni C, et al. Complete mesocolic excision (CME) impacts survival only for Stage III right-sided colon cancer: a systematic review and meta-analysis. Minim Invasive Ther Allied Technol 2024;33(6):323–33.

[34] Dalager T, Jensen PT, Eriksen JR, et al. Surgeons' posture and muscle strain during laparoscopic and robotic surgery. Br J Surg 2020;107(6):756–66.
[35] de'Angelis N, Lizzi V, Azoulay D, Brunetti F. Robotic versus laparoscopic right colectomy for colon cancer: analysis of the initial simultaneous learning curve of a surgical fellow. J Laparoendosc Adv Surg Tech A 2016;26(11):882–92.
[36] van Oostendorp S, Elfrink A, Borstlap W, et al. Intracorporeal versus extracorporeal anastomosis in right hemicolectomy: a systematic review and meta-analysis. Surg Endosc 2017;31(1):64–77.
[37] Sorgato N, Mammano E, Contardo T, et al. Right colectomy with intracorporeal anastomosis for cancer: a prospective comparison between robotics and laparoscopy. J Robot Surg 2021;16(3):655–63.
[38] Rawlings AL, Woodland JH, Vegunta RK, et al. Robotic versus laparoscopic colectomy. Surgical Endoscopy and Other Interventional Techniques 2007;21(10):1701–8.
[39] Weber PA, Merola S, Wasielewski A, et al. Telerobotic-assisted laparoscopic right and sigmoid colectomies for benign disease. Dis Colon Rectum 2002;45(12):1689–96.
[40] Baik SH. Robotic colorectal surgery. Yonsei Med J 2008;49(6):891–6.
[41] D'Annibale A, Morpurgo E, Fiscon V, et al. Robotic and laparoscopic surgery for treatment of colorectal diseases. Dis Colon Rectum 2004;47(12):2162–8.
[42] Papanikolaou IG. Robotic surgery for colorectal cancer. Surg Laparosc Endosc Percutan Tech 2014;24(6):478–83.
[43] Mirkin KA, Kulaylat AS, Hollenbeak CS, et al. Robotic versus laparoscopic colectomy for stage I–III colon cancer: oncologic and long-term survival outcomes. Surg Endosc 2018;32(6):2894–901.
[44] Berger Y, Khajoueinejad N, Imtiaz S, et al. Robotic colorectal resections are associated with less postoperative pain, decreased opioid use, and earlier return to work as compared to the laparoscopic approach. J Robot Surg 2024;18(1):1–10.
[45] Solaini L, Bocchino A, Avanzolini A, et al. Robotic versus laparoscopic left colectomy: a systematic review and meta-analysis. Int J Colorectal Dis 2022;37(7):1497–507.
[46] Dohrn N, Klein MF, Gögenur I. Robotic versus laparoscopic right colectomy for colon cancer: a nationwide cohort study. Int J Colorectal Dis 2021;36(10):2147–58.
[47] Jayne D, Pigazzi A, Marshall H, et al. Robotic-assisted surgery compared with laparoscopic resection surgery for rectal cancer: the ROLARR RCT. Efficacy Mech Eval 2019;6(10):1–140.
[48] Jayne D, Pigazzi A, Marshall H, et al. Effect of robotic-assisted vs conventional laparoscopic surgery on risk of conversion to open laparotomy among patients undergoing resection for rectal cancer: the ROLARR randomized clinical trial. JAMA 2017;318(16):1569–80.
[49] Feng Q, Yuan W, Li T, et al. Robotic vs laparoscopic surgery for middle and low rectal cancer: the REAL randomized clinical trial. JAMA 2025;334(2):136–48.
[50] Laredo JA, Torres-Small S, Patel D, et al. Recent patterns in minimally invasive colectomies: where are we now? Laparosc Endosc Robot Surg 2025;8(1):23–7.
[51] Manisundaram N, Childers CP, Hu CY, et al. Rise in minimally invasive surgery for colorectal cancer is associated with adoption of robotic surgery. Dis Colon Rectum 2025;68(4): 426–36.
[52] Aquina CT, Becerra AZ, Justiniano CF, et al. Surgeon, hospital, and geographic variation in minimally invasive colectomy. Ann Surg 2019;269(6):1109–16.
[53] Awad M, Awad F, Carter F, et al. Consensus views on the optimum training curriculum for advanced minimally invasive surgery: a Delphi study. Int J Surg 2018;53:137–42.
[54] Baek SJ, Kim CH, Cho MS, et al. Robotic surgery for rectal cancer can overcome difficulties associated with pelvic anatomy. Surg Endosc 2015;29(6):1419–24.
[55] Marks JH, Perez RE, Salem JF. Robotic transanal surgery for rectal cancer. Clin Colon Rectal Surg 2021;34(5):317–24.
[56] Jeong M, Kim H, Choi G, et al. Single-port versus multiport robotic total mesorectal excision for rectal cancer: initial experiences by case-matched analysis of short-term outcomes. Ann Surg Treat Res 2023;105(2):99–106.

[57] Brucchi F, Montroni I, Cirocchi R, et al. A systematic review of the Da Vinci® Single-Port system (DVSP) in the context of colorectal surgery. Int J Colorectal Dis 2025;40(1):1–13.
[58] Haas AJ, Feria A, Noubani L, et al. Evolution of robotics in endoscopy—past and future. Dig Dis Interv 2025;09(01):023–9.
[59] Lam K, Chen J, Wang Z, et al. Machine learning for technical skill assessment in surgery: a systematic review. Nature Partner Journals Digital Medicine 2022;5(1):1–16.
[60] Yang GZ, Cambias J, Cleary K, et al. Medical robotics-regulatory, ethical, and legal considerations for increasing levels of autonomy. Sci Robot 2017;2(4):1–2.

Advances in Surgery 60 (2026) 15–28

ADVANCES IN SURGERY

Management of Acute Diverticulitis

Role of Minimally Invasive Surgery versus Nonoperative Management

Sameh Hany Emile, MBBCh, MSc, MD[a],
Steven D. Wexner, MD, PhD (Hon)[b,*]

[a]Ellen Leifer Shulman and Steven Shulman Digestive Disease Center, Cleveland Clinic Florida, Weston, FL, USA; [b]Department of Colorectal Surgery, MedStar Health Georgetown University Hospital, 3800 Reservoir Road NW, Washington, DC 20007, USA

Keywords

• Diverticulitis • Nonoperative management • Laparoscopy • Hinchey classification
• Minimally invasive surgery

Key points

- Most patients with uncomplicated acute diverticulitis can be treated without surgery; routine antibiotics are not required for immunocompetent patients with mild disease.
- CT with IV contrast is the preferred initial imaging test; CT severity correlates with the failure of non-operative management.
- Image-guided percutaneous drainage is generally recommended for diverticular abscesses >3 cm.
- Urgent resection is indicated in generalized peritonitis or failure of non-operative management.
- Minimally invasive options are preferred to laparotomy.

INTRODUCTION

Acute diverticulitis (AD) is a common complication of diverticular disease of the colon, which accounts for over 300,000 annual hospital admissions in the United States. It has been suggested that most complications of diverticular

*Corresponding author. Colorectal Surgery Department, 2950 Cleveland Clinic Boulevard, Weston, FL 33331. *E-mail address:* steven.d.wexner@medstar.net

https://doi.org/10.1016/j.yasu.2026.03.002

Abbreviations

AD	acute diverticulitis
ASCRS	American Society of Colon and Rectal Surgeons
CI	confidence interval
CT	computed tomography
ESCP	European Society of Coloproctology
HIH	hospital-in-home
IV	intravenous
MIS	minimally invasive surgery
WSES	World Society of Emergency Surgery

disease start with microperforation of diverticula, which induces pericolic inflammation of varying degrees. In uncomplicated AD, the inflammation is usually limited and does not progress further, whereas in complicated AD, complications, including abscess, fistula, or free perforation, ensue. Computed tomography (CT)-based classification systems for the severity of AD include the modified Hinchey classification, which grades severity into 5 stages: stage 0 (uncomplicated AD), stage Ia (pericolic phlegmon); stage Ib (confined pericolic abscess); stage II (pelvic, distant intra-abdominal, or retroperitoneal abscess); stage III (purulent peritonitis); and stage IV (fecal peritonitis; Table 1). AD presents with a spectrum of severity from self-limited inflammation to perforation and sepsis [1,2].

Diagnosis and assessment of AD are essential before management. Abdominopelvic CT scans with intravenous (IV) contrast are the standard investigation for suspected AD; however, noncontrast CT scanning may be used in high-risk patients [3]. Contemporary management of AD is essentially dependent on the disease stage and the patients' overall status. Accurate risk stratification is paramount before selecting the treatment modality. Overall, the treatment armamentarium comprises the use of antibiotics, CT-guided drainage of abscesses, and surgery, including minimally invasive surgery (MIS). While management of uncomplicated AD is basically nonoperative

Table 1
Hinchey classification of acute diverticulitis and management options

Stage	Description	Recommended management
0	Uncomplicated diverticulitis	Outpatient care, selective antibiotics, bowel rest, and analgesia
Ia	Pericolic phlegmon	Nonoperative, possible outpatient care
Ib	Confined pericolic abscess	Antibiotics ± percutaneous drainage
II	Pelvic/intra-abdominal abscess	Percutaneous drainage ± antibiotics
III	Purulent peritonitis	Urgent laparoscopic or open resection (primary anastomosis ± diversion vs Hartmann's)
IV	Fecal peritonitis	Urgent resection (primary anastomosis ± diversion vs Hartmann's)

and surgery is used for complicated disease, there is a gray area where either treatment strategy is valid or can be employed.

ROLE OF NONOPERATIVE MANAGEMENT IN ACUTE DIVERTICULITIS

Nonoperative management may be appropriate in patients with either uncomplicated and complicated AD. While nonoperative management is the standard of care for uncomplicated Hinchey 0 to Ia diverticulitis, it is selectively used in complicated Hinchey Ib to II diverticulitis with abscess (Fig. 1).

Nonoperative management of uncomplicated acute diverticulitis

Patients with Hinchey 0 to Ia AD are generally candidates for nonoperative management if they are hemodynamically stable and have mild symptoms that do not warrant urgent surgery [4,5]. The main elements of nonoperative management in these patients are close observation, antibiotics, bowel rest, and pain control. Patients should be closely monitored to assess their disease progression and response to treatment. Failure of response to treatment, increase in pain severity, and/or hemodynamic instability are indications for further interventions, including urgent surgery.

Antibiotics

The role of antibiotics in uncomplicated AD has been debated over the last decade. A selective approach to the use of antibiotics in mild uncomplicated AD has been advocated. This recommendation is supported by a myriad of randomized clinical trials, including the Antibiotika Vid Okomplicerad Divertikulit (AVOD) and Diverticulitis: AntiBiotics Or cLose Observation? (DIABLO) trials, and meta-analyses that found no significant differences in complications, recovery, or recurrence when antibiotics are omitted [6–8]. It has been proposed that antibiotics should be reserved for immunocompromised patients and

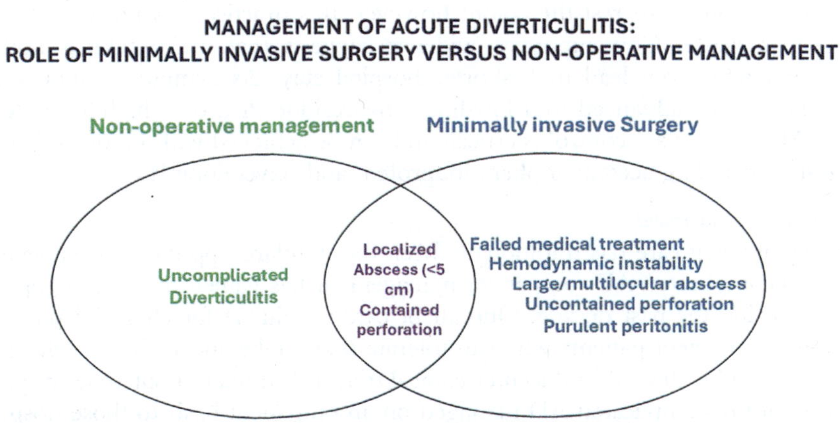

Fig. 1. The role of nonoperative management versus minimally invasive surgery in acute diverticulitis.

patients with medical comorbidities. A meta-analysis with a meta-regression analysis reported similar odds of treatment failure, recurrence of diverticulitis, complications, readmission, and need for surgery ($P = .28$) between the antibiotics and nonantibiotic groups. Furthermore, this meta-analysis found that medical comorbidities were the only factor associated with treatment failure in patients with uncomplicated AD who did not receive antibiotics [9]. Guidelines, including the American Gastroenterological Association (AGA) Clinical Practice Update on Medical Management of Colonic Diverticulitis and American Society of Colon and Rectal Surgeons (ASCRS) practice guidelines, also recommended selective use of antibiotics in uncomplicated AD [10,11]. When indicated, the recommended antibiotic regimens would include metronidazole and fluoroquinolone, whereas amoxicillin–clavulanate is a valid fluoroquinolone-sparing alternative with comparable outcomes and fewer adverse effects [12].

Despite this compelling evidence against the routine use of antibiotics in uncomplicated AD, a survey of members of the Society of American Gastrointestinal and Endoscopic Surgeons (SAGES) and the European Association of Endoscopic Surgery (EAES) in 2018 found that half of the members would not change their practice following the society's recommendation on selective antibiotic use [13,14]. Interestingly, a patient survey study in 2024 found that 62% of respondents were willing to participate in a randomized clinical trial on nonantibiotic management of AD, although they had "complex and varying perceptions of antibiotic use" [15]. The authors favor the use of antibiotics in most patients.

Bowel rest and pain control

Perhaps 2 of the most important elements in nonoperative management of AD are bowel rest and pain control. As with other acute gastrointestinal conditions, resting the gastrointestinal tract is essential for recovery. Historically, patients with AD were advised to have nothing by mouth or just a clear liquid diet during an AD attack to rest the colon; however, this practice was not based on strong evidence. Contemporary evidence suggests that oral intake is both safe and may even lead to a shorter hospital stay. As symptoms improve, the diet can be advanced to a low-fiber, low-residue diet, or a high-fiber diet [16]. Moreover, pain control is crucial and can be achieved with IV or oral analgesics, including acetaminophen, ibuprofen, and oxycodone [17].

Outpatient management

While inpatient care has traditionally been the standard approach for patients with uncomplicated AD, outpatient management has gained increasing popularity during the past decade. Outpatient care is suitable for clinically stable, immunocompetent patients who can tolerate oral intake and maintain reliable follow-up. The DIVER multicenter clinical trial [18] compared outcomes of patients with uncomplicated AD managed on an outpatient basis to those hospitalized, concluding that "outpatient treatment is safe and effective in selected patients." There were no differences in treatment failure or quality of life between the groups; however, outpatient management resulted in lower overall health care costs, with estimated savings of €1124.70 per patient. A systematic review of 21 studies confirmed the safety of outpatient management of AD and reported a pooled failure rate of 4.3% (95% confidence interval [CI] 2.6%–6.3%), which was unaffected by the number of previous AD episodes, comorbidities, presence of pericolic air or intra-abdominal abscess, diabetes mellitus, or type of antibiotic treatment [19]. Hamilton and colleagues [20] examined hospital-in-home (HIH) management in 23 patients with AD within a dedicated HIH unit, reporting no acute complications with only 2 patients experiencing subsequent episodes of AD within 2 months. The HIH management approach was further studied by Boutros and colleagues [21], involving 60 patients compared to 39 hospitalized patients. Overall, 6.6% of HIH patients were eventually hospitalized. Patients in the HIH group required significantly fewer IV narcotics (3.3% vs 64%, $P < .001$) and IV fluids (18.3% vs 100%, $P < .001$). Both groups had similar rates of ED visits without readmission (8.3% vs 0, $P = .168$), readmissions without surgery (3.3% vs 7.7%, $P = .346$), and readmissions with surgery (1.6% vs 5.1%, $P = .351$). These findings support the feasibility and safety of outpatient HIH management for AD.

Nonoperative management of complicated diverticulitis with abscess

Patients with Hinchey Ib to II AD can be nonoperatively treated with antibiotics, with or without image-guided percutaneous drainage, depending on the abscess size and location. Nonoperative management is successful in up to 80% of patients with Hinchey Ib to II AD [22]. The 2020 ASCRS clinical practice guidelines devised a strong recommendation for image-guided percutaneous drainage of AD-related abscesses greater than 3 cm in size in stable patients [11]. It should be noted that the abscess size does not affect the success of percutaneous drainage [11,22]. Conversely, outpatient antibiotic treatment without drainage is usually sufficient for stable patients with abscesses less than 3; however, percutaneous drainage may be required if this approach fails [23].

Drainage of abscesses is best guided by a CT scan to allow for the visualization of nearby structures and enable complex drainage procedures [24]. When CT scanning is not available or contraindicated, ultrasound-guided drainage can be a viable alternative. The drainage catheters are generally percutaneously inserted or, on rare occasions, have been transrectally placed [5]. Although percutaneous drainage is typically used in larger and more complex abscesses, the rates of abscess recurrence are lower after percutaneous drainage (15%–25%) than after antibiotic-only treatment (25%–60%) [25].

According to a systematic review of 42 observational studies, incorporating 8766 patients with Hinchey Ib to II diverticulitis, percutaneous drainage was associated with lower recurrence rates than antibiotics only (15.9% vs 22.2%), and drainage-related complications occurred in 2.5% of patients. Acute surgery was associated with an increased risk of death compared to nonoperative management (12.1% vs 1.1%) [26]. That is why surgery is reserved for patients with worsening sepsis or recurrent abscesses within 30 days and patients with no safe access window for percutaneous drainage. Thankfully, laparoscopic drainage is sufficient in most cases, and surgical resection is reserved for select cases [11,27]. A small case series of 18 patients with Hinchey II AD treated with laparoscopic drainage of abscesses without resection reported that only 3 patients required a resection after follow-up for up to 34 months [28]. A summary of nonoperative management of uncomplicated and complicated AD is shown in Fig. 2.

Assessment and monitoring after the resolution of acute diverticulitis

Upon recovery of AD after nonoperative management, an endoscopic evaluation of the entire colon and rectum is necessary, if it has not been recently performed. This assessment is particularly needed in patients with complicated AD, as they are at a higher risk of harboring an occult malignancy [11]. Several medications have been suggested to prevent recurrence of symptoms after an episode of AD, including anti-inflammatory agents such as mesalazine, broad-spectrum nonabsorbable antibiotics such as rifaximin, and probiotics. According to the European Society of Coloproctology (ESCP) guidelines [29], none of these agents are recommended to prevent recurrent diverticulitis after an episode of AD. The same guidelines found little evidence that a high-fiber diet can prevent the recurrence of AD following nonoperative management. The ASCRS guidelines [11] also did not recommend the use of mesalamine, rifaximin, or probiotics to reduce the risk of AD recurrence, although they may be effective in alleviating chronic symptoms.

ROLE OF MINIMALLY INVASIVE SURGERY IN ACUTE DIVERTICULITIS

Indications for surgery

Patients with AD may require elective or emergency surgery, depending on the disease presentation and severity of symptoms. The most common indications for emergency surgery for AD are diffuse peritonitis (Hinchey III–IV) and failure of initial nonoperative management. Elective surgery maybe indicated for

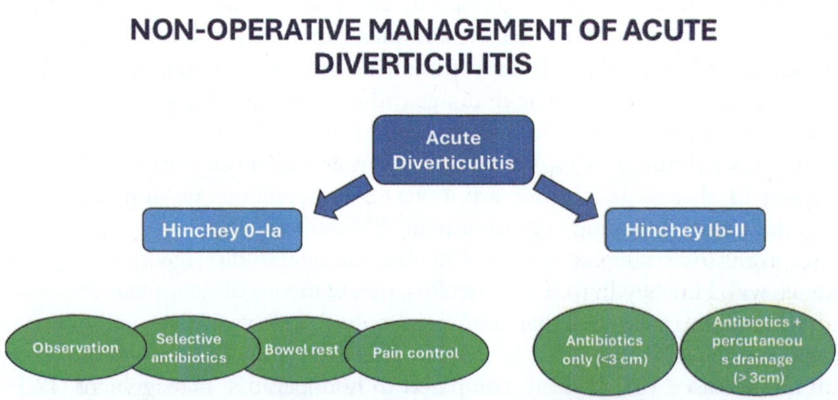

Fig. 2. Nonoperative management of acute Hinchey 0 to Ia and Hinchey Ib to II diverticulitis.

patients with recurrent attacks of AD that significantly impair their quality of life. Historically, a second episode of uncomplicated AD was sufficient to warrant an elective resection to prevent future severe attacks. However, the current practice does not consider the number of episodes of AD per se as an absolute indication for elective surgery. Disease severity, comorbidities, quality of life, and patient preferences should all be considered when making a decision on elective surgery. While the ASCRS guidelines [11] suggest that "elective sigmoid colectomy after recovery from uncomplicated acute diverticulitis should be individualized"; they recommend elective resection after successful nonoperative management of a diverticular abscess and in diverticular disease complicated by fistula, obstruction, or stricture. Conversely, the ESCP guidelines do not recommend routine resection after a conservatively managed episode of complicated AD [29]. The ESCP guidelines justified this recommendation by the little existing evidence that supports routine elective resection after nonoperative management of complicated AD, which is mainly derived from retrospective cohort studies.

Type of surgery

While elective surgery for AD is usually the resection of the affected colonic segment, emergency surgery entails both resection and damage-control interventions, such as peritoneal lavage. Patients with AD presenting with peritonitis are typically managed by resection, which can be either restorative with primary anastomosis or nonrestorative, such as Hartmann's procedure. The DIVERTI trial provided good evidence in favor of primary anastomosis with diverting ileostomy over Hartmann's procedure in patients with AD and peritonitis [30]. Another multicenter randomized clinical trial concluded that primary anastomosis with diverting ileostomy is a better treatment option than Hartmann's procedure in patients with perforated diverticulitis [31]. A meta-analysis of long-term outcomes showed that colonic resection with primary anastomosis reduced the odds of long-term ostomy by 98%, long-term complications by 81%, and incisional hernia by 82%, as compared to Hartmann's procedure [32].

An alternative to colonic resection in complicated AD with peritonitis is laparoscopic peritoneal lavage, which is mainly used for purulent peritonitis, but not for feculent peritonitis [11]. While lavage may be appropriately used by experienced teams for select patients [33], current evidence does not substantiate its role as equivalent or superior to resection [30,34], as it is associated with higher rates of early reintervention and abscess formation. Nonetheless, collective long-term data imply that laparoscopic lavage may be associated with a lower likelihood of long-term ostomy (OR = 0.133, 95% CI: 0.278–0.579) and reoperation (OR = 0.585, 95% CI: 0.365–0.937), yet higher odds of diverticular disease recurrence (OR = 5.8, 95% CI: 2.33–14.42) than colonic resection [32]. The ASCRS guidelines recommend that colectomy is preferred over laparoscopic lavage in patients with purulent peritonitis, whereas the ESCP guidelines regarded laparoscopic lavage as a feasible option in select patients with Hinchey III peritonitis, with resection being an alternative [11,29].

Elective surgery for AD involves a colectomy with primary anastomosis that can be achieved through an open approach or preferably using a minimally invasive operation. Long-term follow-up of randomized trials, such as the DIRECT trial [35], found that almost one-third of patients initially randomized to conservative treatment underwent sigmoid resection within 4 years. Although elective surgery helped prevent the recurrence of AD more than conservative treatment, it was not associated with an improved quality of life. In contrast, a meta-analysis of 3 randomized controlled trials and 6 retrospective cohorts concluded that elective surgery significantly improved long-term quality of life in patients with AD; however, the clinical relevance of the difference in quality-of-life scores was uncertain because of the small effect size [36]. Perhaps, the ongoing Comparison of Surgery and Medicine on the Impact of Diverticulitis trial [NCT04095663] may provide additional evidence on the impact of elective surgery for recurrent AD on the quality of life.

Surgical approach

Traditionally, open surgery was the standard of care for surgery for AD, in both the elective and emergency settings. However, with the advances and growing experience with MIS, a paradigm shift has occurred with laparoscopic and robotic-assisted resections accounting for the majority of surgery for AD in the developed countries. A German study reported a significant increase in the rate of MIS from 67.8% to 86.2% for uncomplicated AD and from 34.6% to 52.9% for complicated cases between 2019 and 2023 [37]. The increased adoption of MIS for AD is attributable to its documented benefits, which include smaller incisions, less postoperative pain, and reduced hospital stays, in addition to long-term benefits such as fewer incisional hernias and adhesion-related complications [38]. The authors support and practice a minimally invasive operative approach.

Minimally invasive surgery in the elective setting

Several randomized clinical trials compared the outcomes of laparoscopic and open sigmoidectomy for diverticular disease. Gervaz and colleagues [39] found that laparoscopic sigmoidectomy was associated with a 30% reduction in postoperative ileus and hospital stay. Kalrenbeek and colleagues [40] reported that laparoscopic sigmoidectomy was associated with a significant reduction in major complications, less pain, better quality of life, and shorter hospital stay than open surgery. Conversely, another randomized trial found that laparoscopy and open surgery had similar morbidity, mortality, and quality of life at 12 months [41]. A meta-analysis [42] supported the use of laparoscopy for the elective surgical treatment of AD, citing lower rates of morbidity, namely ileus, anastomotic leakage, bowel obstruction, surgical site infection, and fascial dehiscence, and shorter hospital in favor of laparoscopy. Given this compelling evidence, current guidelines, including the ASCRS, ESCP, and German national guidelines [11,29,43] recommend a minimally invasive approach to elective resection of AD.

While the role of laparoscopy in elective surgery for AD has been thoroughly studied with robust randomized data existing, robotic surgery has been far less evaluated. The ESCP guidelines [29] described the evidence for the use of a robotic approach in AD as "scarce." It has been presumed that robotic surgery has a role in complex clinical scenarios where traditional laparoscopic surgery is less likely to be successfully completed and conversion to open surgery would be needed. Such settings include colovaginal and colovesical fistulas and male patients with high body mass index and narrow pelvises. The use of robotic surgery may overcome the limitations of the surgical instruments by enhancing the surgeon's visualization and dexterity to reduce conversion [44]. A single-center retrospective study on 83 patients with sigmoid diverticulitis compared the outcomes of laparoscopic and robotic-assisted surgery and reported robotic surgery to be cost-effective and associated with less intraoperative trauma, as shown by lower postoperative C-reactive protein levels than conventional laparoscopy [45]. A systematic review and meta-analysis of 15 cohort studies on robotic resections for diverticular disease found that robotic surgery is a feasible and safe option that was associated with a 43% lower conversion rate than laparoscopic surgery, with similar odds of major complications, yet with longer operating times [46]. However, this meta-analysis did include a cost-effectiveness analysis of the robotic approach, which is crucial when deciding on the optimal approach for any surgical condition. The robotic-assisted Natural orifice IntraCorporeal anastomosis with transrectal Extraction (NICE) procedure was investigated in patients with complicated AD with high body mass index, and the NICE procedure could mitigate some of the challenges associated with traditional MIS. Although patients with high body mass index had a higher rate of 30 day unplanned operations (7.9% vs 1.7%, $P = .034$), there were no significant differences in hospital stay, time to first flatus, or intensive care unit admission between the high and average body mass index groups [47].

Minimally invasive surgery in the emergency setting

Patients presenting with Hinchey III/IV diverticulitis with purulent or feculent peritonitis represent a surgical emergency that necessitates prompt intervention. Upon adequate resuscitation, colonic resection is the cornerstone of the management of AD with peritonitis [11,29]. Resection can be performed using the traditional open approach or alternatively via a minimally invasive approach. While MIS is the preferred approach to elective resections according to the ASCRS guidelines [11], its role in the emergency setting is less clear. The World Society of Emergency Surgery (WSES) 2020 guidelines [2] suggest performing an emergency laparoscopic resection in patients with diffuse peritonitis due to perforated diverticulitis, if technical skills and equipment are available. The guidelines explain this recommendation that laparoscopic sigmoidectomy may be feasible even with purulent and fecal peritonitis as long as the patient is physiologically stable. Vennix and colleagues [48] conducted a systematic review of 5 observational studies with a total of 104 patients who underwent laparoscopic sigmoidectomy for perforated diverticulitis and generalized peritonitis. The review reported that the mean operative time varied between 115 and 200 minutes, with conversion rates up to 19%. Only 2

Table 2
Minimally invasive surgical treatments of acute diverticulitis

Approach	Suggested indications	Benefits	Limitations
Laparoscopic resection	Elective or emergency	Reduced morbidity, shorter stay, and fewer hernias	Requires expertise and risk of conversion to open surgery
Robotic-assisted resection	Complex cases (fistulas, obesity, and narrow pelvis)	Lower conversion rates and better dexterity	Higher cost and longer operative times
Laparoscopic lavage	Hinchey III (purulent peritonitis)	Lower long-term ostomy rates	Higher recurrence rates, need for reintervention

patients needed surgical reintervention, and no anastomotic leakage was reported. The stoma reversal after Hartmann's procedure was 76%. However, given the lack of randomized trials, a definitive conclusion on the safety of emergency laparoscopic resection in Hinchey III diverticulitis cannot be made.

An alternative indication for MIS in diverticulitis peritonitis is laparoscopic lavage. The ESCP guidelines [29] consider lavage feasible in select patients with Hinchey III peritonitis, yet conversely, the ASCRS guidelines [11] recommend against laparoscopic lavage, due to its association with higher rates of secondary intervention than with resection. The WSES guidelines [2] suggested that laparoscopic lavage and drainage should be only performed in very select patients with generalized peritonitis, but not as a first-line treatment.

A systematic review of 19 studies including 871 patients found that the success rate of laparoscopic lavage in diverticular peritonitis was 24.3%. Conversion to laparotomy was required in 1% of patients with Hinchey III diverticulitis and 45% of patients with stage IV diverticulitis. Approximately 5% of patients needed at least 1 postoperative reintervention within 30 days, including 2% who required percutaneous drainage. Moreover, 6% of patients were readmitted after the first hospitalization for recurrent AD, and 69% of them underwent a redo surgery. The authors concluded that laparoscopic lavage may be considered as a "bridge" toward delayed and elective laparoscopic sigmoidectomy to avoid a Hartmann's procedure [49]. The authors do not practice laparoscopic lavage.

Overall, MIS for AD includes laparoscopic resections, robotic-assisted resections, and laparoscopic peritoneal lavage. The suggested indications, benefits, and limitations of each treatment are summarized in Table 2.

FUTURE DIRECTIONS

There remain several questions regarding selection criteria for elective surgery, the impact of surgery on quality of life, comparative cost-effectiveness of robotic versus laparoscopic resection across learning curves, optimal management of chronic disease, and treatment without antibiotics.

CLINICS CARE POINTS

- It is safe to omit routine antibiotics in mild uncomplicated diverticulitis. Immunocompetent patients with Hinchey 0–Ia diverticulitis can often be safely managed without antibiotics.
- Contrast-enhanced CT is not only essential for diagnosis but also for stratifying risk, identifying abscesses, and predicting failure of non-operative management.
- Diverticular abscesses >3 cm should be drained. Image-guided percutaneous drainage is recommended for stable patients with accessible abscesses, whereas smaller abscesses may be treated with antibiotics only.
- Decisions on elective colectomy should be individualized based on symptom burden, quality of life, and patient preferences. The number of diverticulitis episodes alone should not dictate surgery.
- Minimally invasive colectomy is preferred to open surgery, and laparoscopic surgery is the standard approach as it is associated with fewer complications, shorter hospitalization, and quicker recovery.

Disclosure

Dr S.D. Wexner is a consultant for Activ Surgical, Arthex, Baxter, Becton, Dickinson and Co., Glaxo Smith Kline, Intuitive Surgical, Ostomy Secure, Polypid, Seikagaku, and Takeda, has consulting agreements with stock options for consulting with Ostomy Secure and Polypid, and receives royalties from Intuitive Surgical, Karl Storz Endoscopy America Inc., and Unique Surgical Solutions, LLC. Dr S.H. Emile was a consultant for Becton, Dickinson and Co.

References

[1] Carr S, Velasco AL. Colon diverticulitis. In: StatPearls. Treasure Island (FL): StatPearls Publishing; 2025 [Figure, Hinchey Classification of Diverticulitis Contributed by S Carr, DO] Available at: https://www.ncbi.nlm.nih.gov/books/NBK541110/figure/article-19724.image.f1/.

[2] Sartelli M, Weber DG, Kluger Y, et al. 2002 update of the WSES guidelines for the management of acute colonic diverticulitis in the emergency setting. World J Emerg Surg 2020;15:22.

[3] Andeweg CS, Wegdam JA, Groenewoud J, et al. Toward an evidence-based step-up approach in diagnosing diverticulitis. Scand J Gastroenterol 2014;49:775–84.

[4] Boukhili N, Caminsky NG, Sabboobeh S, et al. Nonoperative management of acute complicated diverticulitis: a retrospective cohort needs-assessment study for home-based management. Surgery 2025;186:109537.

[5] Schaffzin DM, Wong WD. Nonoperative management of complicated diverticular disease. Clin Colon Rectal Surg 2004;17(3):169–76.

[6] Chabok A, Påhlman L, Hjern F, et al, AVOD Study Group. Randomized clinical trial of antibiotics in acute uncomplicated diverticulitis. Br J Surg 2012;99:532–9.

[7] Daniels L, Ünlü Ç, de Korte N, et al. Dutch diverticular disease (3D) collaborative study group. Randomized clinical trial of observational versus antibiotic treatment for a first episode of CT-proven uncomplicated acute diverticulitis. Br J Surg 2017;104:52–61.

[8] van Dijk ST, Chabok A, Dijkgraaf MG, et al. Observational versus antibiotic treatment for uncomplicated diverticulitis: an individual-patient data meta-analysis. Br J Surg 2020;107(8):1062–9.

[9] Emile SH, Elfeki H, Sakr A, et al. Management of acute uncomplicated diverticulitis without antibiotics: a systematic review, meta-analysis, and meta-regression of predictors of treatment failure. Tech Coloproctol 2018;22(7):499–509.
[10] Peery AF, Shaukat A, Strate LL. AGA clinical practice update on medical management of colonic diverticulitis: expert review. Gastroenterology 2021;160(3):906–11.e1.
[11] Hall J, Hardiman K, Lee S, et al, Prepared on behalf of the Clinical Practice Guidelines Committee of the American Society of Colon and Rectal Surgeons. The American society of colon and rectal surgeons clinical practice guidelines for the treatment of left-sided colonic diverticulitis. Dis Colon Rectum 2020;63(6):728–47.
[12] Gaber CE, Kinlaw AC, Edwards JK, et al. Comparative effectiveness and harms of antibiotics for outpatient diverticulitis : two nationwide cohort studies. Ann Intern Med 2021;174(6): 737–46.
[13] Koprowski MA, Affleck A, Tsikitis VL. Emerging evidence and recent controversies in diverticulitis: a 5-year review. Ann Gastroenterol 2022;35(1):8–16.
[14] Francis NK, Sylla P, Abou-Khalil M, et al. EAES and SAGES 2018 consensus conference on acute diverticulitis management: evidence-based recommendations for clinical practice. Surg Endosc 2019;33(9):2726–41.
[15] Altman-Merino A, Bonnet K, Schlundt D, et al. Patient perspectives on evolving diverticulitis treatment: an assessment of patient willingness to enroll in a randomized controlled trial. Ann Surg Open 2024;5(3):e476.
[16] van Dijk ST, Rottier SJ, van Geloven AAW, et al. Conservative treatment of acute colonic diverticulitis. Curr Infect Dis Rep 2017;19(11):44.
[17] UpToDate. UpToDate. Available at: https://www.uptodate.com/contents/acute-colonic-diverticulitis-outpatient-management-and-follow-up#:~:text=Initial%20outpatient%20care%20%E2%80%93%20Patients%20are,antibiotic%20treatment%20(Grade%202B). Accessed August 25, 2025.
[18] Biondo S, Golda T, Kreisler E, et al. Outpatient versus hospitalization management for uncomplicated diverticulitis: a prospective, multicenter randomized clinical trial (DIVER trial). Ann Surg 2014;259(1):38–44.
[19] Cirocchi R, Randolph JJ, Binda GA, et al. Is the outpatient management of acute diverticulitis safe and effective? A systematic review and meta-analysis. Tech Coloproctol 2019;23(2): 87–100.
[20] Hamilton J, Crosthwaite G, Montalto M. Hospital in the home-based management of acute diverticulitis: a safe and effective alternative to inpatient care. ANZ J Surg 2021;91(10): 2106–9.
[21] Boutros M, Al Khaldi M, Champagne B, et al. Admitting acute diverticulitis patients to home: results from an established hospital-in-home. Dis Colon Rectum 2025;68(5):e747.
[22] Lambrichts DPV, Bolkenstein HE, van der Does DCHE, et al. Multicentre study of non-surgical management of diverticulitis with abscess formation. Br J Surg 2019;106:458–66.
[23] Brandt D, Gervaz P, Durmishi Y, et al. Percutaneous CT scan-guided drainage vs. antibiotherapy alone for hinchey II diverticulitis: a case-control study. Dis Colon Rectum 2006;49: 1533–8.
[24] Neff CC, vanSonnenberg E. CT of diverticulitis. Diagnosis and treatment. Radiol Clin North Am 1989;27:743–52.
[25] Garfinkle R, Kugler A, Pelsser V, et al. Diverticular abscess managed with long-term definitive nonoperative intent is safe. Dis Colon Rectum 2016;59:648–55.
[26] Gregersen R, Mortensen LQ, Burcharth J, et al. Treatment of patients with acute colonic diverticulitis complicated by abscess formation: a systematic review. Int J Surg 2016;35: 201–8.
[27] Toorenvliet BR, Swank H, Schoones JW, et al. Laparoscopic peritoneal lavage for perforated colonic diverticulitis: a systematic review. Colorectal Dis 2010;12:862–7.
[28] Franklin ME Jr, Dorman JP, Jacobs M, et al. Is laparoscopic surgery applicable to complicated colonic diverticular disease? Surg Endosc 1997;11:1021–5.

[29] Schultz JK, Azhar N, Binda GA, et al. European society of coloproctology: guidelines for the management of diverticular disease of the colon. Colorectal Dis 2020;22(Suppl 2): 5–28.
[30] Bridoux V, Regimbeau JM, Ouaissi M, et al. Hartmann's procedure or primary anastomosis for generalized peritonitis due to perforated diverticulitis: a prospective multicenter randomized trial (DIVERTI). J Am Coll Surg 2017;225(6):798–805.
[31] Oberkofler CE, Rickenbacher A, Raptis DA, et al. A multicenter randomized clinical trial of primary anastomosis or Hartmann's procedure for perforated left colonic diverticulitis with purulent or fecal peritonitis. Ann Surg 2012;256:819–26 [discussion: 826–817].
[32] Horesh N, Emile SH, Khan SM, et al. Meta-analysis of randomized clinical trials on long-term outcomes of surgical treatment of perforated diverticulitis. Ann Surg 2023;278(5): e966–72.
[33] Binda GA, Bonino MA, Siri G, et al. Multicentre international trial of laparoscopic lavage for hinchey III acute diverticulitis (LLO study). Br J Surg 2018;105:1835–43.
[34] Schultz JK, Yaqub S, Wallon C, et al, SCANDIV Study Group. Laparoscopic lavage vs primary resection for acute perforated diverticulitis: the SCANDIV randomized clinical trial. JAMA 2015;314(13):1364–75.
[35] Santos A, Mentula P, Pinta T, et al. Sigmoid resection vs conservative treatment after diverticulitis: prespecified 4-year analysis of the laser randomized clinical trial. JAMA Surg 2025;160(6):615–22.
[36] Kahana N, Horesh N, Emile SH, et al. Meta-analysis and systematic review of long-term quality of life and recurrence following elective surgery versus non-operative management for colonic diverticulitis. Surgery 2025;181:109143.
[37] Kolbe EW, Buciunas M, Krieg S, et al. Minimally invasive versus open surgery for colonic diverticular disease: a nationwide analysis of German hospital data. Tech Coloproctol 2025;29(1):46.
[38] Klarenbeek BR, Bergamaschi R, Veenhof AA, et al. Laparoscopic versus open sigmoid resection for diverticular disease: follow-up assessment of the randomized control sigma trial. Surg Endosc 2011;25:1121–6.
[39] Gervaz P, Inan I, Perneger T, et al. A prospective, randomized, single-blind comparison of laparoscopic versus open sigmoid colectomy for diverticulitis. Ann Surg 2010;252(1):3–8.
[40] Klarenbeek BR, Veenhof AA, Bergamaschi R, et al. Laparoscopic sigmoid resection for diverticulitis decreases major morbidity rates: a randomized control trial: short-term results of the sigma trial. Ann Surg 2009;249(1):39–44.
[41] Raue W, Paolucci V, Asperger W, et al, LAPDIV-CAMIC Trial Group. Laparoscopic sigmoid resection for diverticular disease has no advantages over open approach: midterm results of a randomized controlled trial. Langenbecks Arch Surg 2011;396(7):973–80.
[42] Wu KL, Lee KC, Liu CC, et al. Laparoscopic versus open surgery for diverticulitis: a systematic review and meta-analysis. Dig Surg 2017;34(3):203–15.
[43] Kruis W, Germer CT, Böhm S, et al. German guideline diverticular disease/diverticulitis: part II: conservative, interventional and surgical management. United Eur Gastroenterol J 2022;10:940–57.
[44] Ali F, Raskin E. Robotic surgery for complicated diverticular disease. Clin Colon Rectal Surg 2021;34(5):297–301.
[45] Presl J, Ehgartner M, Schabl L, et al. Robotic surgery versus conventional laparoscopy in sigmoid colectomy for diverticular disease-a comparison of operative trauma and cost-effectiveness: retrospective, single-center analysis. Langenbecks Arch Surg 2024;409(1): 200.
[46] Larkins K, Mohan H, Apte SS, et al. A systematic review and meta-analysis of robotic resections for diverticular disease. Colorectal Dis 2022;24(10):1105–16.
[47] Bistre-Varon J, Gunter R, Del Rio RS, et al. Is the NICE procedure the great equalizer for patients with high BMI undergoing resection for diverticulitis? Surg Endosc 2024;38(12): 7518–24.

[48] Vennix S, Boersema GS, Buskens CJ, et al. Emergency laparoscopic sigmoidectomy for perforated diverticulitis with generalised peritonitis: a systematic review. Dig Surg 2016;33(1):1–7.
[49] Cirocchi R, Trastulli S, Vettoretto N, et al. Laparoscopic peritoneal lavage: a definitive treatment for diverticular peritonitis or a "bridge" to elective laparoscopic sigmoidectomy?: a systematic review. Medicine (Baltim) 2015;94(1):e334.

Advances in Surgery 60 (2026) 29–48

ADVANCES IN SURGERY

Which Is Preferable for Chronic Limb-threatening Ischemia

Bypass versus Endovascular Therapy?

Mohammed Hamouda, MD, Kevin Yei, MD, Mahmoud B. Malas, MD, MHS, RPVI*

Division of Vascular and Endovascular Surgery, Department of Surgery, UC San Diego, La Jolla, CA, USA

Keywords

• Chronic limb-threatening ischemia • Amputation • Bypass • Endovascular therapy • Limb salvage

Key points

- Chronic limb-threatening ischemia is the most advanced stage of peripheral arterial disease and typically requires revascularization to prevent limb-loss.
- The choice of open surgical bypass versus endovascular therapy should be individualized based on patients' anatomy, operative risk, and conduit availability.
- Patients who are suitable candidates for both bypass and endovascular intervention and have an adequate SSGSV should undergo surgical bypass based on level-1 evidence.

INTRODUCTION

Over 200 million people worldwide are estimated to have peripheral arterial disease (PAD) [1]. Chronic limb-threatening ischemia (CLTI) is considered the most advanced stage of PAD, characterized by the presence of ischemic rest pain or tissue loss. According to the Society for Vascular Surgery (SVS) guidelines, patients presenting with CLTI are indicated for lower extremity revascularization in most cases, as the risk of amputation and mortality in untreated patients exceeds 20% within the first year [2,3]. Lower extremity

*Corresponding author. *E-mail address:* mmalas@health.ucsd.edu

https://doi.org/10.1016/j.yasu.2026.03.003

Abbreviations

ABI	ankle-brachial index
AFS	amputation-free survival
BASIL-1	Bypass versus Angioplasty in Severe Ischemia of the Leg
BEST-CLI	Best Endovascular versus Best Surgical Therapy in Patients with Critical Limb Ischemia
BMS	bare metal stents
BWGSV	bypass with GSV
BWPG	bypass with prosthetic graft
CFA	common femoral artery
CI	confidence interval
CLTI	chronic limb-threatening ischemia
ET	endovascular therapy
GLASS	Global Limb Anatomic Staging System
HR	hazard ratio
HRQL	health-related quality of life
MACE	major adverse cardiovascular events
MALE	major adverse limb events
MI	myocardial infarction
PAD	peripheral arterial disease
SFA	superficial femoral artery
SSGSV	single-segment great saphenous vein
SVS	Society for Vascular Surgery
WIfI	Wound, Ischemia, and foot Infection

revascularization is associated with a significant improvement in limb salvage and quality of life [4].

The 2 main revascularization modalities for CLTI are open surgical bypass and endovascular therapy (ET). Although both are considered standard-of-care strategies for CLTI, there is no consensus on which revascularization method is optimal. Surgical bypass has for long considered the gold standard treatment method, however, at the expense of higher risk of postoperative morbidity, wound complications, and prolonged hospitalization. ET, on the other hand, has been advocated as the minimally invasive alternative to open bypass. However, data related to its durability and efficacy compared to a surgical bypass are inconclusive [5].

Currently, 3 major randomized controlled trials have been published comparing bypass surgery and ET in patients with CLTI: Bypass versus Angioplasty in Severe Ischemia of the Leg (BASIL-1), Best Endovascular versus Best Surgical Therapy in Patients with Critical Limb Ischemia (BEST-CLI), and BASIL-2 [6–8]. In this article, we aim to explore the nuances of both revascularization modalities, including their technical and clinical considerations, and to discuss the data comparing their safety and efficacy.

DIAGNOSTIC WORKUP AND IMAGING

CLTI should be suspected in patients with atherosclerotic risk factors who present with characteristic rest pain, tissue loss, or both, usually involving the distal leg or foot. The ischemic pain typically occurs at rest, often in the foot, and tends to worsen when the leg is elevated at night and often awakening the patients from sleep. The discomfort results from a combination of ischemia, ischemic neuropathy, and, when present, tissue loss. In patients with diabetes, foot ulcers are often painless due to underlying peripheral neuropathy. The extent of tissue loss can vary widely, from a small ulcer to areas of gangrene, sometimes complicated by localized infection [9]. On physical examination, patients often lack palpable ankle pulses and may have shiny or thin skin, loss of hair, and delayed capillary refill. Tissue loss most commonly involves the toes, but it can also affect the heel, ankle, or even the calf. If osteomyelitis is suspected, it can usually be confirmed at the bedside by gently probing the wound with a sterile instrument to determine if bone is exposed.

Noninvasive physiologic vascular laboratory tests can be helpful in confirming the diagnosis and localizing the disease. The most common initial test is the ankle-brachial index (ABI), which is calculated as the ratio of highest systolic pressure at the ankle divided by the higher systolic pressure of both arms. ABI can be combined with color duplex scanning of the lower extremity. A normal ABI is generally around 1.0 ± 0.1; an ABI of less than 0.9 is diagnostic of PAD. Roughly, an ABI between 0.4 and 0.9 is present in patients with claudication, while an ABI below 0.4 is compatible with rest pain or tissue loss. An ABI greater than 1.2 may be falsely elevated because of severe arterial calcification, which is seen in diabetes and end-stage renal disease, hence obtaining toe pressures and/or pulse volume recordings might be helpful [10]. A toe-brachial index of less than 0.7 is indicative of significant disease. Toe pressure greater than 40 mm Hg is required to heal any wound. Color duplex ultrasound is consistent of B-Mode imaging and color flow Doppler sampling will determine the location and severity of the disease based on increased velocity of blood or occlusion. For patients who need invasive therapy, further imaging is obtained to show both inflow and outflow arteries (eg, contrast CT, MR angiography, and/or digital subtraction angiography). Vein mapping is typically performed to screen for adequate autogenous vein conduit in cases where an infrainguinal bypass is planned.

INFRAINGUINAL BYPASS

A successful bypass requires an adequate inflow, outflow, and a conduit. Infrainguinal bypasses can originate from the common femoral artery (CFA), superficial femoral artery (SFA), deep femoral artery, or the popliteal artery depending on how extensive the lesion to be bypassed is. The distal target site can be an above-knee or below-knee popliteal, tibial peroneal trunk, or a tibial vessel (dorsalis pedis, posterior tibial, anterior tibial, and common peroneal artery). A good outflow vessel should be the least diseased with continuous flow to the foot. Autogenous vein is always the first-choice conduit for all infrainguinal bypasses. The great saphenous vein, particularly if harvested as a single segment, is the preferred choice and should be evaluated with preoperative duplex vein mapping. If this vein is inadequate, a mapping of alternative veins including small saphenous and upper arm veins (basilic and cephalic arm) is done [11]. The vein should be nondiseased and at least 3 mm in diameter. Vein bypasses can be placed in a reversed, nonreversed, or in situ configuration. Every effort should be made to minimize the time of the harvested vein from not being perfused with the patient's blood. We generally prepare the vein while exposing both proximal and distal inflow and outflow arteries with 2 team approach, so once the vein is harvested, it is ready to be used. We routinely use a tunneler, which is inserted just deep to the sartorius muscle and superficial to the SFA from distal to proximal incision. For below-knee popliteal artery bypass, the graft is pulled from above knee to below knee with an aortic clamp creating a tunnel between the heads of the gastrocnemius muscle to prevent compression. Alternatively, the vein can be tunneled anatomically with careful blunt fingers dissection next to popliteal vessels from below knee to above knee. In tibial bypasses, our preference is to perform the distal anastomosis after inflating a pneumatic tourniquet proximally for adequate hemostasis while avoiding using clamps on the delicate distal arteries. It is generally recommended to have completion duplex imaging to assess both proximal and distal anastomoses. Completion contrast angiography can also be used if there is any question concerning the technical results. It is critical to evaluate the distal pulses by palpation and the use of continuous wave Doppler. The distal foot signal should augment when pinching and releasing the bypass. The groin is then closed with multiple layers of absorbable sutures. The thigh and leg subcutaneous layers are closed in layers using absorbable sutures. Finally, our preference is always approximating the subcutaneous layers using multiple layers of absorbable sutures, followed by 3-0 nylon in an interrupted vertical mattress manner for skin closure. Staples are not recommended due to higher risk of surgical site infections and wound complications [12].

ENDOVASCULAR THERAPY

The first step to an endovascular intervention is to obtain access. A variety of techniques exist by which this can be accomplished. Retrograde CFA access is the most common approach for femoral artery access [13,14]. The femoral bifurcation is identified and accessed using a micropuncture needle under ultrasound guidance. Access should be performed over the lower third of the femoral head. This was traditionally confirmed via fluoroscopy and/or angiography to enable hemostasis via manual pressure. Currently, we use ultrasound exclusively to direct the microneedle into the middle CFA avoiding the bifurcation and staying distal to the external iliac artery marked by the superficial epigastric and superficial circumflex iliac arteries origins. The contralateral femoral artery is selected, and a long sheath is placed up and over the aortic bifurcation. Antegrade CFA access is an alternative approach that affords greater pushability and shorter working length for endovascular interventions. However, this access is more challenging and has been associated with higher odds of access site complications [15]. Retrograde pedal artery access represents an additional option for patients with suitable anatomy. This modality is typically reserved for lesions that are unable to be recanalized from an antegrade approach [16,17].

After access is secured and a diagnostic angiogram obtained, the lesion of interest must be crossed. A wide variety of guidewires and crossing catheters (.035″, .018″, .014″) are available [18]. For chronic total occlusions that cannot be crossed using standard wire and catheter techniques, a variety of crossing and re-entry devices may be employed [19–21]. Once the lesion is crossed, a multitude of interventional options become available [22]. Balloon angioplasty is frequently employed for initial treatment of a stenotic lesion. For femoropopliteal disease, drug-coated balloon angioplasty may reduce the risk of restenosis [23]. The decision of whether or not to stent is driven by patient anatomy, lesion characteristics, and operator experience. For intermediate length (10–20 cm) SFA lesions, bare metal stents (BMS), drug eluting stents, and covered stents have been associated with better patency compared to angioplasty alone [22,24,25]. There are no currently approved stents or drug-coated balloons for use in the tibial arteries. Resorbable tibial scaffolds have shown promising early results as they aim to provide structural support while allowing for long-term remodeling and preserving long-term interventional options [26]. However the long-term data in durability of these stents are limited.

For highly stenotic and/or calcified lesions, preparation of the vessel prior to treatment may be beneficial. Intravascular lithotripsy utilizes sonic pressure waves to modify intimal and medial calcium and has shown promising results in safety and efficacy in the lower extremities [27,28]. A variety of atherectomy devices (directional, orbital, rotational, and laser) exist, which may assist in increasing the size of the vessel lumen [29]. The comparative efficacy of these devices remains to be determined. For long femoropopliteal lesions in patients who are not surgical candidates for open bypass, percutaneous femoropopliteal bypass involving placement of a covered stent conduit from the distal artery into the deep femoral vein, and then back into the proximal femoral artery can be considered [30,31]. For patients without any patent distal target for revascularization, deep venous arterialization involves venous valvular lysis followed by covered stenting from the donor artery into the tibial vein. Initial results have been promising, with additional randomized trials ongoing [32,33].

OPEN SURGICAL BYPASS VERSUS ENDOVASCULAR THERAPY

The choice between open surgical revascularization and ET should be guided by multiple factors, including the patient's anatomic characteristics and overall risk profile (Table 1) [34]. Many surgeons consider open surgical bypass the gold standard for patients presenting with ischemic rest pain or tissue loss. However, ET is increasingly being adopted as the initial treatment approach in many cases. According to the SVS Global CLTI guidelines, the decision between ET and open bypass in average-risk patients (anticipated periprocedural mortality <5% and expected 2 year survival >50%) should be based on 3 major considerations: the anatomic pattern of disease (as defined by the Global Limb

Table 1
Factors that May influence optimal revascularization modality

Anatomy	Strategy for current revascularization considers history of failed previous revascularization procedures (surgical, endovascular, or both) Anatomic characteristics that may favor surgical revascularization include • lesions involving both the common femoral artery and origin of the profunda femoris artery • Multilevel chronic total occlusions • lesions in which endovascular treatment would adversely impact future surgical bypass options • lesions that are long segment, involving the below-knee popliteal and infrapopliteal arteries
Available conduit	Absence of suitable autogenous vein (eg, due to previous harvest for coronary artery bypass surgery) may favor endovascular revascularization
Patient comorbidities	High estimated perioperative risk (eg, coronary ischemia, cardiomyopathy and heart failure, severe lung disease, chronic kidney disease, and frailty) may favor endovascular revascularization
Patient preferences	Patient preference for (surgical or endovascular) over the other, after participating in shared decision-making

From Gornik, H. et al. 2024 ACC/AHA/AACVPR/APMA/ABC/SCAI/SVM/SVN/SVS/SIR/VESS Guideline for the Management of Lower Extremity Peripheral Artery Disease: A Report of the American College of Cardiology/American Heart Association Joint Committee on Clinical Practice Guidelines. J Am Coll Cardiol. null2024, 0 (0). https://doi.org/10.1016/j.jacc.2024.02.013

Anatomic Staging System [GLASS; Fig. 1]), the severity of limb threat (as classified by the SVS Wound, Ischemia, and foot Infection [WIfI] system [Table 2]), and the availability of autologous vein conduit [2,35]. Fig. 2 summarizes the preferred infrainguinal revascularization strategies for average-risk patients with available vein conduit, based on the combination of limb severity (WIfI stage) and the anatomic pattern of disease (GLASS stage) [2]. Given the ongoing debate regarding which strategy offers superior outcomes in CLTI, there was a significant need for randomized controlled trials directly comparing open surgical bypass and endovascular intervention. In the following sections, we will discuss the major clinical trials that have addressed this question, along with data from real-world studies in order to clarify which procedure may be superior. We will also touch base on how patient-related factors, comorbidities, and anatomic characteristics may influence limb salvage and survival outcomes.

LANDMARK RANDOMIZED CONTROLLED TRIALS

Bypass versus Angioplasty in Severe Ischemia of the Leg-1

The first trial to randomize patients with CLTI to bypass versus ET was the BASIL-1 trial. The study was based in the United Kingdom and included a total of 452 patients; 228 randomized to surgery-first and 224 to angioplasty-first

A

0	Mild or no significant (<50%) disease	
1	• Total length SFA disease <1/3 (<10 cm) • May include single focal CTO (< 5 cm) as long as not flush occlusion • Popliteal artery with mild or no significant disease	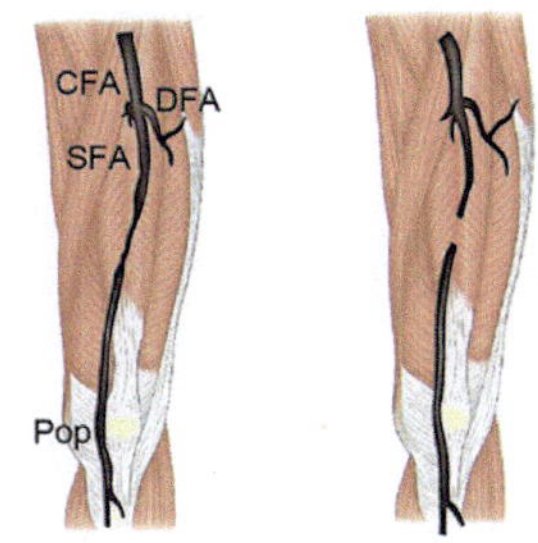
2	• Total length SFA disease 1/3-2/3 (10-20 cm) • May include CTO totaling < 1/3 (10 cm) but not flush occlusion • Focal popliteal artery stenosis <2 cm, not involving trifurcation	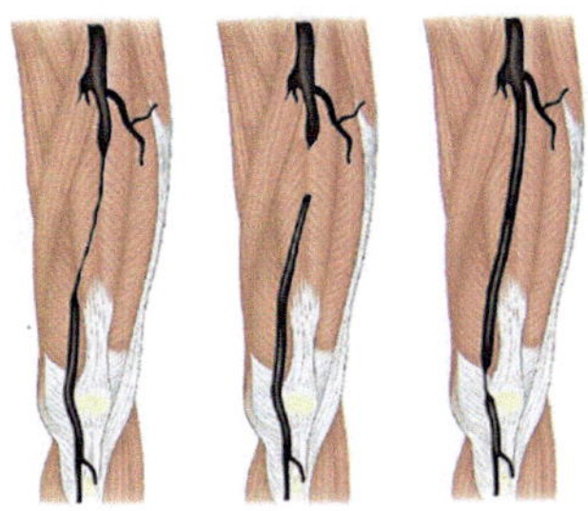
3	• Total length SFA disease >2/3 (>20 cm) length • May include any flush occlusion <20 cm or non-flush CTO 10-20 cm long • Short popliteal stenosis 2-5 cm, not involving trifurcation	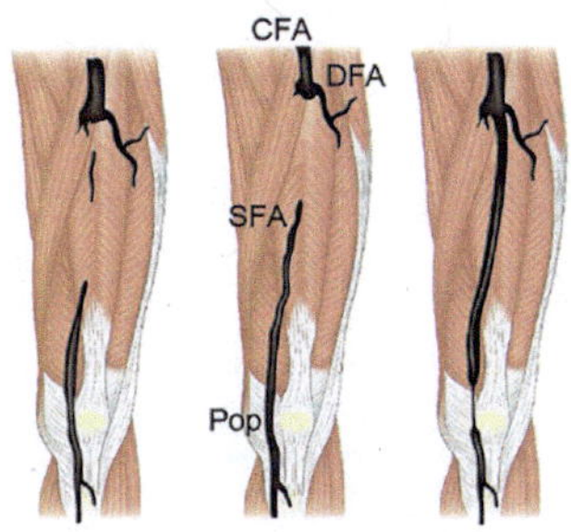
4	• Total length SFA occlusion > 20 cm • Popliteal disease >5 cm or extending into trifurcation • Any popliteal CTO	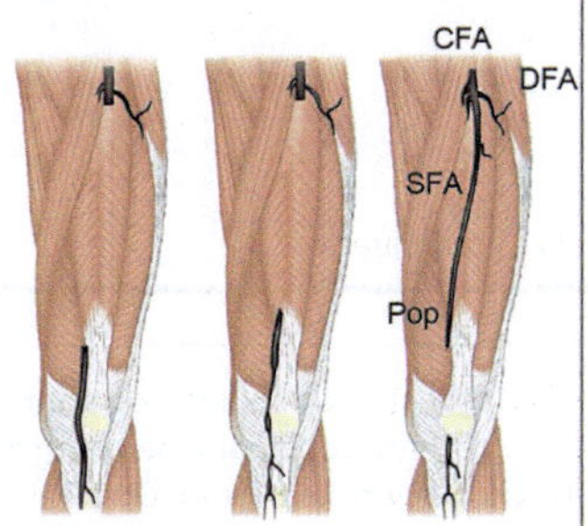

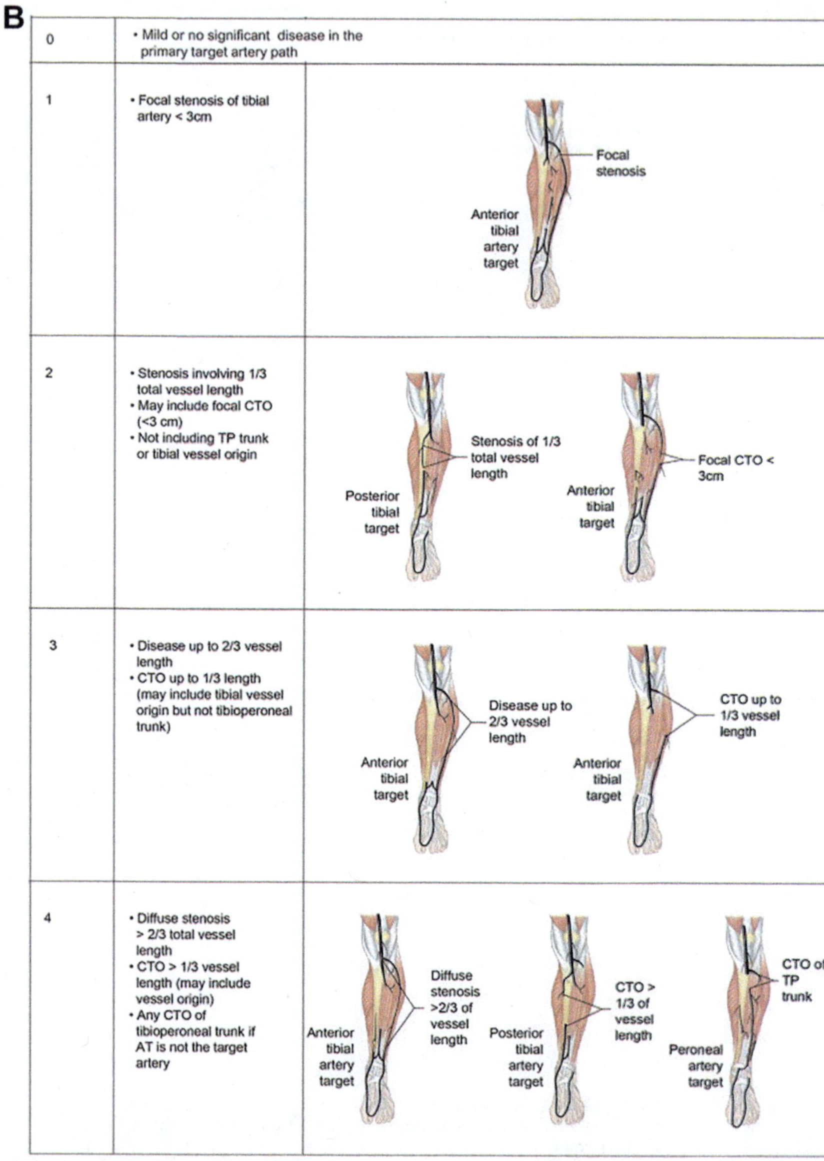

Fig. 1. (*continued*)

Fig. 1. (*A*) Femoropopliteal disease grading in Global Limb Anatomic Staging System (GLASS). (*B*) Infrapopliteal disease grading in GLASS. (*From* Conte MS et al; GVG Writing Group. Global vascular guidelines on the management of chronic limb-threatening ischemia. J Vasc Surg. 2019 Jun;69(6S):3S–125S.e40. https://doi.org/10.1016/j.jvs.2019.02.016. Epub 2019 May 28. Erratum in: J Vasc Surg. 2019 Aug;70(2):662. PMID: 31159978; PMCID: PMC8365864.)

Table 2
Wound, Ischemia, foot Infection classification

Wound			
Ulcer		Gangrene	Grade
None		None	0
Shallow (subcutaneous)		Small ulcer and no gangrene	1
Deep (tendon/muscle)		Limited to digits	2
Extensive (bone)		Extensive	3
Ischemia			
ABI		Toe Pressure (mm Hg)	Grade
≥0.8		≥60	0
0.6–0.79		40–59	1
0.4–0.59		30–39	2
≤0.39		<30	3
Foot infection			
Clinical manifestation			Grade
No signs or symptoms of infection			0
Local infection involving skin and subcutaneous tissue only			1
Local infection extending to deeper layers			2
As above plus systematic inflammatory response			3
WIfI clinical stage	Risk of major limb amputation	WIfI score	
Stage 1	Very Low	W0 I0 fI0,1	W1 I0 fI0,1
		W0 I1 fI0	W1 I1 fI0
Stage 2	Low	W0 I0 fI2	W1 I0 fI2
		W0 I1 fI1	W1 I1 fI1
		W0 I2 fI0,1	W1 I2 fI0
		W0 I3 fI0	W2 I0 fI0,1
Stage 3	Moderate	W0 I0 fI3	W1 I3 fI0,1
		W0 I2 fI1,2	W2 I0 fI2
		W0 I3 fI1,2	W2 I 1 fI0,1
		W1 I0 fI3	W2 I2 fI0
		W1 I1 fI2	W3 I0 fI0,1
		W1 I2 fI1	
Stage 4	High	W0 I1,2,3 fI3	W2 I2 fI1,2,3
		W1 I1 fI3	W2 I3 fI0,1,2,3
		W1 I2,3 fI2,3	W3 I0 fI2,3
		W2 I0 fI3	W3 I1,2,3 fI0,1,2,3
		W2 I1 fI2,3	

Adapted from Mills JL Sr and colleagues; Society for Vascular Surgery Lower Extremity Guidelines Committee. The Society for Vascular Surgery Lower Extremity Threatened Limb Classification System: risk stratification based on wound, ischemia, and foot infection (WIfI). J Vasc Surg. 2014 Jan;59(1):220–34.e1-2. https://doi.org/10.1016/j.jvs.2013.08.003. Epub 2013 Oct 12. PMID: 24126108.

therapy [6]. The trial's primary outcome was time to amputation of the trial leg above the ankle or death from any cause, whichever occurred first (amputation-free survival [AFS]). Secondary outcomes were all-cause mortality, 30 day morbidity and mortality, reinterventions, health-related quality of life

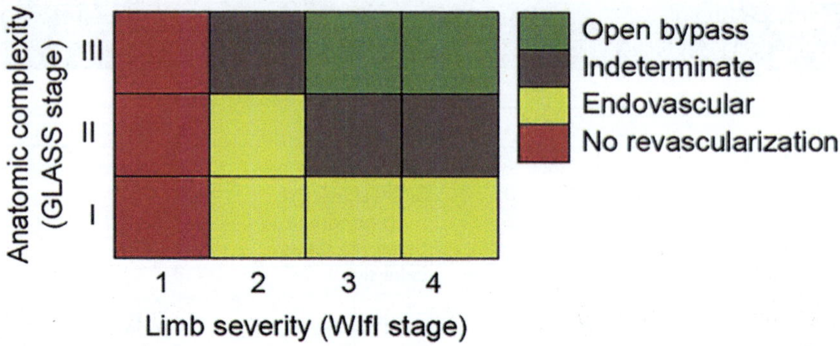

Fig. 2. Preferred initial revascularization strategy for infrainguinal disease in average-risk patients with suitable autologous vein conduit available for bypass. GLASS stage I includes Femoropopliteal (FP) GLASS grade 1 and grade 2, stage II includes FP GLASS grade 3, and stage III includes FP GLASS grade 4. Revascularization is considered rarely indicated in limbs at low risk (Wound, Ischemia, and foot Infection [WIfI] stage 1). Anatomic stage (y-axis) is determined by the Global Limb Anatomic Staging System (GLASS); limb risk (x-axis) is determined by WIfI staging. The dark gray shading indicates scenarios with least consensus (assumptions-inflow disease either is not significant or is corrected; absence of severe pedal disease). (*From* Conte MS et al; GVG Writing Group. Global vascular guidelines on the management of chronic limb-threatening ischemia. J Vasc Surg. 2019 Jun;69(6S):3S–125S.e40. doi: 10.1016/j.jvs.2019.02.016. Epub 2019 May 28. Erratum in: J Vasc Surg. 2019 Aug;70 (2):662. PMID: 31159978; PMCID: PMC8365864.)

(HRQL), and use of hospital resources. Randomization was stratified by center and then categorized into 4 groups by clinical presentation (rest pain only vs tissue loss with or without rest pain) and ankle pressure ($\geq$50 mm Hg vs $\leq$50 mm Hg).

In the surgery-first group, 94% of the bypasses originated from the femoral artery with only 75% performed using autogenous great saphenous vein. About a third of the distal anastomoses were constructed at each of the following sites: above-knee popliteal artery, below-knee popliteal artery, and infrapopliteal arteries (anterior tibial, posterior tibial, or peroneal arteries). In the angioplasty-first group, the SFA was treated in 80% of patients, and more distal vessels underwent angioplasty in 62% of the cohort. Thus, the extent of the lesion that had been bypassed at surgery and recanalized by angioplasty was similar. Technical success was 97% and 80% in the surgery-first and angioplasty-first groups, respectively.

On intention-to-treat analysis, the surgery-first group demonstrated a lower reintervention rate compared with the angioplasty-first group (18% vs 26%; difference 8%, 95% confidence interval [CI] 0.04%–15%), which was more prominent in the as-treated analysis (17% vs 28%; difference 11%, 95% CI 4%–19%). However, the surgery-first group experienced a higher 30 day morbidity rate (57% vs 41%; difference 15.5%, 95% CI 5.8–24.8), primarily related to wound complications, infections, and cardiovascular events. The 30 day mortality rate remained similar between the 2 groups (5% vs 3%). AFS rates at 1 and 3 years after surgery were 68% and 57%; and 71% and 52% for those randomized to angioplasty, respectively (p = NS). A post hoc analysis, done after examination of the survival curves, showed a significantly reduced hazard in AFS (adjusted hazard ratio [HR] 0·37 [95% CI 0.17–0.77], *P*= .008) and all-cause mortality (0.34 [0.17–0.71], *P*= .004) for surgery relative to angioplasty in the period beyond 2 years from randomization.

The 5 year follow-up of the trial patients revealed that autogenous vein bypasses demonstrated superior AFS compared to prosthetic grafts, and those undergoing a secondary bypass after a failed angioplasty had significantly worse AFS than those undergoing primary bypass (20% vs 40% at 5 years, *P*= .006) [36]. These findings indicate that angioplasty-first approach is not without consequences, since subsequent bypass procedures tend to have reduced long-term durability compared with primary bypass. Furthermore, it is important to note that endovascular procedures utilized in the BASIL trial comprised only of balloon angioplasty, while currently bare-metal stents and drug-eluting stents (DES) are used more commonly.

Bypass versus Angioplasty in Severe Ischemia of the Leg-2

BASIL-2 was an open-label, pragmatic, multicenter, randomized trial that enrolled patients with CLTI in the United Kingdom, Sweden, and Denmark between 2014 and 2020 [8]. Eligible patients required infrapopliteal revascularization (with or without additional proximal infrainguinal intervention) to restore limb perfusion, had a life expectancy greater than 6 months, and were deemed suitable for both infrapopliteal vein bypass and ET. Patients were excluded if they had undergone a vascular intervention to the target infrapopliteal artery within the prior 12 months. The primary endpoint was also AFS and the median follow-up was 40 months. A total of 345 patients were randomized, with 172 assigned to vein bypass and 173 to best endovascular treatment.

AFS rate was 53% in the vein bypass group and 63% in the endovascular group (HR 1.35, 95% CI 1.02–1.8, *P*= .037). Thirty-day morbidity (46% vs 42%) and mortality (6% vs 3%) were comparable between the 2 revascularization strategies. Reintervention rates were also similar, occurring in 29% of vein bypass patients and 32% of endovascular patients. Crossover revascularization occurred more frequently in the vein bypass group (27% vs 19%). However, reinterventions using the same modality were less common after vein bypass than after initial ET (5% vs 19%). Rates of major adverse limb events (MALE), major adverse cardiovascular events (MACE), hemodynamic improvements, ischemic pain relief, and HRQL were not significantly different between groups. Overall mortality was 53% in the vein bypass group and 45% in the endovascular group (HR 1.37, 95% CI 1.00–1.87). Based on these findings, the BASIL-2 investigators recommended an endovascular-first approach for patients with CLTI requiring infrapopliteal revascularization.

The BASIL-2 trial has received significant criticism on several fronts. Some have argued that the study was underpowered as it failed to reach its original target enrollment of 600 patients. Concerns were also raised regarding the use of composite or prosthetic grafts instead of vein based on surgeon's discretion, which could dramatically alter the outcomes. There was also underrepresentation of female and non-White patients [37]. Another major criticism was the prolonged recruitment period, attributed to limited equipoise, logistical barriers, and the coronavirus disease 2019 pandemic, which ultimately led to early closure below the planned sample size. The generalizability of BASIL-2 might be questionable, as it included only patients suitable for both infrapopliteal bypass and ET.

Best Endovascular versus Best Surgical Therapy in Patients with Critical Limb Ischemia

BEST-CLI was an international, prospective, randomized, pragmatic, open-label, multicenter, superiority trial, with patients enrolled at 150 sites in the United States, Canada, Finland, Italy, and New Zealand [7]. The trial consisted of 2 parallel studies. Cohort 1 included patients with adequate single-segment great saphenous vein (SSGSV), and Cohort 2 included those without an adequate SSGSV. Both cohorts were stratified by clinical presentation (ischemic rest pain vs tissue loss) and anatomic severity (presence or absence of significant tibial disease). Patients were then randomized to either ET or open bypass, with procedural techniques left to operator judgment. A total of 1830 patients were enrolled between 2014 and 2019, with 1434 in Cohort 1 (718 assigned to bypass and 716 to ET) and 396 in Cohort 2 (197 bypass and 199 ET). Patients were excluded from the trial if they had excessive risk associated with open vascular surgery or less than 2 years life-expectancy. Surgeons selected the bypass approach based on their preference, and all contemporary endovascular modalities were allowed including plain old balloon angioplasty, BMS, DES, drug-coated balloons, and atherectomy. The primary endpoint was MALE or all-cause mortality, where MALE was defined as above-ankle amputation or major reintervention on the index limb such as new bypass, interposition graft, thrombectomy, or thrombolysis. Secondary outcomes included MALE, 30 day mortality, major or minor reinterventions, AFS, hemodynamic or clinical failure, resolution or recurrence of CLTI, MACE, health-related quality-of-life metrics, and cost.

In Cohort 1 patients undergoing bypass, 43% had femoral–popliteal, 38% had femoral–tibial or pedal, and 16% had popliteal–tibial or pedal bypasses, with 85% of procedures performed using an SSGSV. ET involved the SFA in 68% of the cases, the popliteal artery in 53% cases, and the tibial or pedal arteries in 53% of cases as well. Endovascular interventions were performed by vascular surgeons in 73% of cases, by interventional cardiologists in 15%, and by interventional radiologists in 13%. Technical success was achieved in 98% of surgical cases and 85% of endovascular cases. Among the 108 early technical failures in the endovascular group, 66 patients underwent surgical bypass within 30 days. The composite primary outcome of MALE/Death occurred in 42.6% of the surgical group and 57.4% of the endovascular group, corresponding to HR of 0.68 (95% CI, 0.59–0.79; $P < .001$). This benefit for surgery persisted in both per-protocol and as-treated analyses. Major reinterventions were significantly less frequent in the surgical group (9.2%) compared with the endovascular group (23.5%), HR 0.35 (95% CI, 0.27–0.47). Major amputation of the index limb occurred in 10.4% of surgical patients versus 14.9% of endovascular patients (HR, 0.73; 95% CI, 0.54–0.98). Furthermore, the incidence of new or recurrent CLTI events was lower in the surgical group (incidence rate ratio, 0.82; 95% CI, 0.70–0.95). There was no significant difference in mortality (30 day and at last follow-up), MACE, myocardial infarction (MI), or stroke between the 2 groups.

One the other hand in Cohort 2, among 396 patients without a suitable SSGSV, there was no significant difference in MALE/Death (42.8% versus 47.7%; HR, 0.79; 95% CI, 0.58–1.06; $P = .12$), major amputation, MALE, all-cause mortality, MI, stroke, or incidence of new or recurrent CLTI events between the bypass and ET groups. However, major reinterventions were significantly lower in the surgery group (HR, 0.47; 95% CI, 0.29–0.76). These findings were also consistent across subgroups and in per-protocol and as-treated analyses.

The BEST-CLI investigators then concluded that patients with CLTI being considered for limb salvage should first undergo assessment of overall surgical risk and availability of an adequate vein conduit. For those with suitable anatomy and acceptable risk, bypass using SSGSV should be considered a first-line option as part of shared, informed decision-making.

Just like BASIL-2, BEST-CLI also received considerable criticism regarding its design, patient selection, and interpretation of results. Some questioned the choice of MALE/Death as the primary endpoint instead of AFS and the representativeness of enrolled patients to real-world clinical practice. In response, the investigators clarified that MALE captures limb-specific outcomes more accurately than AFS, as the latter often underrepresents limb-related outcomes that directly reflect the effectiveness of revascularization [38]. Additionally, AFS excludes important clinical events such as reinterventions or acute limb ischemia. In contrast, MALE focuses on limb-specific outcomes that are directly impacted by treatment choice.

Others raised concerns about operator skill, the use of suboptimal endovascular techniques, and whether early endovascular failure accounted for the observed differences in outcomes. To address that, all investigators in BEST-CLI underwent credentialing by a multidisciplinary committee that established criteria to balance operator experience with the goal of conducting a real-world trial. To qualify as a surgeon, investigators had to have performed at least 10 infrainguinal bypasses for CLTI (half using vein) to below-knee targets within 2 years. Endovascular operators had to have completed at least 12 below-knee interventions for CLTI in 2 years. Device use reflected guideline-based, real-world practice, and sensitivity analyses confirmed that early technical failures did not explain the superiority of surgical bypass with vein. Overall, BEST-CLI remains the highest quality evidence to date comparing both strategies, reinforcing that open and endovascular revascularization are complementary rather than competing approaches in CLTI management.

SUBANALYSES FROM BEST ENDOVASCULAR VERSUS BEST SURGICAL THERAPY IN PATIENTS WITH CRITICAL LIMB ISCHEMIA

Several post hoc studies from BEST-CLI have been published to put the trial into appropriate context, by elucidating the results of the trial in different patient subgroups of interest. One of the trials prespecified secondary objectives was to assess the effects of revascularization strategy on health-related quality of life (HRQoL). Results from that study indicated that revascularization by either bypass or ET significantly improved HRQoL over baseline across the entire range of quality-of-life metrics used, and the differences between both approaches were below the threshold of clinically meaningful difference [39]. Other studies comparing the incidence of perioperative complications and cardiovascular events between bypass and ET found similar results following either approach. Hence the authors concluded that a concern about the risk of periprocedural cardiovascular complications should not be a deterrent in deciding revascularization strategy. Rather, other factors, including effectiveness in restoring perfusion and patient preference, are more relevant [40,41].

Given the contradictory findings between BASIL-2 and BEST-CLI, an analysis of patients in BEST-CLI with significant infrapopliteal disease was performed to formulate a relevant comparator with the outcomes reported from BASIL-2. Results of that study showed that among patients with suitable SSGSV who underwent infrapopliteal revascularization for CLTI, open bypass surgery was associated with a lower incidence of MALE/Death (HR 0.69; 95% CI [0.54–0.87], $P = .0018$) and major amputation (HR 0.59; 95% CI [0.38–0.92] $P = .0205$) compared with ET [42]. However, all-cause mortality and AFS were similar between the groups. Reasons for proposed differences between both trial results will be discussed in detail later in this article.

Subanalyses focusing on conduit choice, durability of revascularization strategy, and limb salvage outcomes have confirmed a lot of biases among bypass enthusiasts. For instance, the use of a prosthetic conduit was found to be associated with inferior outcomes compared with SSGSV, particularly for infrapopliteal targets [43]. Another analysis highlighted the superior durability following initial treatment with SSGSV as it was associated with a significantly lower hazard of target limb reinterventions compared to ET (major reintervention HR 0.37; [95% CI, 0.28–0.49; $P < .001$]; any reintervention HR, 0.63; [95% CI, 0.53–0.75]; $P < .001$) [44]. Furthermore, SSGSV bypass was found to be more effective than ET at healing wounds, preventing CLTI recurrence, as well as reducing the risk of major amputations [45,46].

Despite being underrepresented in BEST-CLI, female patients had better MALE-free survival and AFS compared with male patients [47]. On the other hand, ethnic disparities in limb-related outcomes were not observed for Hispanic patients in the trial [48]. An interesting spline model analysis investigating the impact of estimated glomerular filtration rate (eGFR) on CLTI outcomes revealed that the hazard of MALE/Death increased sharply at eGFR less than 30, with no difference observed when stratifying by procedure received (surgical or endovascular revascularization) [49]. However, in dialysis-dependent patients, ET was associated with better survival, but twice the risk of reintervention compared with open bypass. Although the trial included patients who have at least 2 years of life expectancy, over 50% of the patients on hemodialysis were dead within 3 years regardless of the treatment received, which was a very sobering finding [50]. Finally, although patients receiving insulin for diabetes management present with worse glucose control and more advanced CLTI, open bypass still was superior to ET regardless of insulin use or hemoglobin A1c (HbA1c) level [51].

BYPASS VERSUS ANGIOPLASTY IN SEVERE ISCHEMIA OF THE LEG-2 VERSUS BEST ENDOVASCULAR VERSUS BEST SURGICAL THERAPY IN PATIENTS WITH CRITICAL LIMB ISCHEMIA

Both BASIL-2 and BEST-CLI trials provided substantial and much-needed evidence comparing open and endovascular revascularization strategies. Despite differences in geography, design, and patient selection, both trials were well-conducted and pragmatic in design, and emphasized that both open and endovascular approaches play essential and complementary roles in limb salvage. However, several factors likely explain their contrasting results. While both trials shared similar technical success rates and baseline medical therapy use, key differences in design, patient populations, and health care systems likely influenced outcomes. BEST-CLI was much larger, included a broader and more diverse population, and enrolled younger patients with better life-expectancy. BASIL-2 on the other hand was limited to patients requiring infrapopliteal revascularization and included older patients with lower life expectancy. This could explain why results appear primarily driven by overall mortality rather than limb-related events in BASIL-2. Ultimately, both trials complement rather than contradict one another, and certainly individualized treatment selection and multidisciplinary expertise remain central to optimal CLTI care.

REAL-WORLD OUTCOMES

Infrainguinal bypass continues to offer durable long-term results for patients with symptomatic PAD, even as ET expands. In one of the contemporary series, we evaluated all patients who underwent infrainguinal bypass with autogenous vein conduits in a single institution. Primary patency at 1, 3, and 5 years was 66%, 59%, and 55%, respectively, and limb salvage rate was 88% after a mean follow-up of 2 ± 1.8 years. We were able to show that patency and limb salvage rates are optimized with careful selection of autogenous conduits and close monitoring of high-risk groups such as patients with diabetes or hyperlipidemia [52].

We have published the first study in the literature that documents femoropopliteal bypass being associated with higher reintervention rates compared with angioplasty and stenting [53]. In this study, we grouped patients into either PTA/stenting of the SFA or femoral-popliteal bypass and compared the overall patency and reintervention rates between both groups. The primary patency at 2 years was better for the endovascular group 67% (95% CI, 0.52–0.78) versus bypass group 49% (95% CI, 0.32–0.64; $P = .05$). The rate of reintervention was higher in the bypass group compared with the ET group (54% vs 31%; $P = .02$). However, since 77% of patients with TASC II A and B lesions underwent ET, whereas 73% of patients with TASC C and D lesions underwent bypass ($P < .01$), we believe that the main reason for this finding is the fact that the bypass patients had significantly more advanced disease. This emphasizes that one must consider the patient population undergoing intervention when comparing revascularization procedures. Coinciding with this study, the BEST-CLI trial at that time started the patient recruitment phase.

Recent real-world practice analysis by our team on over 30,000 patients included in a Medicare-linked database, showed that SSGSV bypass was associated with better overall survival, AFS, and freedom from amputation compared to ET [54]. In this study, 3 cohorts were queried: bypass with GSV (BWGSV: N = 5279, 14.7%), bypass with prosthetic graft (BWPG: N = 2778, 7.7%), and ET (ET: N = 27,977, 77.6%). Propensity score matching produced 2 sets of well-matched cohorts: 4705 pairs of ET versus BWGSV and 2583 pairs of ET versus BWPG. In the matched cohorts of ET versus BWGSV, ET was associated with greater hazards of death (HR = 1.34, 95% CI, 1.25–1.43; $P < .001$), amputation (HR = 1.30, 95% CI, 1.17–1.44; $P < .001$), and amputation/death (HR = 1.32, 95% CI, 1.24–1.40; $P < .001$) up to 4 years. In the matched cohorts of ET versus BWPG, ET was associated with greater hazards of death up to 2 years (HR = 1.11, 95% CI, 1.00–1.22; $P = .042$). In other words, results from our study mirror the outcomes demonstrated by the BEST-CLI trial.

On the contrary, an analysis performed by our team on over 25,000 infrapopliteal revascularization procedures (bypass vs ET) showed conflicting results to BASIL-2. We found superior 1 year outcomes with infrapopliteal bypasses using SSGSV compared with ET in terms of overall survival (HR = 0.73 [95% CI, 0.60–0.88]; $P = .001$) and AFS (HR = 0.84 [95% CI, 0.72–0.97]; $P = .020$) [55]. However, ET was superior to bypass with AC in terms of limb salvage, AFS, and freedom from MALE. We concluded that bypass with SSGSV should be considered first-line therapy for CLTI when there is infrapopliteal involvement. However, when a good-quality SSGSV is not available, ET can offer lower amputation and MALE risk and higher AFS compared with AC.

A recent multi-institutional study from 4 centers in Europe retrospectively evaluated outcomes of patients who underwent first-time infrainguinal bypass or ET [56]. A total of 793 patients met the eligibility criteria, and 236 matched pairs were included in the final analysis with a mean follow-up of 52 months. Among the bypass cohort, 80.5% were autogenous grafts and 64% were infrapopliteal. In the ET group, the treated lesion involved the femoropopliteal segment in 34.3%, combined femoropopliteal and infrapopliteal segments in

42.8%, and isolated infrapopliteal segments in 22.9%. At 5 years, AFS was superior after bypass compared with ET (60.5% vs 35.3%; $P < .001$). Major amputation occurred in 25.8% of bypass patients versus 36.0% of patients with ET (HR 0.66, 95% CI 0.47–0.92; $P = .014$). Wound healing at 6 months was also superior following bypass ($P = .003$). Although the hospital stay was shorter for the ET group (median 4 vs 8 days; $P = .001$), urgent reintervention and readmission rates were comparable between both cohorts. Overall, this study demonstrates that bypass surgery provides significantly better long-term AFS and faster wound healing compared with ET, reaffirming the durable benefits of surgical revascularization in appropriately selected patients.

SUMMARY

CLTI represents the most advanced stage of PAD and typically requires revascularization to prevent limb loss and improve survival. Both open surgical bypass and endovascular intervention are established treatment options, yet randomized trials have shown mixed results due to differences in patient populations, anatomy, and methodology. Overall, current level 1 evidence supports bypass as the preferred first-line revascularization strategy when a suitable SSGSV conduit is available, and the patient can safely undergo an open procedure. However, ET remains an important and less-invasive alternative for patients with high surgical risk or without a suitable vein.

CLINICS CARE POINTS

- The choice between bypass and ET should be individualized based on anatomy, operative risk, and conduit availability.
- Patients with CLTI indicated for revascularization should undergo vein mapping to be screened for an adequate vein conduit.
- Those with acceptable operative risk and a suitable SSGSV, open bypass should be considered.
- Those with high surgical risk or without a suitable SSGSV, ET should be recommended.
- Optimal management of CLTI requires multidisciplinary collaboration between vascular surgeons, interventionalists, and wound care specialists to achieve the best results.

Disclosure

M. Hamouda: None; K. Yei: None; M.B. Malas: Consultant for Bard and Cordis.

References

[1] Fowkes FGR, Rudan D, Rudan I, et al. Comparison of global estimates of prevalence and risk factors for peripheral artery disease in 2000 and 2010: a systematic review and analysis. Lancet 2013;382:1329–40.

[2] Conte MS, Bradbury AW, Kolh P, et al. Global vascular guidelines on the management of chronic limb-threatening ischemia. J Vasc Surg 2019;69(6):3S–125S.e40.
[3] Verwer MC, Wijnand JGJ, Teraa M, et al. Long term survival and limb salvage in patients with non-revascularisable chronic limb threatening ischaemia. Eur J Vasc Endovasc Surg 2021;62(2):225–32.
[4] Shan LL, Yang LS, Tew M, et al. Quality of life in chronic limb threatening ischaemia: systematic review and meta-analysis. Eur J Vasc Endovasc Surg 2022;64(6):666–83.
[5] Cheng TW, Farber A. Surgery or endovascular therapy for chronic limb-threatening ischemia. Adv Surg 2024;58(1):121–33.
[6] Adam DJ, Beard JD, Cleveland T, et al. Bypass versus angioplasty in severe ischaemia of the leg (BASIL): Multicentre, randomised controlled trial. Lancet Lond Engl 2005;366(9501):1925–34.
[7] Farber A, Menard MT, Conte MS, et al. Surgery or endovascular therapy for chronic limb-threatening ischemia. N Engl J Med 2022;387(25):2305–16.
[8] Bradbury AW, Moakes CA, Popplewell M, et al. A vein bypass first versus a best endovascular treatment first revascularisation strategy for patients with chronic limb threatening ischaemia who required an infra-popliteal, with or without an additional more proximal infra-inguinal revascularisation procedure to restore limb perfusion (BASIL-2): an open-label, randomised, multicentre, phase 3 trial. Lancet Lond Engl 2023;401(10390):1798–809.
[9] Farber A. Chronic limb-threatening ischemia. N Engl J Med 2018;379(2):171–80.
[10] Nakhaei P, Hamouda M, Malas MB. The double burden: deciphering chronic limb-threatening ischemia in end-stage renal disease. Ann Vasc Surg 2024;107:105–21.
[11] Hamouda M, Zarrintan S, Vootukuru N, et al. Outcomes of prosthetic and biological grafts compared to arm vein grafts in patients with chronic limb-threatening ischemia. J Vasc Surg 2025;81(3):682–92.
[12] Hamouda M, Rogers UH, Farber A, et al. Impact of skin closure with staples vs sutures on perioperative outcomes following lower extremity bypass surgery. J Vasc Surg 2025;81 (3):743–50.
[13] Rajebi H, Rajebi MR. Optimizing common femoral artery access. Tech Vasc Intervent Radiol 2015;18(2):76–81.
[14] Irani F, Kumar S, Colyer WRJ. Common femoral artery access techniques: a review. J Cardiovasc Med 2009;10(7):517.
[15] Stone PA, Campbell JE. Complications related to femoral artery access for transcatheter procedures. Vasc Endovasc Surg 2012;46(8):617–23.
[16] Bazan HA, Le L, Donovan M, et al. Retrograde pedal access for patients with critical limb ischemia. J Vasc Surg 2014;60(2):375–82.
[17] El-Sayed H, Bennett ME, Loh TM, et al. Retrograde pedal access and endovascular revascularization: a safe and effective technique for high-risk patients with complex tibial vessel disease. Ann Vasc Surg 2016;31:91–8.
[18] Lorenzoni R, Ferraresi R, Manzi M, et al. Guidewires for lower extremity artery angioplasty: a review. EuroIntervention 2015;11(8):799–807.
[19] Khaitovitch B, Cohen I, Gilat EK, et al. Percutaneous recanalization of lower limb chronic total occlusions via tibial artery access using the BeBack^{TM} crossing catheter. Vascular 2024;33(6):1457–62.
[20] Bausback Y, Botsios S, Flux J, et al. Outback catheter for femoropopliteal occlusions: immediate and long-term results. J Endovasc Ther 2011;18(1):13–21.
[21] Sheikh AB, Llanos-Chea F, Jelani QUA, et al. Safety and efficacy outcomes of the pioneer plus catheter in endovascular revascularization of lower extremity chronic total occlusions. J Vasc Surg 2021;74(3):746–55.
[22] Beckman JA, Schneider PA, Conte MS. Advances in revascularization for peripheral artery disease: revascularization in PAD. Circ Res 2021;128(12):1885–912.
[23] Giacoppo D, Cassese S, Harada Y, et al. Drug-coated balloon versus plain balloon angioplasty for the treatment of femoropopliteal artery disease. JACC Cardiovasc Interv 2016;9 (16):1731–42.

[24] Schillinger M, Sabeti S, Dick P, et al. Sustained benefit at 2 years of primary femoropopliteal stenting compared with balloon angioplasty with optional stenting. Circulation 2007;115(21):2745–9.
[25] Dake MD, Ansel GM, Jaff MR, et al. Durable clinical effectiveness with paclitaxel-eluting stents in the femoropopliteal artery. Circulation 2016;133(15):1472–83.
[26] DeRubertis BG, Varcoe RL, Krishnan P, et al. Drug-eluting resorbable scaffold versus balloon angioplasty for below-the-knee peripheral artery disease: 2-year results from the LIFE-BTK trial. Circulation 2025;152(15):1076–86.
[27] Adams G, Shammas N, Mangalmurti S, et al. Intravascular lithotripsy for treatment of calcified lower extremity arterial stenosis: initial analysis of the disrupt PAD III study. J Endovasc Ther 2020;27(3):473–80.
[28] Brodmann M, Holden A, Zeller T. Safety and feasibility of intravascular lithotripsy for treatment of below-the-knee arterial stenoses. J Endovasc Ther 2018;25(4):499–503.
[29] Akkus NI, Abdulbaki A, Jimenez E, et al. Atherectomy devices: technology update. Med Dev Evid Res 2014;8:1–10.
[30] Krievins DK, Halena G, Scheinert D, et al. One-year results from the DETOUR I trial of the PQ bypass DETOUR system for percutaneous femoropopliteal bypass. J Vasc Surg 2020;72(5):1648–58.e2.
[31] Lyden SP, Soukas PA, De A, et al. DETOUR2 trial outcomes demonstrate clinical utility of percutaneous transmural bypass for the treatment of long segment, complex femoropopliteal disease. J Vasc Surg 2024;79(6):1420–7.e2.
[32] Yan Q, Prasla S, Carlisle DC, et al. Deep venous arterialization for chronic limb threatening ischemia in atherosclerosis patients – a meta-analysis. Ann Vasc Surg 2022;81:1–21.
[33] Clair DG, Mustapha JA, Shishehbor MH, et al. Promise I: early feasibility study of the LimFlow system for percutaneous deep vein arterialization in no-option chronic limb-threatening ischemia: 12-Month results. J Vasc Surg 2021;74(5):1626–35.
[34] Gornik HL, Aronow HD, Goodney PP, et al. ACC/AHA/AACVPR/APMA/ABC/SCAI/SVM/SVN/SVS/SIR/VESS guideline for the management of lower extremity peripheral artery disease: a report of the American college of Cardiology/American Heart Association Joint Committee on clinical practice Guidelines. Circulation 2024;149(24):e1313–410.
[35] Mills JL, Conte MS, Armstrong DG, et al. The society for vascular surgery lower extremity threatened limb classification system: risk stratification based on wound, ischemia, and foot infection (WIfI). J Vasc Surg 2014;59(1):220–34.e2.
[36] Bradbury AW, Adam DJ, Bell J, et al. Bypass versus angioplasty in severe ischaemia of the leg (BASIL) trial: an intention-to-treat analysis of amputation-free and overall survival in patients randomized to a bypass surgery-first or a balloon angioplasty-first revascularization strategy. J Vasc Surg 2010;51(5 Suppl):5S–17S.
[37] Popplewell MA, Bradbury AW. Responses to the main critiques of the bypass versus angioplasty in severe ischemia of the leg (BASIL)-2 trial. Ann Vasc Surg 2024;107:43–7.
[38] D'Angelo O, Menard MT, Farber A. Common criticisms and rebuttals of the best endovascular versus best surgical therapy in patients with chronic limb-threatening ischemia (BEST-CLI) trial. Ann Vasc Surg 2024;107:93–100.
[39] Menard MT, Farber A, Powell RJ, et al. Quality of life in patients with chronic limb-threatening ischemia treated with revascularization. Circulation 2024;149(16):1241–53.
[40] Siracuse JJ, Farber A, Menard MT, et al. Perioperative complications following open or endovascular revascularization for chronic limb-threatening ischemia in the BEST-CLI trial. J Vasc Surg 2023;78(4):1012–20.e2.
[41] Siracuse JJ, Menard MT, Rosenfield K, et al. Characterization of cardiovascular serious adverse events after bypass or endovascular revascularization for limb-threatening ischemia in the BEST-CLI trial. J Vasc Surg 2024;80(3):774–9.
[42] Giles KA, Farber A, Menard MT, et al. Surgery or endovascular therapy for patients with chronic limb-threatening ischemia requiring infrapopliteal interventions. J Vasc Surg 2024;80(5):1515–24.

[43] Farber A, Menard MT, Conte MS, et al. Prosthetic conduits have worse outcomes compared with great saphenous vein conduits in femoropopliteal and infrapopliteal bypass in patients with chronic limb-threatening ischemia. J Vasc Surg 2025;81(2):408–16.e2.
[44] Conte MS, Azene E, Doros G, et al. Secondary interventions following open vs endovascular revascularization for chronic limb threatening ischemia in the BEST-CLI trial. J Vasc Surg 2024;79(6):1428–37.e4.
[45] Venermo MA, Farber A, Schanzer A, et al. Editor's choice – reduction of major amputations after surgery versus endovascular intervention: the BEST-CLI randomised trial. Eur J Vasc Endovasc Surg 2024;68(5):590–7.
[46] Menard MT, Farber A, Doros G, et al. The impact of revascularization strategy on clinical failure, hemodynamic failure, and chronic limb-threatening ischemia symptoms in the BEST-CLI trial. J Vasc Surg 2024;80(6):1755–65.e4.
[47] McGinigle KL, Doros G, Alabi O, et al. Female patients have fewer limb amputations compared to male patients in the BEST-CLI trial. J Vasc Surg 2025;81(2):366–73.e1.
[48] Ulloa JG, Alabi O, McGinigle K, et al. Outcomes for Hispanic patients undergoing open bypass in BEST-CLI. J Vasc Surg 2025;81(6):1420–9.
[49] Malas MB, Hamouda M, Farber A, et al. Outcomes of chronic limb-threatening ischemia revascularization in patients with chronic kidney disease in the BEST-CLI trial. J Vasc Surg 2025;81(4):945–56.e3.
[50] Malas MB, Hamouda M, Farber A. Reply. J Vasc Surg 2025;81(6):1531–2.
[51] Alameddine D, Hamouda M, Doros G, et al. Insulin therapy and outcomes of revascularization procedures for chronic-limb threatening ischemia in the BEST-CLI trial. J Vasc Surg 2025;83(1):246–55.e3.
[52] Reifsnyder T, Arhuidese IJ, Hicks CW, et al. Contemporary outcomes for open infrainguinal bypass in the endovascular era. Ann Vasc Surg 2016;30:52–8.
[53] Malas MB, Enwerem N, Qazi U, et al. Comparison of surgical bypass with angioplasty and stenting of superficial femoral artery disease. J Vasc Surg 2014;59(1):129–35.
[54] Zarrintan S, Hamouda M, Mills JL, et al. Bypass versus endovascular therapy for elective infrapopliteal interventions in chronic limb-threatening ischemia: propensity score-matched analyses of vascular quality initiative registry. Ann Surg 2025;282(3):494–502.
[55] Zarrintan S, Rahgozar S, Ross EG, et al. Endovascular therapy versus bypass for chronic limb-threatening ischemia in a real-world practice. J Vasc Surg 2024;80(4):1169–81.
[56] Ricco JB, Roiger RJ, Schneider F, et al. Editor's choice - infra-inguinal endovascular revascularisation and bypass surgery for chronic limb threatening ischaemia: a retrospective european multicentre cohort study with propensity score matching. Eur J Vasc Endovasc Surg 2023;66(4):531–40.

Advances in Surgery 60 (2026) 49–64

ADVANCES IN SURGERY

Omission of Axillary Surgery for Low-Risk Breast Cancer

Kate R. Pawloski, MD, MPH, Andrea V. Barrio, MD*

Breast Service, Department of Surgery, Memorial Sloan Kettering Cancer Center, New York, NY, USA

Keywords

- Low-risk breast cancer • Sentinel lymph node biopsy
- Omission of axillary surgery • SOUND • INSEMA

Key points

- Sentinel lymph node biopsy (SLNB) can be safely omitted in clinically node-negative, postmenopausal patients with small, low-risk, luminal breast cancer undergoing upfront breast-conserving surgery (BCS).
- SLNB should still be performed in premenopausal patients with HR+/HER2-negative breast cancer, and most patients with triple-negative and HER2-positive breast cancer undergoing BCS.
- SLNB should still be performed in patients with early-stage breast cancer undergoing mastectomy.
- De-escalation of axillary surgery should be performed with multidisciplinary consensus, with the understanding that SLNB should be performed if knowledge of pathologic nodal status will impact systemic therapy decisions.

HISTORICAL PERSPECTIVE OF AXILLARY SURGERY FOR BREAST CANCER

For most of the 20th Century, axillary lymph node dissection (ALND) represented the standard of care for both staging and treatment of breast cancer. The Halsted radical mastectomy was regarded as the curative surgical approach for breast cancer in the early 1900s, involving en bloc resection of the breast, pectoralis muscles, and level I-III axillary lymph nodes. The rationale and procedural steps of this operation were described by William Stewart Halsted in 1894, who theorized that cancer spread in a contiguous fashion from the breast

*Corresponding author. *E-mail address:* barrioa@mskcc.org

https://doi.org/10.1016/j.yasu.2026.03.004

Abbreviations

ACOSOG	American College of Surgeons Oncology Group
ALND	axillary lymph node dissection
BCS	breast-conserving surgery
CI	confidence interval
HR	hormone receptor
INSEMA	Intergroup-Sentinel-Mamma
MSKCC	Memorial Sloan Kettering Cancer Center
NSABP	National Surgical Adjuvant Breast and Bowel Project
SLN	sentinel lymph node
SLNB	sentinel lymph node biopsy
SOUND	Sentinel Node versus Observation After Axillary Ultra-Sound

to regional lymph nodes, then systemically [1]. Halsted presumed that curative resection of the primary tumor and regional lymph nodes, representing barriers to systemic spread, was necessary to achieve locoregional control irrespective of the disease presentation and clinical nodal status.

Following decades of routine ALND for all patients with breast cancer, Halsted's principle was challenged by a growing recognition that breast cancer is a systemic disease at presentation. Initiated by Bernard Fisher in 1971, the National Surgical Adjuvant Breast and Bowel Project (NSABP) B-04 randomized trial was designed to test whether less-extensive surgery in the breast and axilla resulted in similar survival as radical mastectomy. Results of B-04 demonstrated equivalence in disease-free and overall survival among 1079 clinically node-negative patients randomized to radical mastectomy or total mastectomy with or without chest and regional nodal irradiation at 25 years of follow-up [2]. NSABP B-04 was unique in that none of the patients received systemic therapy, allowing for an understanding of the natural history of untreated nodal disease in the cohort of patients treated without ALND (ie, the total mastectomy cohort). In the trial, approximately 40% of clinically node-negative patients who underwent radical mastectomy had positive nodes at the time of ALND. Presumably, 40% of the patients randomized to total mastectomy without ALND also had positive nodes, and yet only 18% of patients subsequently developed a clinically apparent axillary recurrence during the follow-up period in the absence of systemic therapy (Fig. 1) [2]. Notably, axillary failures were early events, occurring within the first 2 years after surgery. NSABP B-04 was a landmark trial because it was the first successful surgical de-escalation trial and because it demonstrated that not all untreated nodal disease results in axillary failure, laying the groundwork for future trials of surgical de-escalation in the axilla.

ADOPTION OF SENTINEL LYMPH NODE BIOPSY IN LIEU OF AXILLARY LYMPH NODE DISSECTION FOR CLINICALLY NODE-NEGATIVE PATIENTS

Sentinel lymph node biopsy (SLNB), which involves selectively removing only the first draining axillary node(s), replaced ALND as the standard method to

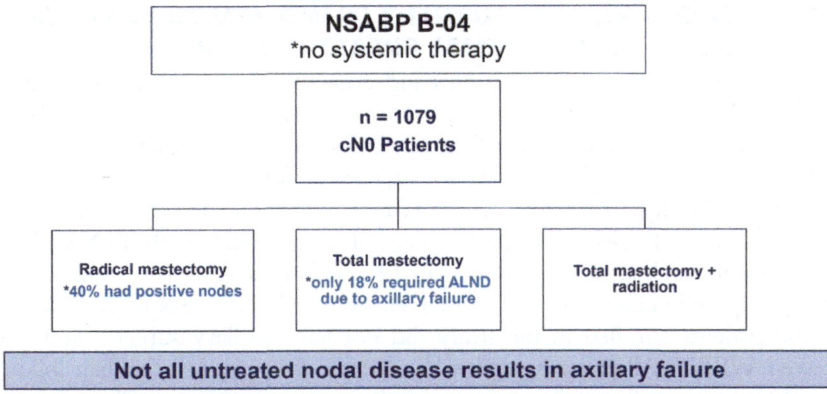

Fig. 1. NSABP B-04 randomized controlled trial design. ALND, axillary lymph node dissection; NSABP, National Surgical Adjuvant Breast and Bowel Project.

stage the axilla in clinically and pathologically node-negative patients in the mid-1990s to late-1990s; this de-escalated axillary staging approach minimized arm and shoulder morbidity without compromising survival [3–6]. As systemic therapy for breast cancer improved in the late 1990s and early 2000s, the benefit of ALND in patients with limited nodal disease in the axilla was questioned. The American College of Surgeons Oncology Group (ACOSOG) Z0011 trial and the European Organisation for Research and Treatment of Cancer 10981-22023 AMAROS trial randomized women with cT1-2, cN0 breast cancer with 1 to 2 positive sentinel lymph nodes (SLNs) undergoing breast-conserving surgery (BCS)-only (Z0011), or BCS or mastectomy (AMAROS), to ALND versus SLNB alone (Z0011) or SLNB plus axillary radiation (AMAROS) [7,8]. All patients received appropriate systemic therapy and whole-breast radiotherapy (WBRT) after BCS. In the Z0011 and AMAROS trials, 27% and 33% of patients in the ALND cohorts, respectively, had additional positive nodes on final pathology; however, this did not translate into an increased risk of axillary failure in patients treated without ALND. In Z0011, the 10-year rate of axillary recurrence was 0.5% following ALND versus 1.5% following SLNB alone ($P = .28$) [9]. In AMAROS, the 10-year cumulative incidence of axillary recurrence was 0.93% after ALND versus 1.82% after SLNB plus regional nodal irradiation (hazard ratio 1.71, 95% confidence interval [CI] 0.67 to 4.39) [10]. Omission of ALND in both trials did not result in worse survival [10,11]. Both the Z0011 and AMAROS trials confirmed that residual microscopic disease in the undissected axilla can be adequately treated with systemic therapy and RT, precluding the need for ALND.

Both ACOSOG Z11 and AMAROS demonstrated that leaving microscopic residual disease in the undissected axilla does not result in worse outcomes.

OMISSION OF AXILLARY SURGERY IN WOMEN 70 YEARS OF AGE OR OLDER WITH LUMINAL BREAST CANCER

The favorable tumor biology and more judicious use of systemic chemotherapy in women 70 years of age or older with luminal (ie, hormone receptor-positive [HR+]/human epidermal growth factor 2 [HER2]-negative) cancers resulted in early adoption of omission of axillary surgery in this group of patients. The CALGB 9343 randomized trial was primarily conducted to assess whether omission of RT after BCS in women 70 years of age or older with T1N0, HR+ breast cancer resulted in worse survival [12]. Axillary staging with ALND was initially required in the trial, with subsequent removal of this requirement. Overall, 400 patients enrolled in the study did not have axillary surgery, and half received WBRT. All patients received endocrine therapy. At a median follow-up of 12.6 years, axillary failures among patients treated without axillary surgery were uncommon (0% radiation therapy [RT]; 3% no RT). Unlike CALGB, the IBCSG 10-93 trial was specifically designed to assess outcomes between postmenopausal patients 60 years of age or older with cN0, HR+ breast cancer treated with endocrine therapy with or without ALND [13]. In this cohort, most (55%) underwent BCS, with more than half receiving RT and 45% undergoing mastectomy. At 6 years of follow-up, nodal recurrence was observed in 1% of the ALND group and 3% of the no-axillary surgery group. Finally, a randomized trial conducted by Martelli and colleagues randomized women age 65 to 80 years with clinical T1N0 tumors undergoing BCS to either ALND or no axillary surgery [14]. At a median follow-up of 15 years, axillary recurrence was observed in 6% of patients in whom ALND was omitted, and there were no axillary recurrences in patients who underwent ALND.

Given the lack of benefit to axillary staging in women 70 years of age or older, the Society of Surgical Oncology Choosing Wisely guidelines recommended in 2016 that SLNB should not routinely be performed in cN0 women in this age group with early-stage HR+ invasive breast cancer [15]. Despite this recommendation, adoption of these guidelines has been slow. A National Cancer Database analysis from 2017 to 2020 found that SLNB was omitted in only 21% of eligible patients 70 years of age or older, with SLNB omission occurring more frequently in academic centers compared with community practices [16]. Continued efforts should focus on moving away from routine axillary staging in this group of patients, in whom the risks of axillary surgery outweigh the benefits.

> SLNB should not be routinely offered to women 70 years of age or older with small, clinically node-negative HR+/HER2-negative breast cancer undergoing lumpectomy.

TUMOR BIOLOGY PREDICTS PROGNOSIS AND GUIDES SYSTEMIC THERAPY

Nodal status in breast cancer was once the primary determinant of prognosis and the need for chemotherapy, with limited use of receptor status for decision making. Over the years, we have gained a deeper understanding of tumor biology and its impact on systemic therapy decisions and prognosis. We now know that there are distinct molecular subtypes of breast cancer (Luminal A, Luminal B, HER2-enriched, and Basal-like), and that prognosis varies by subtype. While nodal status remains important for treatment decisions in HER2-positive and triple-negative breast cancer, this information has become increasingly less relevant in luminal cancers with the emergence of genomic assays. While several validated genomic assays are available to assess recurrence risk (Oncotype DX, Mammaprint, PAM-50) [17–20], the 21-gene recurrence score (Oncotype DX; Exact Sciences, Madison, WI) provides prognostic information specifically in patients with HR+/HER2-negative (luminal) breast cancer, with high-risk scores (>25) predictive of response to chemotherapy, and low-risk scores (0–10) prognostic for excellent distant recurrence-free survival with endocrine therapy alone [21,22]. The TAILORx trial, which randomized 6711 women with HR+/HER2-negative node-negative breast cancer with a recurrence score of 11 to 25 to chemoendocrine therapy versus endocrine therapy alone, demonstrated no difference in 9-year invasive disease-free survival (iDFS) between the two groups (84.3% [chemoendocrine] vs 83.3% [endocrine]) or distant recurrence-free survival (95.0% vs 94.5%, respectively) [22]. This landmark trial provided further evidence that chemotherapy is not indicated in node-negative patients with a recurrence score of less than or equal to 25.

With an increased understanding of tumor biology and genomic risk came the recognition that there may be a subset of node-positive women with luminal breast cancer who do not benefit from systemic chemotherapy. This hypothesis was tested by the RxPONDER trial, which randomized 5083 women with luminal breast cancer and 1 to 3 positive lymph nodes with a recurrence score less than or equal to 25 to chemoendocrine therapy versus endocrine therapy alone [23]. Among postmenopausal patients (n = 3350), there was no benefit to chemotherapy in the node-positive group with a recurrence score less than or equal to 25 (5-year iDFS: 91.3% [chemoendocrine therapy] vs 91.9% [endocrine therapy alone]). Conversely, for "younger" premenopausal, node-positive women younger than 50 years of age, there was a benefit to chemotherapy across all recurrence scores, although many postulate that this benefit was secondary to the ovarian suppression from chemotherapy. Although nodal status remains important for systemic chemotherapy decisions in premenopausal women younger than 50 years of age with luminal cancers, it has become relatively inconsequential for systemic chemotherapy decisions in postmenopausal women with negative nodes or limited nodal disease where genomic risk is the primary determinant of treatment, suggesting that axillary surgery in this subset of patients could be omitted.

With consideration of omission of axillary surgery in clinically node-negative postmenopausal women, concern arose regarding the possibility of missing patients with a heavy nodal burden (≥4 positive nodes) in whom chemotherapy would still be recommended irrespective of genomic risk. However, most studies have demonstrated that the likelihood of a heavy nodal burden in postmenopausal women with cN0, HR+/HER2-negative breast cancer is uncommon, with a 3.5% (92/2639) prevalence of 4 or more positive nodes observed in retrospective study from Memorial Sloan Kettering Cancer Center (MSKCC) [24], and a 2.2% likelihood in a study utilizing the National Cancer Database [25], confirming that the risk of chemotherapy undertreatment in this subset with axillary surgery omission is negligible.

There is no benefit to chemotherapy in node-negative or postmenopausal node-positive (1-3 positive nodes) women with HR+/HER2-negative breast cancer and a recurrence score of less than or equal to 25.

OMISSION OF AXILLARY SURGERY FOR LOW-RISK BREAST CANCER

Considering the lack of benefit with ALND for women enrolled in ACOSOG Z0011 and AMAROS despite the presence of residual microscopic disease in approximately one-third of those treated without ALND, as well as evidence supporting SLNB omission in elderly, low-risk women, contemporary randomized trials sought to determine whether SLNB can be safely omitted in women with early, clinically node-negative breast cancer. The completed and ongoing trials are listed in Table 1 [26–29].

The SOUND [*Sentinel Node versus Observation After Axillary Ultra-Sound*] trial was a prospective non-inferiority phase 3 randomized clinical trial that accrued patients between February 2012 and June 2017 [26]. Enrolled patients had invasive breast cancer up to 2 cm (cT1), were clinically node-negative, planned for BCS and RT, and had a normal preoperative axillary ultrasound. If nodes were indeterminate on ultrasound, patients could enroll on trial with a negative fine-needle aspiration. Patients were randomized to SLNB versus no axillary surgery. All patients in the SLNB cohort with a positive SLN underwent completion ALND.

The analysis cohort included 1405 women, of whom 708 underwent SLNB and 697 had no axillary surgery. The median age was 60 years, median tumor size was 1.1 cm, and 88% of patients had HR+/HER2-negative breast cancer. Among patients who were randomized to SLNB, 13.7% had positive sentinel nodes (5.1% macrometastases, 8.6% micrometastases). Importantly, only 0.6% of patients had 4 or more positive nodes, even lower than the percentage observed in the retrospective MSKCC trial, likely due to the requirement of a negative axillary ultrasound in SOUND. The proportion of patients who received chemotherapy (approximately 20%) and radiation (approximately 98%) was similar between groups. Over 80% of patients received WBRT, 11% received partial-breast irradiation with intraoperative electron RT (ELIOT), and a small proportion had intraoperative RT boost

Table 1
Randomized Trials of Omission of Axillary Surgery in Early-Stage Breast Cancer

Trial	Country	N	Inclusion	Randomization Arms	Study Endpoints
SOUND (Gentilini et al. [26] 2023) (2012–2021) Active, not recruiting	Italy	1560	cT1N0 BCS + RT	Observation vs SLNB	5-y DDFS
INSEMA (Reimer et al. [28] 2025) (2015–2024) Active, not recruiting	Germany	5505	cT1-2N0 BCS + RT	Observation vs SLNB	5-y IDFS
BOOG 2013–08 (van Roozendaal et al. [29] 2017) (2015–2027) Active, recruiting	Netherlands	1644	cT1-2N0 BCS + RT	Observation vs SLNB	10-y regional recurrence
NAUTILUS (Jung et al. [27] 2022) (2020–2027) Active, recruiting	Korea	1734	cT1-2N0 BCS + RT	Observation vs SLNB	5-y IDFS

Abbreviations: BCS, breast-conserving surgery; DDFS, distant disease-free survival; IDFS, invasive disease-free survival; RT, radiation therapy; SLNB, sentinel lymph node biopsy.

followed by hypofractionated WBRT, with no difference in RT type between groups.

At a median follow-up of 5.8 years, there was no difference in 5-year distant disease-free survival between the SLNB group (97.7%) and the no-axillary-surgery group (98.0%, $P = .67$). The 5-year cumulative incidence of axillary recurrence was 0.4% in both groups (Gray $P = .91$) Although the SOUND trial demonstrated that omission of axillary surgery was non-inferior to SLNB in patients with small breast cancer and a negative axillary ultrasound, its authors emphasized that nodal status remains important for systemic therapy decisions in young (age <50 years) premenopausal patients with HR+/HER2-negative breast cancer, and in all triple-negative and HER2-positive breast cancer patients, and therefore axillary surgery should not be omitted in these populations. In postmenopausal patients with small HR+/HER2-negative breast cancers with a normal axillary ultrasound who are undergoing BCS and RT, axillary surgery can be safely omitted.

Following the publication of the SOUND trial, results from the INSEMA [*Intergroup-Sentinel-Mamma*] trial, a prospective, randomized, non-inferiority trial further support the omission of axillary surgery for patients with early-stage breast cancer [28]. Between September 2015 and April 2019, INSEMA randomized patients 18 years of age or older with early-stage breast cancer (including patients with tumors up to 5 cm) with a negative axillary ultrasound and undergoing lumpectomy to SLNB versus no axillary surgery. Patients were randomized in a 4:1 fashion ($n = 3896$ SLNB vs $n = 962$ no axillary surgery). The median age of the cohort was 62 years, 98.5% were HR+, 96.4% were HER2 negative, and fewer than 4% had grade 3 tumors. While INSEMA allowed enrollment of patients with larger tumors up to 5 cm, only 10% of patients enrolled had tumors between 2 and 5 cm, with a median tumor size of 1.1 cm. In patients undergoing SLNB, 15% had positive sentinel nodes, with fewer than 0.2% having 4 or more positive nodes.

At a median follow-up of 6.1 years, omission of axillary surgery was noninferior to SLNB with no difference in iDFS (hazard ratio 0.91, 95% CI 0.73–1.14). The 5-year iDFS was 91.9% (95% CI 89.9–93.5) for no axillary surgery compared to 91.7% (95% CI 90.8–92.6) for SLNB, with no difference in 5-year overall survival. Axillary recurrence was rare in both groups, observed in 0.3% of patients undergoing SLNB compared with 1.0% of patients in whom axillary surgery was omitted.

In addition to demonstrating no oncologic benefit to SLNB in patients with early-stage breast cancer, both SOUND and INSEMA demonstrated improved quality of life in patients when axillary surgery was omitted. SOUND patients randomized to SLNB experienced worse postoperative ipsilateral arm physical function in the early postoperative period compared with those having no axillary surgery [30]. Long-term follow-up of INSEMA demonstrated a lower incidence of lymphedema (1.8% vs 5.7%), restriction of arm or shoulder mobility (2.0% vs 3.5%), and pain associated with arm or shoulder movement (2.0% vs 4.2%) with SLNB omission [31]. Although the frequency of postoperative complications with SLNB is low overall, given the substantial number of patients currently undergoing SLNB, early adoption of these trials into clinical practice will substantially reduce arm morbidity for a significant number of breast cancer survivors. Two additional trials evaluating omission of axillary surgery include the Netherlands-BOOG 2013-08 trial [29] and the South Korea-NAUTILUS trial [27], with both expected to result in the coming years.

In 2025 the American Society of Clinical Oncology updated its guidelines on axillary staging in early-stage breast cancer, recommending omission of routine SLNB in select postmenopausal patients 50 years of age or older with small ($\leq$2 cm), grade 1 to 2, cN0 HR+/HER2-negative breast cancer with a negative axillary ultrasound who are planning to undergo BCS [32]. These guidelines lend strong support to the early adoption of axillary surgery omission in women with low-risk breast cancer given the lack of benefit observed with axillary staging.

SLNB should be omitted in postmenopausal women 50 years of age or older with small ($\leq$2 cm), grade 1 to 2, HR+/HER2-negative breast cancer and a normal preoperative axillary ultrasound who are planning for lumpectomy and RT.

ADOPTION OF SOUND AND INSEMA INTO CLINICAL PRACTICE

When planning adoption of the SOUND and INSEMA trials into clinical practice, it is important to consider the clinical characteristics of the patients enrolled in the two trials. Most patients were 50 years of age or older, and postmenopausal, with small (cT1) tumors less than or equal to 2 cm that were mostly of ductal histology, mostly grade 1 to 2, and predominantly HR+/HER2-negative (Table 2) [26,28]. Importantly, in this subset of patients, decisions regarding adjuvant systemic chemotherapy are primarily based on genomic risk, as highlighted by the fact that chemotherapy administration did not differ in SOUND between groups (20.1% SLNB vs 17.5% no SLNB, $P = .22$). In INSEMA, the difference in chemotherapy administration was statistically different but not clinically meaningful (12.9% SLNB vs 10.4% no SLNB; OR 0.78, 95% CI 0.62–0.98). SLNB omission should likely not be implemented in patients in whom nodal status is still an important determinant of systemic chemotherapy decisions (ie, premenopausal HR+/HER2-negative, any HER2-positive, and any triple-negative breast cancer patient). SLNB omission should also not be applied to early-stage breast cancer patients undergoing mastectomy, as decisions for PMRT are currently based on nodal status. Caution should be exercised when applying SLNB omission to patients with larger tumors (ie, cT2, 2–5 cm), as these patients were not included in SOUND and were under-represented in the INSEMA study population (~10% of the

Table 2
Comparison of Patient and Tumor Characteristics Between SOUND and INSEMA Study Populations

	SOUND (Gentilini et al. [26] 2023) N = 1405	INSEMA (Reimer et al. [28] 2025) N = 4858	Patient Characteristics
Age (years, median)	60	62	> 50 y, postmenopausal
Tumor size (cm, median)	1.1	1.1	Small (≤2 cm) tumors
Clinical T2 tumors	Excluded	10%	Mostly cT1 tumors
Ductal histology	78%	73%	Mostly ductal
Grade 3	18%	<4%	Mostly grade 1–2
HR+/HER2-negative	88%	95%	Mostly HR+/HER2-negative
Positive SLNs	13.7%	17%	Low nodal burden
≥ 4 positive SLNs	0.6%	0.8%	
Partial-breast irradiation	11%	Not allowed	Most treated with whole-breast radiation
Adjuvant chemotherapy	18.8%	12.4%	

Abbreviations: HER2, human epidermal growth factor receptor 2; HR, hormone receptor; SLN, sentinel lymph node.

cohort). In addition, multidisciplinary consensus is necessary for the successful implementation of SLNB omission. Figure 2 outlines our multidisciplinary approach for the implementation of SLNB omission at MSKCC.

THE IMPACT OF SENTINEL LYMPH NODE BIOPSY OMISSION ON ELIGIBILITY FOR CDK4/6 INHIBITORS

Both SOUND and INSEMA accrued patients before the routine use of adjuvant cyclin-dependent kinase (CDK) 4/6 inhibitors for patients with high-risk stage II-III HR+/HER2-negative breast cancer. Both abemaciclib and ribociclib were approved for the treatment of "high-risk" early-stage HR+/HER2-negative breast cancer in 2021 and 2024, respectively, following trial data demonstrating an oncologic benefit to the addition of these drugs to endocrine therapy [33,34]. The monarchE trial enrolled 5637 patients with HR+/HER2-negative breast cancer with either 4 or more positive axillary lymph nodes, or 1 to 3 positive nodes with either grade 3 disease, or a tumor size greater than or equal to 5 cm (cohort No. 1), or 1 to 3 positive nodes with Ki-67 greater than or equal to 20% (cohort No. 2). Patients were randomized in a 1:1 ratio to abemaciclib 150 mg orally twice daily for 2 years plus endocrine therapy for up to 10 years or endocrine therapy alone for up to 10 years. The addition of abemaciclib to endocrine therapy in this "high-risk" node-positive cohort resulted in a 5-year iDFS benefit of 7.6% [35].

Following the monarchE trial, results from the NATALEE trial broadened the eligibility for CDK 4/6 inhibitors to include patients with pathologically negative nodes, provided they had other high-risk features, adding further nuance to the multidisciplinary management of early-stage, HR+/HER2-negative breast cancer

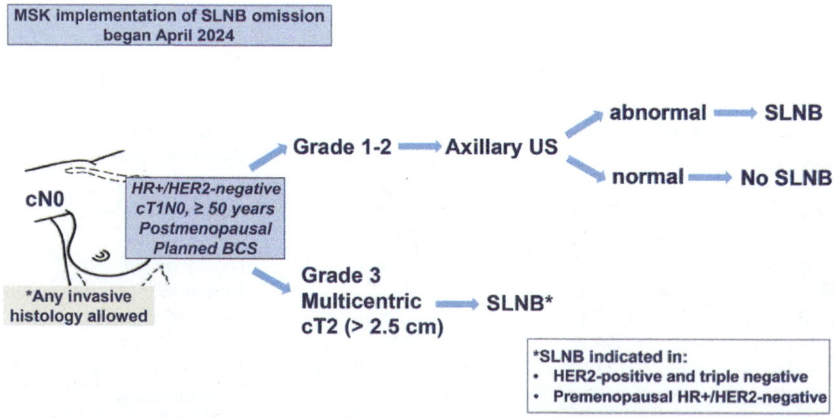

Fig. 2. Implementation of the SOUND trial into clinical practice: MSKCC guidelines. BCS, breast-conserving surgery; HER2, human epidermal growth factor receptor 2; HR, hormone receptor; LVI, lymphovascular invasion; MSKCC, Memorial Sloan Kettering Cancer Center; SLNB, sentinel lymph node biopsy; US, ultrasound.

patients [36]. Overall, 5101 patients with stage II or III HR+/HER2-negative early breast cancer were randomized 1:1 to 3 years of ribociclib plus aromatase inhibitor or an aromatase inhibitor alone. Patients were eligible for enrollment if they had at least one positive axillary lymph node. Patients with tumors >2 cm and negative nodes were eligible if they had grade 3 tumors, grade 2 tumors with Ki67 greater than 20%, or high genomic risk (recurrence score >25). The addition of ribociclib to aromatase inhibitor resulted in a 3-year iDFS benefit of 3.1%; this benefit was consistent across prespecified node-positive and node-negative subgroups.

Patients selected for SLNB omission have "low-risk" breast cancer, and therefore, the overlap between patients eligible for CDK4/6 inhibitors and those eligible for SLNB omission is minimal. SLNB should be performed in instances where omission of axillary surgery would result in a high probability of undertreatment with CDK 4/6 inhibitors–specifically, patients with grade 3 tumors or tumors larger than 5 cm. In patients who are initially suspected to have low/intermediate grade tumors and/or small tumors, and who are subsequently identified on final pathology to have grade 3 tumors or substantially larger tumors, a return to the operating room for SLNB is indicated if the finding of a positive node would change recommendations for CDK4/6 inhibitors. In patients with small (≤2 cm), grade 1 to 2 tumors, SLNB can be safely omitted with a low risk of undertreatment.

OMISSION OF AXILLARY SURGERY AND RADIATION THERAPY CONSIDERATIONS

In the INSEMA trial, WBRT was mandated by the protocol, whereas regional nodal irradiation and high tangents were not allowed [28]. In the SOUND trial, radiation after lumpectomy was required, but the dose and modality were not specified. Notably, most patients received WBRT, with only 11% of patients enrolled in SOUND treated with partial-breast irradiation utilizing intraoperative RT [26]. As most patients eligible for SLNB omission have low-risk disease, this group would be ideal candidates for treatment with partial-breast irradiation, which may not be considered in patients with uncertain nodal status because the randomized trials demonstrating oncologic equivalence between WBRT and partial-breast irradiation included patients who had axillary staging [37–40]. The lack of pathologic nodal information could therefore result in potential "overtreatment" with WBRT for low-risk patients otherwise suitable for partial-breast irradiation. Of equal concern is the risk of undertreatment for unrecognized patients with occult nodal disease. Approximately 9% to 11% of patients in SOUND and INSEMA had nodal macrometastases, and may have received regional nodal irradiation based on evidence from the MA.20 and EORTC 22922/10,925 trials demonstrating improved survival with the use of regional nodal irradiation in node-positive breast cancer patients [41,42]. Notably, the benefit of nodal irradiation in biomarker "low-risk" node-positive patients remains uncertain and is currently being investigated in the TAILOR RT trial [43].

Table 3
Clinical Characteristics of Patients Eligible for Radiotherapy Omission

	IDEA (Jagsi et al. [44] 2024) N = 200	LUMINA (Whelan et al. [45] 2023) N = 500
Age (years, median)	63	67
Tumor size	1 cm (mean)	1 cm (median)
Histology	12% lobular or mixed	Lobular or mixed excluded
Grade 3	3%	Excluded
Lymphovascular invasion	14.5%	LVI excluded
Extensive intraductal component	Allowed	EIC excluded
pN0	100%	100%
Low-risk assay	RS $\leq$ 18	Ki-67 $\leq$ 13.25%
Endocrine therapy adherence	85%	83%
5-y local recurrence	1%	2.3%

Abbreviation: RS, recurrence score.

While RT is consistently associated with a lower risk of local recurrence, there is an impetus to de-escalate treatment in carefully selected favorable-risk HR+/HER2-negative breast cancer patients to avoid short- and long-term toxicities associated with RT, such as skin effects, fibrosis, suboptimal cosmesis, lymphedema, and rare secondary malignancies. Currently, 2 prospective, single-arm trials–IDEA and LUMINA–evaluated RT omission after lumpectomy in younger postmenopausal women with low-risk HR+/HER2-negative breast cancer [44,45]. The clinical characteristics of the study cohorts were similar, with an Oncotype DX recurrence score of less than or equal to 18 considered low-risk in IDEA, and a Ki-67 less than or equal to 13.25% considered low risk in LUMINA. Performance of an SLNB with pathologically negative nodes was required in both studies, and endocrine therapy adherence exceeded 80% in both trials (Table 3) [44,45]. Five-year local recurrence rates were 1% in IDEA and 2.3% in LUMINA.

While the initial prospective data are promising, randomized trials supporting the safety of RT omission have not been reported, precluding routine implementation of RT omission in younger postmenopausal women. Importantly, the ongoing randomized DEBRA trial requires SLNB with pathologically negative nodes for study entry [46], and therefore the question of whether both RT and axillary surgery can be omitted in postmenopausal patients with low-risk early breast cancer will not be answered by this trial.

SUMMARY

With improvements in systemic therapy and an increased understanding of tumor biology as the main driver of prognosis, our reliance on nodal status for prognostic information and treatment decisions has decreased, particularly in luminal breast cancer patients. While removal of the primary breast tumor remains mandatory for cure and for subsequent treatment decision making in early-stage cancer patients, staging the axilla in low-risk breast cancer patients does not contribute to cure and can be safely avoided in the majority of postmenopausal breast cancer patients with HR+/HER2-negative low-risk breast cancer.

CLINICS CARE POINTS

- SLNB can be safely omitted in clinically node-negative, postmenopausal patients with small, low-risk, luminal breast cancer undergoing upfront breast-conserving surgery.
- SLNB should still be performed in premenopausal patients with HR+/HER2-negative breast cancer, and most patients with triple-negative and HER2-positive breast cancer undergoing breast-conserving surgery.
- SLNB should still be performed in patients with early-stage breast cancer undergoing mastectomy.
- De-escalation of axillary surgery should be performed with multidisciplinary consensus, with the understanding that SLNB should be performed if knowledge of pathologic nodal status will impact systemic therapy decisions.

Disclosures

Dr. A. V. Barrio reports professional services with Novartis and MSD. Dr. K. R. Pawloski has no conflicts of interest to disclose.

References

[1] Halsted WSI. The results of operations for the cure of cancer of the breast performed at the Johns Hopkins Hospital from June, 1889, to January, 1894. Ann Surg 1894;20(5): 497–555.
[2] Fisher B, Jeong JH, Anderson S, et al. Twenty-five-year follow-up of a randomized trial comparing radical mastectomy, total mastectomy, and total mastectomy followed by irradiation. N Engl J Med 2002;347(8):567–75.
[3] Giuliano AE, Kirgan DM, Guenther JM, et al. Lymphatic mapping and sentinel lymphadenectomy for breast cancer. Ann Surg 1994;220(3):391–8 [discussion: 398–01.
[4] Krag DN, Anderson SJ, Julian TB, et al. Sentinel-lymph-node resection compared with conventional axillary-lymph-node dissection in clinically node-negative patients with breast cancer: overall survival findings from the NSABP B-32 randomised phase 3 trial. Lancet Oncol 2010;11(10):927–33.
[5] Krag DN, Weaver DL, Alex JC, et al. Surgical resection and radiolocalization of the sentinel lymph node in breast cancer using a gamma probe. Surg Oncol 1993;2(6):335–9 [discussion: 340].
[6] Veronesi U, Viale G, Paganelli G, et al. Sentinel lymph node biopsy in breast cancer: ten-year results of a randomized controlled study. Ann Surg 2010;251(4):595–600.
[7] Donker M, van Tienhoven G, Straver ME, et al. Radiotherapy or surgery of the axilla after a positive sentinel node in breast cancer (EORTC 10981-22023 AMAROS): a randomised, multicentre, open-label, phase 3 non-inferiority trial. Lancet Oncol 2014;15(12):1303–10.
[8] Giuliano AE, Hunt KK, Ballman KV, et al. Axillary dissection vs no axillary dissection in women with invasive breast cancer and sentinel node metastasis: a randomized clinical trial. JAMA 2011;305(6):569–75.

[9] Giuliano AE, Ballman K, McCall L, et al. Locoregional recurrence after sentinel lymph node dissection with or without axillary dissection in patients with sentinel lymph node metastases: long-term Follow-up from the American College of Surgeons Oncology Group (Alliance) ACOSOG Z0011 randomized trial. Ann Surg 2016;264(3):413–20.
[10] Bartels SAL, Donker M, Poncet C, et al. Radiotherapy or surgery of the axilla after a positive sentinel node in breast cancer: 10-Year results of the randomized controlled EORTC 10981-22023 AMAROS trial. J Clin Oncol 2023;41(12):2159–65.
[11] Giuliano AE, Ballman KV, McCall L, et al. Effect of axillary dissection vs No axillary dissection on 10-Year overall survival among women with invasive breast cancer and sentinel node metastasis: the ACOSOG Z0011 (alliance) randomized clinical trial. JAMA 2017;318(10):918–26.
[12] Hughes KS, Schnaper LA, Bellon JR, et al. Lumpectomy plus tamoxifen with or without irradiation in women age 70 years or older with early breast cancer: long-term follow-up of CALGB 9343. J Clin Oncol 2013;31(19):2382–7.
[13] Rudenstam CM, Zahrieh D, Forbes JF, et al. Randomized trial comparing axillary clearance versus no axillary clearance in older patients with breast cancer: first results of international breast cancer study group trial 10-93. J Clin Oncol 2006;24(3):337–44.
[14] Martelli G, Boracchi P, Ardoino I, et al. Axillary dissection versus no axillary dissection in older patients with T1N0 breast cancer: 15-year results of a randomized controlled trial. Ann Surg 2012;256(6):920–4.
[15] Grossi S, Le J, Armani A. Omitting axillary staging in selected patients: rationale of choosing wisely in breast cancer treatment. Surgery 2023;174(2):413–5.
[16] Whitrock JN, Pratt CG, Long SA, et al. Implementation of choosing wisely guidelines: omission of lymph node surgery. Surgery 2025;179:108843.
[17] Cardoso F, van't Veer LJ, Bogaerts J, et al. 70-Gene signature as an aid to treatment decisions in early-stage breast cancer. N Engl J Med 2016;375(8):717–29.
[18] Nielsen T, Wallden B, Schaper C, et al. Analytical validation of the PAM50-based prosigna breast cancer prognostic gene signature assay and nCounter analysis system using formalin-fixed paraffin-embedded breast tumor specimens. BMC Cancer 2014;14:177.
[19] Paik S, Shak S, Tang G, et al. A multigene assay to predict recurrence of tamoxifen-treated, node-negative breast cancer. N Engl J Med 2004;351(27):2817–26.
[20] Paik S, Tang G, Shak S, et al. Gene expression and benefit of chemotherapy in women with node-negative, estrogen receptor-positive breast cancer. J Clin Oncol 2006;24(23):3726–34.
[21] Albain KS, Barlow WE, Shak S, et al. Prognostic and predictive value of the 21-gene recurrence score assay in postmenopausal women with node-positive, oestrogen-receptor-positive breast cancer on chemotherapy: a retrospective analysis of a randomised trial. Lancet Oncol 2010;11(1):55–65.
[22] Sparano JA, Gray RJ, Makower DF, et al. Adjuvant chemotherapy guided by a 21-Gene expression assay in breast cancer. N Engl J Med 2018;379(2):111–21.
[23] Kalinsky K, Barlow WE, Gralow JR, et al. 21-Gene assay to inform chemotherapy benefit in node-positive breast cancer. N Engl J Med 2021;385(25):2336–47.
[24] Lee MK, Montagna G, Pilewskie ML, et al. Axillary staging is not justified in postmenopausal clinically node-negative women based on nodal disease burden. Ann Surg Oncol 2023;30(1):92–7.
[25] Amlicke MJ, Park J, Agala CB, et al. Prevalence of pathologic N2/N3 disease in postmenopausal women with clinical N0 ER+/HER2- breast cancer. Ann Surg Oncol 2022;29(12):7662–9.
[26] Gentilini OD, Botteri E, Sangalli C, et al. Sentinel lymph node biopsy vs no axillary surgery in patients with small breast cancer and negative results on ultrasonography of axillary lymph nodes: the SOUND randomized clinical trial. JAMA Oncol 2023;9(11):1557–64.

[27] Jung JG, Ahn SH, Lee S, et al. No axillary surgical treatment for lymph node-negative patients after ultra-sonography [NAUTILUS]: protocol of a prospective randomized clinical trial. BMC Cancer 2022;22(1):189.
[28] Reimer T, Stachs A, Veselinovic K, et al. Axillary surgery in breast cancer - primary results of the INSEMA trial. N Engl J Med 2025;392(11):1051–64.
[29] van Roozendaal LM, Vane MLG, van Dalen T, et al. Clinically node negative breast cancer patients undergoing breast conserving therapy, sentinel lymph node procedure versus follow-up: a Dutch randomized controlled multicentre trial (BOOG 2013-08). BMC Cancer 2017;17(1):459.
[30] Gentilini O, Botteri E, Dadda P, et al. Physical function of the upper limb after breast cancer surgery. Results from the SOUND (sentinel node vs. observation after axillary Ultra-souND) trial. Eur J Surg Oncol 2016;42(5):685–9.
[31] Reimer T, Stachs A, Veselinovic K, et al. Patient-reported outcomes for the Intergroup Sentinel Mamma study (INSEMA): a randomised trial with persistent impact of axillary surgery on arm and breast symptoms in patients with early breast cancer. eClinicalMedicine 2023;55:101756.
[32] Park KU, Somerfield MR, Anne N, et al. Sentinel lymph node biopsy in early-stage breast cancer: ASCO guideline update. J Clin Oncol 2025;43(14):1720–41.
[33] Johnston SRD, Harbeck N, Hegg R, et al. Abemaciclib combined with endocrine therapy for the adjuvant treatment of HR+, HER2-node-positive, high-risk, early breast cancer (monarchE). J Clin Oncol 2020;38(34):3987–98.
[34] Royce M, Osgood C, Mulkey F, et al. FDA approval summary: abemaciclib with endocrine therapy for high-risk early breast cancer. J Clin Oncol 2022;40(11):1155–62.
[35] Rastogi P, O'Shaughnessy J, Martin M, et al. Adjuvant abemaciclib plus endocrine therapy for hormone receptor-positive, human epidermal growth factor receptor 2-negative, high-risk early breast cancer: results from a preplanned monarche overall survival interim analysis, including 5-year efficacy outcomes. J Clin Oncol 2024;42(9):987–93.
[36] Slamon D, Lipatov O, Nowecki Z, et al. Ribociclib plus endocrine therapy in early breast cancer. N Engl J Med 2024;390(12):1080–91.
[37] Coles CE, Griffin CL, Kirby AM, et al. Partial-breast radiotherapy after breast conservation surgery for patients with early breast cancer (UK IMPORT LOW trial): 5-year results from a multicentre, randomised, controlled, phase 3, non-inferiority trial. Lancet 2017;390(10099):1048–60.
[38] Meattini I, Marrazzo L, Saieva C, et al. Accelerated partial-breast irradiation compared with whole-breast irradiation for early breast cancer: long-term results of the randomized phase III APBI-IMRT-Florence trial. J Clin Oncol 2020;38(35):4175–83.
[39] Vicini FA, Cecchini RS, White JR, et al. Long-term primary results of accelerated partial breast irradiation after breast-conserving surgery for early-stage breast cancer: a randomised, phase 3, equivalence trial. Lancet 2019;394(10215):2155–64.
[40] Whelan TJ, Julian JA, Berrang TS, et al. External beam accelerated partial breast irradiation versus whole breast irradiation after breast conserving surgery in women with ductal carcinoma in situ and node-negative breast cancer (RAPID): a randomised controlled trial. Lancet 2019;394(10215):2165–72.
[41] Poortmans PM, Collette S, Kirkove C, et al. Internal mammary and medial supraclavicular irradiation in breast cancer. N Engl J Med 2015;373(4):317–27.
[42] Whelan TJ, Olivotto IA, Parulekar WR, et al. Regional nodal irradiation in early-stage breast cancer. N Engl J Med 2015;373(4):307–16.
[43] Canadian Cancer Trials Group. Tailor RT: a randomized trial of regional radiotherapy in biomarker low-risk node positive and T3N0 breast cancer. Available at: https://clinicaltrials.gov/study/NCT03488693. Accessed November 2, 2025.
[44] Jagsi R, Griffith KA, Harris EE, et al. Omission of radiotherapy after breast-conserving surgery for women with breast cancer with low clinical and genomic risk: 5-year outcomes of IDEA. J Clin Oncol 2024;42(4):390–8.

[45] Whelan TJ, Smith S, Parpia S, et al. Omitting radiotherapy after breast-conserving surgery in luminal a breast cancer. N Engl J Med 2023;389(7):612–9.
[46] NRGOncology. A phase III clinical trial evaluating De-Escalation of breast radiation for conservative treatment of stage I, hormone sensitive, HER-2 negative, Oncotype Recurrence Score Less Than or Equal to 18 Breast Cancer. Available at: https://clinicaltrials.gov/study/NCT04852887. Accessed November 2, 2025.

Advances in Surgery 60 (2026) 65–83

ADVANCES IN SURGERY

Current Management of Extremity Lymphedema

Marco Pappalardo, MD, MSc, PhD[a],
Ming-Huei Cheng, MD, MBA[b,*]

[a]Division of Plastic and Reconstructive Surgery, Department of Medical and Surgical Sciences, University of Modena and Reggio Emilia, Italy; [b]A+ Surgery Clinic, Taipei, Taiwan

Keywords

• Extremity lymphedema • Lymphedema diagnosis • Lymphatic microsurgery • Lymphedema grading system • Lymphoscintigraphy

Key points

- The key challenge for managing extremity lymphedema is how to early diagnose the lymphedema, stage the severity correctly, and select appropriate surgical intervention for individual patient.
- The natural progression of extremity lymphedema includes 5 pathologic events: (1) accumulation of protein-rich interstitial fluid, (2) chronic inflammatory of the tissues, (3) recurrent episodes of cellulitis, (4) progressive adipogenesis, and (5) progressive fibrosis.
- Clinical staging in combination with functional staging (Taiwan Lymphoscintigraphy Staging) and indocyanine green (ICG) lymphography identify surgical candidacy and appropriate surgical procedures.
- Complex decongestive therapy remains foundational across stages, but physiologic microsurgery should be considered when edema persists/progresses or cellulitis recurs despite adequate conservative treatment.
- Stage-match physiologic surgery: lymphovenous anastomosis is indicated for partial obstruction with patent lymphatic ducts on ICG lymphography, whereas vascularized lymph node transfer is preferred for advanced total obstruction with diffuse dermal backflow.

*Corresponding author. A+ Surgery Clinic, 3F, 337, Fuxing North Road, Songshan District, Taipei, Taiwan 105. *E-mail address:* minghueicheng@gmail.com

https://doi.org/10.1016/j.yasu.2026.03.016

Abbreviations

CDT	Complex Decongestive Therapy
CT	Computed Tomography
ICG	Indocyanine Green Lymphography
ISL	International Society of Lymphology
LVA	Lymphovenous Anastomosis
VLNT	Vascularized Lymph Node Transfer
VSLN	Vascularized Submental Lymph Node
VTLN	Vascularized Thoracic Lymph Node

INTRODUCTION

Extremity lymphedema is a common and frequently underrecognized condition encountered by health care practitioners and surgeons in daily clinical practice [1]. Its incidence continues to rise as a consequence of improved oncologic survival, more aggressive lymph node dissections, adjuvant radiotherapy, obesity, and the aging population [2–10]. Despite its growing impact, extremity lymphedema is still often misdiagnosed, undertreated, or referred too late for effective intervention [11,12].

Historically, lymphedema management has been relegated almost exclusively to conservative measures, primarily complex decongestive therapy (CDT) with lifelong compression garments [13,14]. These approaches are effective in controlling symptoms but do not address the underlying lymphatic dysfunction or prevent disease progression.

Over the last 2 decades, advances in lymphatic imaging and microsurgery/supermicrosurgery have fundamentally changed the therapeutic landscape for extremity lymphedema [15–26]. Accurate assessment of lymphatic function now allows treatment to be selected according to the stage of disease rather than applied empirically. Management is no longer limited to compression therapy; it now includes diagnostic and therapeutic methods that depend on accurate clinical and functional evaluations.

For health care practitioners, the key challenge is no longer how to manage swelling, but how to recognize lymphedema early, stage it correctly, and identify patients who may benefit from appropriate surgical intervention before irreversible tissue changes occur.

This article provides a practical framework for the evaluation and management of extremity lymphedema, emphasizing accurate diagnostic workup, integrated staging system, and selection of appropriate surgical treatments for both upper and lower extremities.

NATURAL PROGRESSION OF EXTREMITY LYMPHEDEMA

Lymphedema is a progressive disorder resulting from impaired lymphatic transport capacity, leading to chronic accumulation of protein-rich interstitial fluid [27]. Contrary to the common misconception that lymphedema is "fluid retention," the condition represents a dynamic pathologic process that evolves from reversible lymphatic dysfunction to irreversible tissue transformation.

Rather than being a static condition, extremity lymphedema follows a predictable natural progression driven by persistent lymph stasis and its biologic consequences.

The natural progression of extremity lymphedema can be described in 5 sequential pathologic events: (1) lymphatic transport failure with accumulation of protein-rich interstitial fluid, (2) chronic inflammatory state of the tissues due to persistent lymph stasis, (3) recurrent episodes of cellulitis that further damage lymphatic ducts, (4) progressive adipose deposition (adipogenesis) leading to limb enlargement in addition to fluid accumulation, and (5) progressive fibrosis with loss of tissue softness and irreversible structural remodeling [28,29]. This sequence explains why limb enlargement over time is increasingly driven by adipose and fibrotic changes rather than fluid alone, and why compression therapy becomes progressively less effective as the disease advances.

CLINICAL DIAGNOSIS AND DIFFERENTIAL DIAGNOSIS

Extremity lymphedema remains primarily a clinical diagnosis, yet it is frequently confused with other causes of limb enlargement [30]. Patients typically present with progressive limb swelling, heaviness, tightness, and reduced mobility. In the early stages, edema is soft and pitting, and may fluctuate throughout the day. As the disease advances, the limb becomes firm, nonpitting, and progressively enlarged due to adipose and fibrotic tissue deposition rather than simple fluid accumulation [31].

Several clinical signs are characteristic, such as the Stemmer sign (inability to pinch the skin at the base of the second toe or finger), asymmetrical limb circumference, skin thickening, loss of normal skin folds, recurrent episodes of cellulitis, and progressive resistance to elevation and compression. Cellulitis deserves special attention because it is both a complication and a marker of worsening lymphatic dysfunction, and its frequency correlates with greater lymphatic obstruction severity on lymphoscintigraphy [32].

However, many conditions mimic lymphedema and may cause delayed or incorrect management. Distinguishing these entities is fundamental for health care practitioners involved in limb care (Table 1). In doubtful cases, functional imaging is decisive to confirm lymphatic dysfunction and differentiate lymphedema from its mimics. Lymphoscintigraphy remains the most widely adopted tool to confirm diagnosis and characterize obstruction (including deep lymphatic vessels), whereas indocyanine green (ICG) lymphography provides real-time mapping of superficial lymphatics that is particularly useful for planning lymphovenous anastomosis (LVA) [33].

SEVERITY STAGING SYSTEM: COMBINED CLINICAL AND FUNCTIONAL ASSESSMENT

One of the major reasons for suboptimal lymphedema management is the historical reliance on clinical staging alone. Clinical appearance reflects tissue consequences of lymphatic failure but does not accurately describe the functional

Table 1
Differential diagnosis of limb enlargement

Conditions	Features	Distribution	Stemmer sign	Imaging findings
Lymphedema	Progressive swelling, skin thickening, cellulitis	Often asymmetric, distal to proximal	Positive	Abnormal lymphatic findings in lymphoscintigraphy and ICG lymphography
Lipedema	Pure adipose deposition	Bilateral, symmetric, spares feet	Negative	Normal lymphatics
Chronic venous insuficiency	Varicosities, hyperpigmentation, ulcers	Distal legs	Negative	Venous insufficiency in Doppler
Cardiac/renal edema	Pitting, systemic signs, no local etiology	Bilateral	Negative	Normal lymphatics

status (severity) of the lymphatic system, which is the true determinant of surgical candidacy.

For broad clinical communication, the International Society of Lymphology (ISL) staging system is widely used to describe disease severity (stage 0: latent/subclinical; stage I: spontaneously reversible; stage II: spontaneously irreversible; stage III: lymphostatic elephantiasis with skin changes) [34,35]. However, ISL staging is primarily clinical and does not directly quantify lymphatic transport failure or the objective severity of obstruction, limiting its usefulness for selecting appropriate microsurgical strategies [36].

Cheng's lymphedema grading (clinical staging)

Cheng's lymphedema grading system classifies lymphedema based on physical examination and limb characteristics. In practice, Cheng's grading provides an objective measure of clinical severity using the circumferential difference between the affected and contralateral limb (Grade 0 <9%, Grade I 10%–19%, Grade II 20%–29%, Grade III 30%–39%, Grade IV >40%), enabling standardized documentation and longitudinal follow-up [37]. Compared with ISL staging, Cheng's Grading offers greater resolution for measuring severity and reporting outcomes, particularly in surgical series.

Taiwan lymphoscintigraphy staging (functional staging)

Taiwan Lymphoscintigraphy Staging (TLS) evaluates the lymphatic drainage obstruction and dermal backflow patterns. TLS classifies lymphatic drainage into 3 patterns: normal drainage (L-0), partial obstruction (P-1, P-2, P-3), and total obstruction (T-4, T-5, T-6), using hierarchical lymphoscintigraphic criteria that include proximal and/or intermediate lymph node visualization, lymphatic duct morphology, and dermal backflow distribution [32,38,39]. This functional stratification is clinically meaningful: higher TLS stages are associated with greater limb circumferential difference, greater computed tomography (CT) volumetric difference, and increased cellulitis frequency [32,38].

Indocyanine green lymphography (functional staging)

ICG lymphography has become a useful tool in recent years for assessing lymphatic anatomy and function [40,41]. This imaging modality can visualize superficial lymphatic vessels in a finer manner in real time, even during surgery, without radiation exposure [42]. ICG lymphography showed good efficacy, especially for diagnosing subclinical and early-stage lymphedema. However, ICG lymphography cannot be used to observe proximal lymph nodes and lymphatic ducts deeper than 1 cm in the subcutaneous tissue.

Accordingly, ICG lymphography should be considered complementary to lymphoscintigraphy: it provides high-resolution mapping of superficial functional lymphatics and dermal backflow patterns for operative planning.

Why the combination is more accurate

Modern management requires the combination of Clinical staging, which describes tissue changes (Cheng's Lymphedema Grading), and functional staging, describing lymphatic drainage obstruction (TLS, supported by ICG lymphography) [32]. Their combination directly determines the appropriate treatment (Table 2).

A patient may present with Cheng Grade II appearance but TLS P-1 or P-2, and it is still an excellent LVA candidate. Instead, a patient with a Cheng Grade II appearance but TLS P-3 LVA cannot be performed, and vascularized lymph node transfer (VLNT) is indicated. This explains why surgical results in

Table 2
Integrated clinico-functional staging system to select appropriate procedures

Clinical severity	Cheng's grade	Circumferential difference (%)	TLS	ICG lymphography	Preferred managements
Subclinical	0	1–9	L-0	Patent collectors	CDT
Mild	I	10–19	P1–P2	Patent collectors	LVA
Moderate	II (early)	20–29	P1–P2	Patent collectors	LVA
Moderate	II (late)	20–29	P3/T-4 to T-5	Diffuse dermal backflow	VLNT
Advanced	III	30–39	P-3 or T-4 to T-6	Diffuse dermal backflow	VLNT ± liposuction
Advanced	IV	> 40	T5–T6	Diffuse dermal backflow	VLNT with liposuction

Abbreviations: CDT, complex decongestive therapy; ICG, indocyanine green lymphography; LVA, lymphovenous anastomosis; TLS, Taiwan lymphoscintigraphy staging; VLNT, vascularized lymph node transfer.

Marco Pappalardo, Ming-Huei Cheng, 6 - Lymphoscintigraphy Interpretation, Staging, and Lymphedema Grading, Principles and Practice of Lymphedema Surgery, 2nd Edition, Elsevier, 2022.

the literature are inconsistent when staging is based only on clinical findings (see Table 2). This combined approach transforms lymphedema treatment from empirical decision-making into a stage-driven algorithm.

The rationale for combining systems is supported by validation work showing a strong correlation between TLS and objective limb severity (including circumferential and CT volumetric differences) and a substantial correlation between TLS and Cheng grading [32]. Similarly, in cancer-related lower extremity lymphedema, total obstruction stages are the most significant factors associated with clinical severity measures, strengthening the importance of functional staging in treatment selection [38].

DIAGNOSTIC WORKUP ALGORITHM

Once extremity lymphedema is clinically suspected, the goal of the diagnostic workup is to confirm lymphatic dysfunction and define its functional severity with appropriate imaging. A standardized diagnostic pathway reduces misdiagnosis, documents baseline severity, and supports consistent longitudinal follow-up.

Step 1—clinical suspicion

Patients presenting with progressive limb swelling, heaviness or tightness, positive Stemmer sign, history of lymph node dissection, radiotherapy, trauma, infection, or congenital onset and/or recurrent cellulitis should be considered for lymphatic evaluation. Symptoms such as heaviness, tightness, or exertional swelling may precede objective enlargement and warrant evaluation when risk factors are present.

Step 2—exclude common mimics

Venous insufficiency, lipedema, systemic edema, and obesity-related enlargement should be ruled out through history, examination, and, when necessary, venous Doppler studies. When systemic edema is suspected, a basic evaluation for cardiac, renal, hepatic, or medication-related causes is appropriate to avoid delayed diagnosis (see Table 1).

Step 3—functional lymphatic imaging

All patients with suspected lymphedema should undergo lymphoscintigraphy (to determine TLS stage) and ICG lymphography (to map superficial functional lymphatics and dermal backflow). These 2 examinations provide complementary information: lymphoscintigraphy evaluates lymphatic obstruction, including deep lymphatic pathways and proximal nodal visualization, whereas ICG identifies useable superficial lymphatic ducts and dermal backflow patterns relevant to surgical planning. When available, cross-sectional imaging (eg, CT or MRI) may be used to quantify volume and characterize fat and fibrosis, but it does not replace functional imaging for staging lymphatic transport impairment.

CONSERVATIVE TREATMENT

In spite of advances in microsurgery, conservative therapy remains the foundation of lymphedema management and is the appropriate first-line treatment in many patients [13,14]. CDT consists of manual lymphatic drainage, multilayer compression bandaging, compression garments, skin care, exercise, and weight control. In clinical practice, CDT is delivered in 2 phases: an intensive phase focused on volume reduction (typically with multilayer bandaging), followed by a maintenance phase that includes compression garments, self-management, exercise, and ongoing skin care.

Indications for conservative management alone include patients with Cheng's Grade 0 and TLS L-0/P-1, minimal symptoms, good response to compression, no recurrent cellulitis, and stable limb volume. These patients may be successfully managed without surgery. In these early stages, tissue changes are minimal, and edema can often be effectively controlled with compression therapy alone. Conservative management is also appropriate in patients who decline operative intervention or are not medically suitable candidates, provided that symptoms and limb volume remain stable.

Adjunctive conservative strategies include weight optimization, treatment of coexisting venous disease when present, and meticulous skin care to reduce the risk of cellulitis. Patient education, along with adherence are central determinants of success.

Limitations of conservative therapy

However, CDT does not restore the structural integrity of the lymphatic vessels needed to transport fluid to the thoracic duct, venous system, and right heart. It controls symptoms but does not prevent disease progression in many patients. Over time, persistent lymph stasis leads to inflammatory and fibrotic changes that reduce the effectiveness of compression garments. This is the critical moment when timely referral becomes essential.

When to refer for microsurgical evaluation

Referral for specialized evaluation should be considered when edema continues despite adequate compression, limb volume progressively increases, or recurrent cellulitis occurs. Referral is appropriate when functional imaging demonstrates clinically significant lymphatic obstruction (eg, TLS P-2 or higher), or when the patient becomes increasingly compression-dependent to maintain limb stability.

PHYSIOLOGIC MICROSURGERY: LYMPHOVENOUS ANASTOMOSIS

LVA is a supermicrosurgical procedure that diverts lymphatic fluid directly into the venous circulation through anastomoses between functioning lymphatic vessels and small venules. Its success depends on the presence of patent lymphatic ducts identifiable with functional imaging. Technically, LVA is a supermicrosurgical operation performed under high magnification, typically connecting lymphatic ducts (≈0.5–0.8 mm) to subdermal venules (≈0.6–1.0 mm), and is facilitated by ICG lymphography for lymphatic mapping and intraoperative patency assessment [16,43].

Mechanism of action

In early lymphedema, lymphatic vessels are still structurally present but unable to transport lymph effectively due to proximal obstruction. By creating a bypass into the venous system, LVA restores outflow, reduces interstitial fluid accumulation, and re-establishes tissue homeostasis. When performed at the correct stage, LVA addresses the primary functional defect before irreversible adipose and fibrotic transformation occurs. In obstructive disease, retrograde lymph flow is often present; therefore, anastomotic configurations that allow efficient shunting (including bidirectional drainage) are conceptually advantageous [16].

Indications

LVA is indicated in patients with Cheng Grade I, early Cheng Grade II, TLS P-1 and P-2, visible linear lymphatic ducts on ICG lymphography, and persistent edema despite adequate compression therapy. These patients have useable lymphatics, which is the single most important criterion for success.

Technical considerations and anastomotic configuration

LVA may be performed as end-to-end, end-to-side, or side-to-end anastomosis. In a comparative series of 58 patients with early-grade unilateral extremity lymphedema (upper and lower extremity) treated with a single anastomosis, both end-to-end and side-to-end configurations demonstrated clinical benefit, but side-to-end achieved greater improvement in circumferential difference at approximately 16.5 months follow-up [16]. Immediate patency was confirmed intraoperatively using ICG lymphography and dye testing.

Side-to-end anastomosis may provide more effective lymph drainage because it can shunt both proximal and distal lymph flow through a single anastomosis, whereas end-to-end is unidirectional and may require more proximal anastomoses for comparable drainage.

In a recent viewpoint, we pointed out the importance of the lymphovenous pressure gradient and reported an intraoperative strategy to mitigate venous-to-lymphatic reflux by temporarily clamping and subsequently ligating the distal recipient vein. This maneuver effectively converted an end-to-side configuration to an end-to-end LVA, improved venous washout, and increased apparent lymphatic inflow on ICG assessment [44].

Expected outcomes

When correctly indicated, LVA can reduce limb circumferential difference, especially when side-to-end technique is performed, reduce episodes of cellulitis, improve limb softness, and improve quality of life. The greatest benefit is seen when performed early, before structural tissue changes dominate the clinical picture. These data reinforce 2 practical points: (1) careful patient selection (patent lymphatics and partial obstruction) is essential and (2) technique/configuration can influence drainage efficacy (Table 3).

Table 3
Lymphovenous anastomosis: configuration-focused practical summary

Configuration	Flow concept	Potential advantages	Limitations
End-to-end (E-E)	Unidirectional drainage into recipient venule.	Simple geometry	Sacrifices continuity of the lymphatic; require additional/ proximal bypasses
End-to-side (E-S)	Unidirectional; venous flow continues in recipient vein.	Preserves venous continuity; flexible orientation.	Higher risk of venous-to-lymphatic reflux if venous pressure exceeds lymphatic pressure
Side-to-end (S-E)	Shunt bidirectional lymph flow into a single venule via one bypass.	Provide higher drainage efficiency; can accommodate proximal and distal lymph flow through one anastomosis;	Technically demanding; requires suitable lymphatic caliber and wall quality

PHYSIOLOGIC MICROSURGERY: VASCULARIZED LYMPH NODE TRANSFER

VLNT involves transplanting healthy lymph nodes with their vascular supply into the affected limb, acting as a lymphatic pump, and draining the lymph into pedicle vein of the transferred lymph nodes. In the senior author's practice, VLNT is most often selected for moderate-to-advanced lymphedema when functional imaging demonstrates absent or severely compromised lymphatic ducts with adipose deposition, and fibrosis.

Mechanism of action

Transferred lymph nodes function through "pump/catchment" effect in which the transferred lymph node unit absorbs interstitial lymph and facilitates lymphaticovenous drainage at the flap level [45]. Other surgeons addressed the issue by focusing on lymphangiogenesis suggesting that the spontaneous reconnection between transferred nodes and recipient lymphatics helps to improve lymphatic drainage.

In our view, the pump/catchment mechanism is particularly important in VLNT. The transferred lymph node unit can function as a "vacuum-like" pump that actively recruits lymph from surrounding tissues ("catchment effect") and reroutes it into the venous system through intrinsic lymphovenous channels within the flap [17,18,46–48]. Distal (nonanatomic) placement may enhance clearance by leveraging gravity-driven movement of lymph toward the flap ("gravity effect"), helping address persistent distal stagnation when proximal lymphatic pumping is impaired. Intraoperative and experimental ICG observations demonstrating fluorescence appearing in the recipient vein after injection into the flap/lymph nodes support this lymphovenous clearance concept.

Indications

VLNT is indicated in patients with late Cheng Grade II–IV, TLS P-3, T-4 to T-6, and diffuse dermal backflow on ICG lymphography. Patients with active infection/cellulitis at the intended recipient site should undergo medical optimization and delayed surgical intervention, because local infection increases post-operative complications and undermines early flap integration [49].

Donor sites

Multiple donor sites are described in the literature: groin (superficial inguinal), submental, supraclavicular, thoracic, and omentum (Table 4). Each donor site has advantages and disadvantages regarding lymph node yield, donor-site morbidity, and ease of harvest. A widely discussed controversy is the balance between lymph node yield and donor-site safety, particularly the risk of iatrogenic donor-site lymphedema when peripheral nodal basins are harvested [50].

Groin (vascularized groin lymph node): widely used with reliable outcomes since 2 decades ago, and may be harvested with concealed scarring; however, risk of donor-site lymphedema remains a major concern, and reverse lymphatic mapping has been advocated to reduce this risk by avoiding nodes that drain the lower extremity [17,19]. When performed in conjunction with autologous breast reconstruction, it represents a highly efficient option for simultaneous treatment [51–55].

Submental (vascularized submental lymph node; VSLN), preferred in the senior author's practice. The VSLN flap offers greater number of sizable lymph nodes, reliable vascular anatomy, minimal risk of donor-site lymphedema, and concealed scarring, proving it an excellent option in experienced hands [18,21,56]. The VSLN flap also provides an adequate pedicle length and diameter, while maintaining a minimal risk of iatrogenic extremity lymphedema compared with peripheral nodal basin. Potential limitations comprise the learning curve and the need to protect the marginal mandibular nerve under microscope.

Supraclavicular (vascularized supraclavicular lymph node): thin flap and concealed scar; drawbacks include less lymph node number, potential risk of chyle leakage due to the thoracic duct injury and upper chest wall sensory changes [57].

Thoracic (vascularized thoracic lymph node; VTLN): The VTLN flap is based on the thoracodorsal or lateral thoracic artery and can include level I axillary lymph nodes. It offers a favorable lymph node yield, a generous soft-tissue component and an adequate pedicle for microsurgical transfer [58]. The main limitation is the potential risk of iatrogenic upper extremity lymphedema because the donor basin is axillary; therefore, reverse lymphatic mapping is recommended to improve harvest safety [50]. Additional considerations include small pedicle artery, possible thoracodorsal nerve sacrifice, and, in some designs, the need for 2 sets of anastomoses. A skin paddle may be incorporated for monitoring or coverage when required.

Omentum (greater omental lymph node flap): potentially great number of lymph nodes, minimal risk of extremity donor-site lymphedema, and

Table 4
Comparisons of common donor sites for vascularized lymph node transfer

Donor site	Advantages	Main limitations/risks	Typical scenario
Groin (VGLN)	First introduced. Concealed scar; can be combined with DIEP flap; consistent node basin.	Risk of donor-site lower extremity lymphedema, suggest to combinedly use reverse lymphatic mapping; short/small pedicle (SCIA); bulk may limit distal inset.	When concomitant breast reconstruction and meticulous donor-site protection.
Submental (VSLN)	Reliable vascular anatomy; not-reported donor site lymphedema; greater number of node basin.	Learning curve; protection of marginal mandibular nerve.	When achieving maximum functional recovery is a priority and suitable for distal recipient placement.
Supraclavicular (VScLN)	Thin flap; concealed scar; favorable esthetics.	Lower node basin; risk of thoracic duct injury, chyle leak; possible supraclavicular nerve injury.	When a thin flap and easy inset are priorities and modest node yield is acceptable.
Thoracic (VTLN)	Includes level I axillary nodes; favorable node yield with generous soft tissue.	Potential iatrogenic upper-extremity lymphedema. Reverse lymphatic mapping is recommended; pedicle variability; may require 2 sets of anastomoses.	When additional soft tissue is helpful (scar release/dead space) and reverse mapping can be ensured with minimal donor site lymphedema.
Omentum	Good but smaller node basin, no donor-site lymphedema; possible laparoscopic harvest; 2 sets of pedicle veins.	Intra-abdominal operative risks (visceral injury/adhesions); no skin paddle for monitoring; limited long-term donor sequelae data.	When greater node yield is desired and peripheral nodal basins are limited/undesirable (eg, bilateral or severe lymphedema).

Abbreviations: DIEP, deep inferior epigastric perforator; GOLF, greater omental lymph node flap; SCIA, superficial circumflex iliac artery; VGLN, vascularized groin lymph node; VScLN, vascularized supraclavicular lymph node; VSLN, vascularized submental lymph node; VTLN, vascularized thoracic lymph node.

concealed incisions when harvested laparoscopically; disadvantages include intra-abdominal operative risks such as pancreatitis, high venous pressure and lack of a skin paddle for monitoring [59].

Recipient site considerations

Recipient-site selection is still debated (proximal/anatomic vs distal/non-anatomic). Proximal placement (axilla/groin) may facilitate scar release in previously dissected fields. In contrast, distal placement (wrist/ankle) corresponds to the "pump/catchment" concept and may enhance functional drainage with gravity-assisted clearance. In practice, recipient site selection is individualized based on functional versus cosmetic considerations [45].

Expected outcomes

VLNT can reduce limb volume, improve softness, reduce fibrosis, and significantly reduce the frequency of cellulitis episodes over time. Reported series demonstrate improvements in objective limb measurements and patient-reported outcomes [17–19,22–26,60–62], with many patients reducing or discontinuing compression over time, particularly when VLNT is performed in distal recipient site.

Improvement is gradual because 10% of arterial blood still becomes lymph every day. Because VLNT recovery is progressive, outcomes should be assessed longitudinally (eg, cellulitis episodes, limb measurements, and quality-of-life instruments), rather than expecting immediate postoperative volume reduction.

In recent years, several authors have proposed combining LVA and VLNT in the same patient, assuming that the 2 procedures may have additive or synergistic effects. This strategy is frequently justified by the concept that LVA may provide earlier decompression, whereas VLNT may contribute to delayed, longer term improvement as lymphangiogenesis and integration occur [63]. However, interpreting the additive benefit is challenging because postoperative outcomes reflect multiple simultaneous interventions (eg, scar release, variable compression adherence, different numbers of bypasses, and heterogeneous follow-up) [63]. Therefore, while these series support that physiologic microsurgery is beneficial overall, they do not definitively establish that performing both procedures concurrently provides superior outcomes. Combining LVA and VLNT may increase operative time and morbidity without added benefit, and confuse postoperative outcome assessment. In our practice, we favor a simplified, stage-driven strategy. This philosophy improves reproducibility, reduces unnecessary complexity, and yields clearer outcome assessment.

SPECIAL SITUATIONS (PRIMARY, PEDIATRIC, BILATERAL, CELLULITIS, OBESITY)

Primary lymphedema

Primary lymphedema shares the same staging principles as secondary lymphedema. Despite congenital origin, treatment selection must still be guided by functional imaging rather than etiology. This concept is supported by clinical series on primary lymphedema demonstrating that outcomes improve when physiologic microsurgery is selected based on functional lymphoscintigraphy staging and ICG findings [64]. Because primary lymphedema may involve diffuse lymphatic dysplasia, counseling should emphasize that surgical goals often include restore local lymphatic drainage in extremity lymphedema, reduction in cellulitis frequency, and casting off compression garments rather than complete normalization.

Pediatric lymphedema

Pediatric patients benefit particularly from early staging as treatments before adipose deposition and fibrosis may alter the natural progression of the disease. In children, care should emphasize long-term outcome, and preventing progression. Early surgical interventions, as mentioned earlier, may have better outcome when the adipogenesis, fibrosis and infection are not severe.

Bilateral lymphedema

Bilateral lymphedema requires independent staging of each limb, as functional severity may differ and treatment must be limb-specific. This limb-specific strategy is supported by published bilateral series in which different physiologic procedures were selected for the different limbs based on severity and functional imaging findings [24,65].

Recurrent cellulitis

Recurrent cellulitis is not only a complication but a marker of disease progression within the natural history of lymphedema and represents a strong indication for surgical evaluation. Each episode may worsen lymphatic function and accelerate progression, supporting the requirement for proactive prevention (skin care, treatment of feet fungal infection, prompt antibiotics when indicated, and patient education on early symptoms). Elective microsurgery should be deferred during active infection; patients should be optimized with antibiotics with infection-free before intervention.

Obesity

Obesity accelerates adipogenesis and increasing lymph production, worsening the natural progression. Weight reduction should be considered a core component of lymphedema care because obesity increases limb volume, impairs mobility, and may increase the burden of quality of life. Referral to structured weight-management or nutrition services can be beneficial, and even modest weight reduction medications may decrease lymphedema symptoms including the risk of cellulitis.

Elderly patients and comorbidity

Age alone should not exclude the patients from physiologic lymphedema surgery. In elderly patients with secondary upper extremity lymphedema, VLNT has been associated with considerable improvements in limb measurements, reduced cellulitis, and improved quality of life [25]. For elderly patients, preoperative evaluation of comorbidity, perioperative risk reduction, and realistic goal-setting are the key steps for a successful physiologic lymphedema procedure.

PATIENT COUNSELING AND OUTCOMES

Patients should be counseled that the goal of modern lymphedema treatment is not simply to reduce limb size, but to reverse the natural progression of the disease.

Functional improvements including the reduction episodes of cellulitis, casting off the compression garments, improved tissue softness, are more clinically meaningful than circumferential change alone. Patients should also be informed that improvements may be multi-dimensional: some patients experience early symptom relief (heaviness, tightness), while objective volume reduction may be modest but clinically meaningful, particularly in advanced extremity lymphedema with severe adipogenesis and fibrosis. Improvements after VLNT are gradual and continuous for 12 to 24 months because lymph production is ongoing, estimated at 500 cc for the upper limb and 1000 cc for the lower limb per day. Longitudinal follow-up is recommended, documenting cellulitis episodes, limb measurements, and, when available, validated patient-reported outcome measures (Table 5).

Table 5
Objective outcomes tracking after physiologic/reductive surgeries for extremity lymphedema

Outcomes	What to measure	How often	Why it matters
Limb size/ volume	Circumference at standardized levels; or water displacement or CT volume if available	Baseline, 3–6 mo, 12 mo, then yearly	Objective disease burden and response trend
Cellulitis/ infections	Episodes of cellulitis/year; antibiotic courses; hospitalizations	Each visit	Reflects disease control
Tissue Softness	fibrosis/softness from Grade 1–4	Baseline, each visit	Fibrosis tracking
Quality of life (PROs)	LYMQOL, LLIS	Baseline, 6–12 mo, yearly	Captures patient-perceived outcome
Imaging responses	ICG pattern change (linear vs dermal backflow); lymphoscintigraphy	Baseline; selectively at 12–24 mo	Objective outocme assessment

Each patient should be recorded the clinical symptoms/signs, complications of surgery, and compliance of compression garments.

ROLE OF LIPOSUCTION/DEBULKING

Liposuction does not restore lymphatic function, but it can improve limb contour in selected patients. In advanced stages where fibroadipose deposition predominates, reductive procedures such as liposuction may be considered as adjunctive treatments. These techniques are best viewed as contour-reduction and volume-reduction strategies for limbs in which tissue composition (fat and fibrosis) limits the effectiveness of physiologic procedures alone. The order of physiologic procedures and liposuction is still debated. In our opinion, the physiologic procedures take priority, with liposuction performed 1 year later, as this approach removes the need for compression garments following the index procedure.

FUTURE DIRECTIONS

Advances in ICG lymphography and earlier detection of lymphatic dysfunction may allow intervention before the onset of adipogenesis and fibrosis.

Earlier diagnosis and stage-driven treatment have the potential to change the natural progression of extremity lymphedema rather than control its symptoms. Future progress will depend on (1) standardization of imaging protocols and reporting, (2) increased adoption of validated objective outcome measures and patient-reported outcomes, and (3) higher quality comparative studies that clarify which interventions provide the greatest benefit at each functional stage. Ultimately, shifting lymphedema care toward earlier detection and physiologic interventions offer the best opportunity to prevent progression to recurrent cellulitis, adipose deposition, and fibrosis.

DISCUSSION

The contemporary management of extremity lymphedema has shifted from symptom control to stage-driven physiologic interventions. The main practical concept is that clinical grading systems (ISL or Cheng Lymphedema Grading) reflect fat tissue consequences, whereas functional imaging (TLS and ICG) defines lymphatic transport capacity. In early disease with useable collectors (typically TLS P-1/P-2 with linear ducts on ICG), LVA can restore lymph outflow before severe adipogenesis and fibrosis. In contrast, once functional collectors are absent or advanced stages (eg, TLS P-3/T stages with diffuse dermal backflow in ICG lymphography), VLNT is the preferred physiologic procedure through a pump mechanism, catchment and gravity effects.

SUMMARY

Extremity lymphedema is a progressive disease including lymph stasis, inflammation, recurrent cellulitis, adipogenesis, and fibrosis. Modern management of extremity lymphedema includes early diagnosis with lymphoscintigraphy and ICG lymphography, application of a severity staging system, and selection of appropriate physiologic procedures, with or without liposuction. LVA is indicated for partial obstruction with healthy lymphatic ducts in ICG lymphography, while VLNT is effective for advanced extremity lymphedema, often allowing patients to eliminate the need for compression garments.

CLINICS CARE POINTS

- Confirm diagnosis and exclude mimics early: venous insufficiency, lipedema, systemic edema, and obesity-related enlargement; use Doppler/systemic workup when indicated.
- Clinical staging may be combined with TLS system and ICG lymphography to define functional severity and select the surgical procedures.
- Cellulitis as a progression marker: recurrent episodes of cellulitis correlate with more severe obstruction and warrant surgical evaluation when appropriate.
- CDT is not curative: persistent progression despite compression garments, increasing limb volume or fibrosis.
- Stage-match physiologic surgeries: LVA for TLS P-1/P-2 with linear lymphatic ducts; VLNT for TLS P-3/T stages with diffuse dermal backflow.
- Avoid unnecessary combined 2 or 3 procedures: when severity staging is accurate, the correct operation is usually adequate to manage the extremity lymphedema.
- Outcomes include improvement of lymphatic function, circumference reduction, cellulitis reduction, tissue softening, symptom/function improvement, and quality of life.
- Liposuction improves contour/volume in fibroadipose disease but does not restore lymphatic function; compression often is still necessary in liposuction alone.
- Reduction of risks: weight reduction, and avoidance of infection may reduce complications of extremity lymphedema.

Disclosures

M-H. Cheng received textbook royalties from Elsevier, Inc.

References

[1] Pappalardo M, Chang DW, Masia J, et al. Summary of hands-on supermicrosurgery course and live surgeries at 8th world symposium for lymphedema surgery. J Surg Oncol 2020;121(1):8–19.
[2] Cemal Y, Pusic A, Mehrara BJ. Preventative measures for lymphedema: separating fact from fiction. J Am Coll Surg 2011;213(4):543–51.
[3] Földi M, Földi E, editors. Foldi's textbook of lymphology for physicians and lymphedema therapists. Elsevier GmbH, Munich, Germany: Mosby Elsevier; 2006.
[4] Rockson SG, Rivera KK. Estimating the population burden of lymphedema. Ann N Y Acad Sci 2008;1131:147–54.
[5] Rebegea L, Firescu D, Dumitru M, et al. The incidence and risk factors for occurrence of arm lymphedema after treatment of breast cancer. Chirurgia (Bucur) 2015;110(1):33–7.
[6] Zhu YQ, Xie YH, Liu FH, et al. Systemic analysis on risk factors for breast cancer related lymphedema. Asian Pac J Cancer Prev 2014;15(16):6535–41.
[7] McLaughlin SA, Wright MJ, Morris KT, et al. Prevalence of lymphedema in women with breast cancer 5 years after sentinel lymph node biopsy or axillary dissection: objective measurements. J Clin Oncol 2008;26(32):5213–9.
[8] Ohba Y, Todo Y, Kobayashi N, et al. Risk factors for lower-limb lymphedema after surgery for cervical cancer. Int J Clin Oncol 2011;16(3):238–43.

[9] Kim JH, Choi JH, Ki EY, et al. Incidence and risk factors of lower-extremity lymphedema after radical surgery with or without adjuvant radiotherapy in patients with FIGO stage I to stage IIA cervical cancer. Int J Gynecol Cancer 2012;22(4):686–91.
[10] Ryan M, Stainton MC, Slaytor EK, et al. Aetiology and prevalence of lower limb lymphoedema following treatment for gynaecological cancer. Aust N Z J Obstet Gynaecol 2003;43 (2):148–51.
[11] Baccarani A, Pappalardo M, Starnoni M, et al. Plastic surgeons in the middle of the coronavirus disease 2019 pandemic storm in Italy. Plast Reconstr Surg Glob Open 2020;8(5): e2889; https://doi.org/10.1097/GOX.0000000000002889.
[12] Starnoni M, Baccarani A, Pappalardo M, et al. Management of personal protective equipment in plastic surgery in the era of coronavirus disease. Plast Reconstr Surg Glob Open 2020;8(5):e2879; https://doi.org/10.1097/GOX.0000000000002879.
[13] Cormier JN, Rourke L, Crosby M, et al. The surgical treatment of lymphedema: a systematic review of the contemporary literature (2004-2010). Ann Surg Oncol 2012;19(2):642–51.
[14] Bergmann A, Baiocchi JMT, de Andrade MFC. Conservative treatment of lymphedema: the state of the art. J Vasc Bras 2021;20:e20200091; https://doi.org/10.1590/1677-5449.200091.
[15] Chang DW, Suami H, Skoracki R. A prospective analysis of 100 consecutive lymphovenous bypass cases for treatment of extremity lymphedema. Plast Reconstr Surg 2013;132(5): 1305–14.
[16] AlJindan FK, Lin CY, Cheng MH. Comparison of outcomes between side-to-end and end-to-end lymphovenous anastomoses for early-grade extremity lymphedema. Plast Reconstr Surg 2019;144(2):486–96.
[17] Lin CH, Ali R, Chen SC, et al. Vascularized groin lymph node transfer using the wrist as a recipient site for management of postmastectomy upper extremity lymphedema. Plast Reconstr Surg 2009;123(4):1265–75.
[18] Cheng M, Huang J, Nguyen D, et al. A novel approach to the treatment of lower extremity lymphedema by transferring a vascularized submental lymph node flap to the ankle. Gynecol Oncol 2012;126:93–8.
[19] Cheng MH, Chen SC, Henry SL, et al. Vascularized groin lymph node flap transfer for postmastectomy upper limb lymphedema: flap anatomy, recipient sites, and outcomes. Plast Reconstr Surg 2013;131(6):1286–98.
[20] Ito R, Lin MC, Cheng MH. Simultaneous bilateral submental lymph node flaps for lower limb lymphedema post leg charles procedure. Plast Reconstr Surg Glob Open 2015;3(9):e513; https://doi.org/10.1097/GOX.0000000000000489.
[21] Poccia I, Lin CY, Cheng MH. Platysma-sparing vascularized submental lymph node flap transfer for extremity lymphedema. J Surg Oncol 2017;115(1):48–53.
[22] Gustafsson J, Chu SY, Chan WH, et al. Correlation between quantity of transferred lymph nodes and outcome in vascularized submental lymph node flap transfer for lower limb lymphedema. Plast Reconstr Surg 2018;142(4):1056–63.
[23] Engel H, Lin CY, Huang JJ, et al. Outcomes of lymphedema microsurgery for breast cancer-related lymphedema with or without microvascular breast reconstruction. Ann Surg 2018;268(6):1076–83.
[24] Cheng MH, Tee R, Chen C, et al. Simultaneous ipsilateral vascularized lymph node transplantation and contralateral lymphovenous anastomosis in bilateral extremity lymphedema with different severities. Ann Surg Oncol 2020; https://doi.org/10.1245/s10434-020-08720-2.
[25] Francis EC, Kim BS, Lin MC, et al. Vascularized lymph node transfer improved outcomes of elderly patients with secondary upper extremity lymphedema. Ann Surg Oncol 2022;29 (12):7868–78.
[26] Ho OA, Lin CY, Pappalardo M, et al. Comparisons of submental and groin vascularized lymph node flaps transfer for breast cancer-related lymphedema. Plast Reconstr Surg Glob Open 2018;6(12):e1923.

[27] Executive Committee of the International Society of Lymphology. The diagnosis and treatment of peripheral lymphedema: 2020 consensus document of the International Society of Lymphology. Lymphology 2020;53(1):3–19.
[28] Pappalardo M, Lin CY, Lin C, et al. Improvement of the natural progression of extremity Lymphedema treated with lymphatic microsurgery. Ann Surg 2025;282(4):639–49.
[29] Hsiao HY, Liu JW, Pappalardo M, et al. The impacts of lymph on the adipogenesis of adipose-derived stem cells. Plast Reconstr Surg 2023;151(5):1005–15.
[30] Greene AK, Goss JA. Diagnosis and staging of lymphedema. Semin Plast Surg 2018;32(1):12–6.
[31] Cheng M-H, Chang DW, Patel K. Principles and practice of lymphedema surgery. 2nd edition. Philadelphia (PA): Elsevier; 2021.
[32] Cheng MH, Pappalardo M, Lin C, et al. Validity of the novel Taiwan lymphoscintigraphy staging and correlation of cheng lymphedema grading for unilateral extremity lymphedema. Ann Surg 2018;268(3):513–25.
[33] Pappalardo M, Starnoni M, Franceschini G, et al. Breast cancer-related lymphedema: recent updates on diagnosis, severity and available treatments. J Pers Med 2021;11(5); https://doi.org/10.3390/jpm11050402.
[34] International Society of Lymphology. The diagnosis and treatment of peripheral lymphedema. 2009 consensus document of the international Society of Lymphology. Lymphology 2009;42(2):51–60.
[35] International Society of Lymphology. The diagnosis and treatment of peripheral lymphedema: 2013 consensus document of the international Society of Lymphology. Lymphology 2013;46(1):1–11.
[36] Pappalardo M, Cheng M-H. Lymphoscintigraphy interpretation, staging, and lymphedema grading. In: Principles and practice of lymphedema surgery. 2nd edition. St. Louis, Missouri: Elsevier; 2021. p. 39–49.
[37] Patel KM, Lin CY, Cheng MH. A prospective evaluation of lymphedema-specific quality-of-life outcomes following vascularized lymph node transfer. Ann Surg Oncol 2015;22(7):2424–30.
[38] Pappalardo M, Lin C, Ho OA, et al. Staging and clinical correlations of lymphoscintigraphy for unilateral gynecological cancer-related lymphedema. J Surg Oncol 2020;121(3):422–34; https://doi.org/10.1002/jso.25817.
[39] Pappalardo M, Cheng MH. Lymphoscintigraphy for the diagnosis of extremity lymphedema: current controversies regarding protocol, interpretation, and clinical application. J Surg Oncol 2020;121(1):37–47; https://doi.org/10.1002/jso.25526.
[40] Mihara M, Hara H, Araki J, et al. Indocyanine green (ICG) lymphography is superior to lymphoscintigraphy for diagnostic imaging of early lymphedema of the upper limbs. PLoS One 2012;7(6):e38182.
[41] Yamamoto T, Yamamoto N, Doi K, et al. Indocyanine green-enhanced lymphography for upper extremity lymphedema: a novel severity staging system using dermal backflow patterns. Plast Reconstr Surg 2011;128(4):941–7.
[42] Yamamoto T, Yamamoto N, Ishiura R. Evaluation of the upper limb lymphatic system: a prospective lymphoscintigraphic study in melanoma patients and healthy controls. Plast Reconstr Surg 2017;139(4):1028e–9e.
[43] Ito R, Wu CT, Lin MC, et al. Successful treatment of early-stage lower extremity lymphedema with side-to-end lymphovenous anastomosis with indocyanine green lymphography assisted. Microsurgery 2016;36(4):310–5.
[44] Pappalardo M, Blessent CGF, Baccarani A, et al. Eliminating venous-to-lymphatic reflux by converting end-to-side to end-to-end lymphovenous bypass with ligation of the distal vein. Plast Reconstr Surg Glob Open 2025;13(6):e6929.
[45] Pappalardo M, Patel K, Cheng MH. Vascularized lymph node transfer for treatment of extremity lymphedema: an overview of current controversies regarding donor sites, recipient sites and outcomes. J Surg Oncol 2018;117(7):1420–31.

[46] Cheng MH, Huang JJ, Wu CW, et al. The mechanism of vascularized lymph node transfer for lymphedema: natural lymphaticovenous drainage. Plast Reconstr Surg 2014;133(2):192e–8e.
[47] Ito R, Zelken J, Yang CY, et al. Proposed pathway and mechanism of vascularized lymph node flaps. Gynecol Oncol 2016;141(1):182–8.
[48] Patel KM, Lin CY, Cheng MH. From theory to evidence: long-term evaluation of the mechanism of action and flap integration of distal vascularized lymph node transfers. J Reconstr Microsurg 2015;31(1):26–30.
[49] De Santis G, Saxena B, Starnoni M, et al. Efficacy of vascularized submental lymph node transfer with decongestive therapy and antibiotics for early-stage lower limb filarial lymphedema. Plast Reconstr Surg 2023;151(5):850e–6e.
[50] Dayan JH, Dayan E, Smith ML. Reverse lymphatic mapping: a new technique for maximizing safety in vascularized lymph node transfer. Plast Reconstr Surg 2015;135(1):277–85.
[51] Baccarani A, Starnoni M, Pappalardo M, et al. Early venous congestion after diep flap breast reconstruction: case report of a successful management. Acta Biomed 2022;93(S1):e2022180.
[52] Ho OA, Lin YL, Pappalardo M, Cheng MH. Nipple-sparing mastectomy and breast reconstruction with a deep inferior epigastric perforator flap using thoracodorsal recipient vessels and a low lateral incision. J Surg Oncol 2018;118(4):621–9.
[53] Starnoni M, Pappalardo M, Malmassari C, et al. Outcome of breast implant replacement after radiation therapy: a single-centre retrospective comparative study. J Plast Reconstr Aesthet Surg 2026;115:402–11.
[54] Baccarani A, Blessent CGF, Marra C, et al. Two-stage prepectoral breast reconstruction with expander and acellular dermal matrix: why and when. Plast Reconstr Surg Glob Open 2024;12(4):e5774.
[55] Baccarani A, Pappalardo M. Applications of the fold flap in breast reconstruction. Plast Reconstr Surg Glob Open 2026;14(1):e7359.
[56] Masia J, Pons G, Pomata C, et al. Surgical management of lower limb lymphedema after pelvic/perineal resections. In: Kosutic D, editor. Perineal reconstruction. Cham: Springer; 2023; https://doi.org/10.1007/978-3-030-97691-0_18.
[57] Maldonado AA, Chen R, Chang DW. The use of supraclavicular free flap with vascularized lymph node transfer for treatment of lymphedema: a prospective study of 100 consecutive cases. J Surg Oncol 2017;115(1):68–71.
[58] Barreiro GC, Baptista RR, Kasai KE, et al. Lymph fasciocutaneous lateral thoracic artery flap: anatomical study and clinical use. J Reconstr Microsurg 2014;30(6):389–96.
[59] Brown S, Mehrara BJ, Coriddi M, et al. A prospective study on the safety and efficacy of vascularized lymph node transplant. Ann Surg 2022;276(4):635–53.
[60] Koide S, Lin CY, Cheng MH. Delayed primary retention suture for inset of vascularized submental lymph node flap for lower extremity lymphedema. J Surg Oncol 2019; https://doi.org/10.1002/jso.25520.
[61] Koide S, Lin CY, Chen C, et al. Long-term outcome of lower extremity lymphedema treated with vascularized lymph node flap transfer with or without venous complications. J Surg Oncol 2019; https://doi.org/10.1002/jso.25602.
[62] Sachanandani NS, Chu SY, Ho OA, et al. Lymphedema and concomitant venous comorbidity in the extremity: comprehensive evaluation, management strategy, and outcomes. J Surg Oncol 2018;118(6):941–52.
[63] Beederman M, Garza RM, Agarwal S, et al. Outcomes for physiologic microsurgical treatment of secondary lymphedema involving the extremity. Ann Surg 2022;276(4):e255–63.
[64] Cheng MH, Loh CYY, Lin CY. Outcomes of vascularized lymph node transfer and lymphovenous anastomosis for treatment of primary lymphedema. Plast Reconstr Surg Glob Open 2018;6(12):e2056.
[65] Cheng MH. ASO author reflections: simultaneous ipsilateral vascularized lymph node transplantation and contralateral lymphovenous anastomosis in bilateral different-severities extremity lymphedema. Ann Surg Oncol 2020; https://doi.org/10.1245/s10434-020-08810-1.

Advances in Surgery 60 (2026) 85–97

ADVANCES IN SURGERY

Neoadjuvant Therapy for Melanoma

Margaret H. O'Connor, MD, PhD[a], Isabel DeLaura, MD[b], Georgia M. Beasley, MD, MHS[a,*]

[a]Department of Surgery, Duke University Medical Center, Durham, NC, USA; [b]Department of Surgery, Duke University, Durham, NC, USA

Keywords

• Melanoma • Neoadjuvant therapy • Immune checkpoint inhibitor • Targeted therapy

Key points

- Treatment of melanoma has transformed dramatically in the past 13 years with 11 new therapeutic agents approved by the US Food and Drug Administration since 2011 for patients with advanced melanoma in the form of immune checkpoint inhibitors and targeted immune therapies.
- Neoadjuvant treatment with these agents is rapidly evolving with many trials showing the superiority of neoadjuvant over adjuvant treatment.
- The benefits of neoadjuvant therapy are numerous but include the ability to determine pathologic responses to treatment before decisions on next steps in therapy allowing for personalized care.
- Further studies will determine optimal treatment strategies, regimens, and combinations.

CLINICAL BACKGROUND

Treatment of melanoma has transformed dramatically in the past 13 years with 11 new therapeutic agents approved by the US Food and Drug Administration since 2011 for patients with advanced melanoma [1]. Specifically, systemic therapy with immune checkpoint inhibitors (ICI) including anti-programmed cell death protein 1 (anti-PD-1), anti-cytotoxic T-lymphocyte-associated protein 4

*Corresponding author. Duke University Medical Center, Box 3966, 10 Bryan Searle Drive, 466G Seeley G. Mudd Building, Durham, NC 27710. *E-mail address:* Georgia.Beasley@duke.edu

https://doi.org/10.1016/j.yasu.2026.03.005

Abbreviations

anti-PD-1	anti-programmed cell death protein 1
CTLA-4	cytotoxic T-lymphocyte-associated protein 4
EFS	event free survival
ICI	immune checkpoint inhibitors
MPR	major pathologic response
pPR	pathologic partial response
RFS	relapse-free survival
TLND	therapeutic lymph node dissection
T-VEC	Talimogene laherparepvec

(CTLA-4), and anti-lymphocyte-activation gene 3 therapies, as well as targeted therapies (proto-oncogene B-Raf [BRAF]/mitogen-activated protein kinase kinase [MEK] inhibitors, [BRAFi/MEKi]) has dramatically improved outcomes for many patients with advanced cutaneous metastatic melanoma [2,3]. Shortly after approval for metastatic disease, investigation began into using these agents as adjuvant and neoadjuvant strategies around the timing of surgery. Adjuvant therapy and neoadjuvant therapy can be used to treat clinically occult disease and thereby decrease recurrence risk [4]. The success of adjuvant therapy in treating clinically occult disease led to further work in the neoadjuvant setting. In this article, we will provide an overview of the advances of neoadjuvant therapy in melanoma and highlight select clinical trials supporting its use, while discussing its present applications and exploring unanswered questions limiting its broader utilization.

IMMUNE CHECKPOINT INHIBITORS ENTER THE NEOADJUVANT SETTING

Table 1 is a comprehensive list of neoadjuvant trials. In this article, we will review key trials.

Building on smaller initial studies, a larger randomized trial was performed, SWOG S1801, which explored the efficacy of neoadjuvant pembro in resectable Stage III or IV melanoma [5]. This Phase II study included patients with Stage IIIB to IVC melanoma, who were randomized into two groups: one receiving neoadjuvant pembro followed by surgery and adjuvant pembro, and the other receiving surgery followed by standard of care adjuvant pembro monotherapy [5]. Importantly the total therapy (18 total cycles in each arm) and surgery were exactly the same in each group, the only difference was timing of ICI therapy. Results showed that the neoadjuvant–adjuvant group had significantly longer event-free survival (EFS) compared to the adjuvant-only group, with a 2 year EFS of 72% versus 49% [5] (see Table 1). This trial is considered practice changing and helped in establishing neoadjuvant therapy as the newest standard of care for patients with clinically detectable stage III and higher melanoma amenable to surgical resection.

The OpACIN trial was the first to test the combination of anti-PD-1 (nivo) and anti-CTLA-4 (ipi) therapies in the neoadjuvant treatment of Stage III

Table 1
Neoadjuvant trials in melanoma

Trial	Population	Treatment	Path response	EFS/RFS	Grade 3 AEs
High-Dose Interferon-Alfa-2b (HDI) [10]	Stage IIIB-C resectable melanoma or recurrent clinical regional lymphadenopathy	HDI neoadjuvant treatment 20 million units/m^2 5 d per week for 4 wk	Clinical response: 55% path response: 15%	Not reported	Grade 3–4 adverse events: 25%
HDI + ICI [11]	Clinically detectable locally and/or regionally advanced melanoma	2 doses neoadjuvant ipi (3 or 10 mg/kg), surgery, then 2 doses adjuvant with possible additional 4 more doses ipi. HDI was given concurrently neoadjuvant and adjuvant	pCR: 32% 11 patients relapsed with 5/11 with death due to disease	Not reported	Grade 3–4 toxicity below standard range
Huang et al [12] 2019	Stage IIIB/C or IV melanoma	Single dose of neoadjuvant pembro followed by surgery 3 wk later and adjuvant therapy	MPR: 29.6%	Not reported	Not higher than 30%, the prespecified safety end point
SWOG S1801 [5]	Resectable stage III/IV melanoma	Neoadjuvant + adjuvant pembro vs adjuvant pembro only	pCR: 21% neoadj arm	24 mo EFS: 72% neoadj vs 49% adj.	Grade 3–4 toxicity: neoadj 12% vs adj 14%

(*continued on next page*)

Table 1
(*continued*)

Trial	Population	Treatment	Path response	EFS/RFS	Grade 3 AEs
OPACIN [6]	Macroscopic stage III melanoma	Neoadjuvant + adjuvant ipi + nivo vs adjuvant ipi + nivo only	MPR: 67%	5 y RFS: 70% (neoadjuvant–adjuvant) vs 60% (adjuvant only); 5 y OS: 90% vs 70%	
OPACIN-neo [6]	Macroscopic stage III melanoma	3 dosing schedules of neoadjuvant ipi + nivo	pRR: 77%	3 y RFS: 95.3% (responding) vs 36.8% (non-responding)	Grade 3–4: 20%
PRADO [7]	Clinical stage IIIB–D nodal melanoma	Neoadjuvant ipi + nivo, tailored post-treatment based on pathologic response	pRR: 72% MPR: 61%	24 mo RFS: 93% (MPR) vs 64% (pPR) vs 71% (pNR)	Not specified
Amaria Nivo-Rela [13]	Resectable Stage III or oligometastatic Stage IV disease	2 cycles of neoadjuvant nivo and rela at fixed doses, followed by surgical resection, and then 10 doses of adjuvant nivo/rela	pCR: 57%	The 12 and 24 mo RFS: In pPR 100% and 92% In nPR: 88% and 55%	No grade 3–4 adverse events were observed
Neo-MEL-T [14]	Clinical stage IIIB-D melanoma	2 cycles of neoadjuvant anti-PD-1 Dostarlimab (Dostar) or Dostar plus anti-TIM-3 Cobolimab (Cobo) then surgery and adjuvant Dostar	MPR: Combo dostar and cobo: 51.9% dostar alone: 33.3%	RFS: combo: 87% Single agent: 82% both higher than historical average 63%	Grade 3 or higher irAEs Dostar alone (16.7%) and Dostar + Cobo (14.9%)

NADINA [8]	Macroscopic stage III melanoma with at least one pathologically proven, clinically detectable lymph node	2 cycles of neoadjuvant ipi + nivo then TLND. In the case of pathologic partial response or non-response, surgery will be followed by adjuvant nivo (11 cycles) or adjuvant dabrafenib + trametinib (46 wk) if BRAFV600-mutation is present. Patients in adjuvant arm undergo upfront TLND followed by 12 cycles of adjuvant nivo	MPR: Neoadj 58.0%	12 mo EFS rates of 83.7% neoadj vs 57.2% adj	Grade 3 or higher irAEs: Neoadj: 29.7% Adj: 14.7%
Miura et al. [15] 2025	Clinical stage IIB/C melanoma	Single dose of neoadjuvant pembro 3 wk prior to WLE and SLNB followed by 1 y adjuvant pembro	Reported SLN metastasis rate in the neoadj group was 27%.	The 2 y RFS in neoadj was 84%	22% with 14% irAEs

(continued on next page)

Table 1
(*continued*)

Trial	Population	Treatment	Path response	EFS/RFS	Grade 3 AEs
CAP 03-NEO [16]	Resectable Stage II/III acral melanoma	2 cycles of neoadjuvant camrelizumab, apatinib, and temozolomide, followed by surgery and 15 cycles of adjuvant camrelizumab	MPR: 42.9% pRR: 57.1% including: 25.0% with pCR, 17.8% with near pCR, and 16% with pPR.	12 mo EFS: 74.1%	No grade 4 AEs.
Amaria BRAF [17]	Resectable stage IIIB-C or oligometastatic stage IV BRAF mutant melanoma	Neoadjuvant plus adjuvant dabrafenib and trametinib (8 wk neoadjuvant and 44 wk adjuvant vs upfront surgery and consideration for adjuvant therapy (standard of care group)	Not reported	EFS: Neoadj: 19.7 mo vs 2.9 mo adj.	No grade 4 toxicities, 15% grade 3 (colitis)
NeoCombi [18]	Resectable Stage IIIB-C BRAF-mutant melanoma	12 wk of neoadjuvant dabrafenib plus trametinib followed by 40 wk of adjuvant therapy	pCR: 46%	Not reported	Grade 3–4 adverse events: 29%

NeoACTIVATE [19]	Clinically evident resectable Stage III melanoma	12 wk of neoadjuvant vemurafenib, cobimetinib, and atezolizumab (BRAF mutated) or cobimetinib and atezolizumab (BRAF-wild-type) followed by TLND and 24 wk of adjuvant atezolizumab	MPR: In neoadj triple therapy arm: 66.7% in *BRAF*-mutated 33.3% in *BRAF*-wild-type	Not reported	Mostly dermatologic and occurred in 63% during neoadjuvant treatment
Dummer et al. TVEC [20]	Resectable stage IIIB to IVM1a melanoma with 1 or more injectable cutaneous, subcutaneous, or nodal lesions	6 doses of neoadjuvant T-VEC then surgery vs immediate surgery alone with adjuvant therapy per SOC	pCR of the T-VEC group was 17.1% at 3 y	Not reported	Not reported
NIVEC [21]	Resectable stage IIIB–IVA melanoma with injectable lesion	4 doses of intralesional T-VEC and 3 doses of nivo neoadjuvant followed by surgery	MPR: 65%	1 y EFS: 75%	Grade 3 AEs in 9%, no grade 4

Abbreviations: adj, adjuvant; AE, adverse event; Cobo, Cobolimab; Dostar, Dostarlimab; EFS, event-free survival; HDI, high-dose interferon-alfa-2b; ICI, immune checkpoint inhibitors; ipi, ipilimumab; irAE, immune related adverse event; MPR, major pathologic response; neoadj, Neoadjuvant; nivo, nivolumab; nPR, pathologic non response; pCR, pathologic complete response; pembro, pembrolizumab; pPR, pathologic partial response; pRR, pathologic response rate; rela, relatlimab; RFS, relapse-free survival; SLN, sentinel lymph node; SOC, standard of care; TLND, total lymph node dissection; TVEC, talimogene laherparepvec.

melanoma, comparing it with the same combination in the adjuvant setting. This was a Phase Ib randomized trial of 20 patients Stage IIIB/C melanoma randomized to receive either 2 cycles of neoadjuvant ipi plus nivo then 2 cycles adjuvant, or 4 cycles of adjuvant with the same regimen. In the neoadjuvant group, 7 of 9 (78%) patients achieved a pathologic response, with 3 patients having pCR, 3 patients near-pCR, and 1 patient pPR, and there was an 80% relapse-free survival (RFS) rate. Moreover, neoadjuvant treatment was shown to expand tumor-resident T cells in the peripheral circulation, again supporting the hypothesis that turning tumor in situ could generate a more robust immune response. The 2023 update showed an estimated 5 year progression free survival (PFS) and overall survival (OS) of 70% and 90% in patients in the neoadjuvant arm and 60% and 70% in the adjuvant arm, respectively [6].

The (neoadjuvant ipilimumab (ipi) + nivolumab (nivo) in macroscopic stage III melanoma [OpACIN])-neo was a multicenter, Phase II randomized trial that investigated the safety and efficacy of different nivo and ipi dosing regimens in the neoadjuvant setting. The results demonstrated that a flip-dose (arm B) ipi regimen (nivo 3 mg/kg and ipi 1 mg/kg) achieved a 77% pathologic response rate with only 20% incidence of grade 3 to 4 irAEs [6]. Over a median follow-up of 46.8 months, patients with a pathologic response had a 3 year RFS rate of 95.3%, whereas those without a pathologic response had a significantly lower RFS rate of 36.8% (see Table 1) [6]. Both OpACIN and OpACIN-neo confirmed the durability of responses to neoadjuvant ICI in high-risk Stage III melanoma, demonstrating that pathologic response is a reliable surrogate marker for long-term outcomes such as RFS and OS.

Based on the findings in the OpACIN-neo trial, the (Personalized Response-driven ADjuvant cOmbination therapy [PRADO trial]) was created as an extension of this cohort to focus on the personalization of neoadjuvant therapy based on pathologic response [7]. Those with major pathologic response (MPR) of the index lymph node resulted in the omission of further therapy, pathologic partial response (pPR) involved therapeutic lymph node dissection (TLND), and non-response required TLND plus adjuvant therapy [7]. The trial demonstrated a high pathologic response rate (72%), significant survival benefits, and reduced surgical morbidity for patients with MPR who did not undergo TLND (see Table 1) [7]. Importantly, for the 60 patients with an MPR who did not undergo TLDN, there were only 4 regional recurrences during a median follow-up of 28 months. This led to the failure to meet primary RFS end point (if had more than 1 recurrence was not considered significant based on trial criteria). These 4 patients went on to delayed TLND and 1 patient later developed distance recurrence. Thus, while de-escalating surgery led to improved morbidity, further work must be done to identify which patients can safely forego TLND without comprising oncologic outcomes.

The most recent, and most impactful Phase III trial that tailored individual therapy based on pathologic response to neoadjuvant treatment was the

NADINA trial (NCT04949113). This Phase III, multicenter, randomized study compared the efficacy of neoadjuvant ipi plus nivo to standard adjuvant nivo in patients with macroscopic resectable Stage III melanoma [8]. Patients in the neoadjuvant arm received 2 cycles of ipi/nivo followed by TLND and then further adjuvant therapy was determined after pathologic assessment [8]. If pathology showed there was an MPR then the patient did not receive adjuvant treatment. If the pathology showed either pPR (11%–50% residual viable tumor) or non-response (>50% residual viable tumor), surgery was followed by adjuvant nivo (11 cycles). If a BRAFV600-mutation was detected, patients in arm A with greater than 10% viable tumor (partial or non-responders) were treated with adjuvant dabrafenib plus trametinib (46 weeks). Patients in arm B (adjuvant only) underwent upfront TLND followed by 12 cycles of nivo [9]. At a median follow-up of 9.9 months, the estimated 12 month EFS was 83.7% in the neoadjuvant group and 57.2% in the adjuvant group [9]. The MPR in the neoadjuvant group was 59.0% [9]. Grade 3 or higher adverse events related to systemic treatment occurred in 29.7% of the patients in the neoadjuvant group and 14.7% in the adjuvant group (see Table 1) [9]. These data clearly support that neoadjuvant ipi plus nivo followed by surgery and response-driven adjuvant therapy was superior in terms of prolonged EFS when compared to surgery followed by adjuvant nivo. This was the first study to omit adjuvant therapy after an MPR and again represents a major advancement in care.

BRAF/MEK INHIBITOR NEOADJUVANT THERAPIES

In all clinical cases of melanoma, about 50% harbor BRAF mutations [22]. BRAF/MEK inhibition is an established therapy for patients with BRAF mutations [23,24]. This combination therapy was subsequently trialed in the neoadjuvant setting by Amaria and colleagues in Stage IIIB-C or oligometastatic Stage IV BRAF mutant melanoma [17]. Patients were randomized to prior standard of care (surgery and adjuvant therapy) or neoadjuvant plus adjuvant dabrafenib and trametinib (8 weeks neoadjuvant, 44 weeks adjuvant) [17]. The trial was terminated early due to significantly longer progression-free survival in the neoadjuvant group (71% vs 0% at 18.6 months) [17] (see Table 1). There is a new Phase II trial, NeoACTIVATE (NCT03554083), for patients with Stage III melanoma who were randomized to receive either 12 weeks of neoadjuvant vemurafenib, cobimetinib, and atezolizumab (atezo; anti-PD-L1) (BRAF-mutated, Cohort A, $n = 15$), or cobimetinib and atezo (BRAF-wild-type, Cohort B, $n = 15$) followed by TLND and 24 weeks of adjuvant atezo. The neoadjuvant results were published in 2024 showing that based on intent to treat analysis, pathologic response ($\leq$50% viable tumor) and MPR (complete or near-complete, $\leq$10% viable tumor) were observed in 86.7% and 66.7% of BRAF-mutated and 53.3% and 33.3% of BRAF-wild-type patients, respectively (primary endpoint). Grade 3 and higher toxicities, primarily dermatologic, occurred in 63% during neoadjuvant treatment (secondary endpoint) which is notably higher than in similar studies.

NEOADJUVANT TALIMOGENE LAHERPAREPVEC AND OTHER ONCOLYTIC VIRUSES

Intralesional injectable therapies, such as Talimogene laherparepvec (T-VEC), a modified HSV-1 virus, have been utilized in the treatment of advanced melanoma [25]. In a randomized, open-label, Phase II trial (NCT02211131), Dummer and colleagues explored the efficacy of neoadjuvant T-VEC plus surgery versus surgery alone for stage IIIB–IVA melanoma [20]. This group reported a 2 year RFS of 29.5% in the T-VEC followed by surgery group versus 16.5% in the surgery alone group. Furthermore, the pCR of the T-VEC group was 17.1% at 3 years (see Table 1). Further, Zijlker and colleagues [21] conducted the NIVEC trial, a Phase II single-arm trial (NCT04330430), investigating the safety and efficacy of combining nivo with T-VEC as neoadjuvant therapy in 24 patients with resectable Stage IIIB-IVA melanoma. The primary outcome, pathologic response rate, was observed in 74% of patients, with 65% achieving an MPR [21]. Treatment-related adverse events were mostly grade 2 (29%), with only 8% experiencing grade 3 events. The 1 year EFS was 75% [21]. This group concluded that their combination has an acceptable safety profile and induces significant pathologic responses in regionally metastasized melanoma.

CURRENT PRACTICE

For patients presenting with Clinical Stage III disease amenable to surgical resection, the neoadjuvant approach should be presented to the patient as the best chance for a successful outcome from disease and improved disease-free survival. However, some patients may have severe auto-immune diseases, may be transplant recipients, or may have other contraindications for which surgery alone may still be indicated. Historically, surgery alone could benefit up to 30% of patients [26]. ICI should be considered as first line, or the superior regimen given data on durable disease control. In pooled analysis, from the international melanoma consortium, the 2 year RFS for neoadjuvant ICI therapy was 96% compared to 79% for targeted therapy [27]. Targeted therapy may be a better choice if patients are symptomatic or for whom reduction in tumor is necessary as BRAF/MEK response will be more rapid. However, the main concern of BRAFi/MEKi is long-term resistance, so care must be taken when using this approach. For patients with isolated local recurrences for whom systemic therapy risks may be severe (frail patients), neoadjuvant approaches with T-VEC or other clinical trials of intra-lesional agents should also be considered.

FUTURE DIRECTIONS AND UNANSWERED QUESTIONS

The question of whether a patient needs adjuvant therapy after having received neoadjuvant therapy remains unanswered. At present, the International Neoadjuvant Melanoma Consortium recommends that neoadjuvant clinical trials include a conventional postoperative adjuvant phase, which may or may not include the drug(s) under investigation, to complete a total duration of 1 year of systemic therapy as has been the prior standard of care [28]. Trials like NADINA provide additional data to help dictate adjuvant therapy decisions since this trial did not give additional adjuvant therapy to patients with an MPR (<10% viable residual tumor) [8,29]. For patients achieving an MPR, foregoing any adjuvant treatment can be considered especially if there are ongoing side effects.

The decision between single agent ICI and dual checkpoint therapy is complex. Dual checkpoint therapy leads to higher pathologic response rates but significantly increases risk of serious toxic side effects and some side effects are not reversible [30]. For patients with short disease-free intervals, larger tumor burden, and high-performance status, dual checkpoint therapy may be optimal for best chance at pathologic response [31]. However, single agent checkpoint therapy is a good strategy for many patients especially small volume disease. Therapy can be escalated if tumor responses are not observed.

Another question to explore deals with the de-escalation of surgery, most notably the ability to forego lymph node dissection in favor of targeted lymph node excision, after neoadjuvant therapy. This has yet to be standardized. For patients with more than 1 lymph node involved on imaging, performing single node excision should be cautioned since those patients had lymph node recurrence in the PRADO study [7]. Placing a marker in the node, then doing a single node excision, and then doing a third procedure (TLND) if the patient does not have a favorable pathologic response can also be logistically and financially challenging for some patients. For patients where TLND may carry greater risk of side effects (eg, obesity increases the risk of lymphedema) [32], the option for selective dissection should be considered.

SUMMARY

As melanoma therapy continues to evolve, neoadjuvant therapy stands out with an ability to transform patient management and outcomes. However, current real-world practices are not standardized, and several critical questions persist [33]. Surgeons should continue to be highly engaged in the multidisciplinary care of patients with advanced melanoma and can continue to lead groundbreaking clinical trials in neoadjuvant trials.

CLINICS CARE POINTS

- Neoadjuvant therapy for locally advanced melanoma should now be considered standard of care.
- The regimen for therapy should be a multi-disciplinary discussion.
- Pathologic response can provide information about the need for additional therapies.

Disclosures

G.M. Beasley has received clinical trial funding paid to Duke University from Delcath, Istari, Replimune, Oncosec, Checkmate. G.M. Beasley has done

one-time advisory board for Cardinal Health, Regeneron, Bristol-Myers-Squibb. M.H. O'Connor and I. DeLaura have nothing to disclose.

Funding
M.H. O'Connor: 1F32CA294631-02.

References

[1] Institute NC. Drugs approved for Melanoma. National Institutes of Health; 2024.
[2] Tawbi HA, Schadendorf D, Lipson EJ, et al, RELATIVITY-047 Investigators. Relatlimab and nivolumab versus nivolumab in untreated advanced melanoma. N Engl J Med 2022;386: 24–34, PMC9844513.
[3] Atkins MB, Lee SJ, Chmielowski B, et al. Combination dabrafenib and trametinib versus combination nivolumab and ipilimumab for patients with advanced BRAF-mutant melanoma: the DREAMseq Trial-ECOG-ACRIN EA6134. J Clin Oncol 2023;41:186–97, PMC9839305.
[4] Lee AY, Brady MS. Neoadjuvant immunotherapy for melanoma. J Surg Oncol 2021;123: 782–8, PMC8366312.
[5] Patel SP, Othus M, Chen Y, et al. Neoadjuvant–adjuvant or adjuvant-only pembrolizumab in advanced melanoma. N Engl J Med 2023;388:813–23.
[6] Versluis JM, Menzies AM, Sikorska K, et al. Survival update of neoadjuvant ipilimumab plus nivolumab in macroscopic stage III melanoma in the OpACIN and OpACIN-neo trials. Ann Oncol 2023;34:420–30.
[7] Reijers ILM, Menzies AM, van Akkooi ACJ, et al. , Blank CU: personalized response-directed surgery and adjuvant therapy after neoadjuvant ipilimumab and nivolumab in high-risk stage III melanoma: the PRADO trial. Nat Med 2022;28:1178–88.
[8] Lucas MW, Lijnsvelt J, Pulleman S, et al. The NADINA trial: a multicenter, randomised, phase 3 trial comparing the efficacy of neoadjuvant ipilimumab plus nivolumab with standard adjuvant nivolumab in macroscopic resectable stage III melanoma. J Clin Oncol 2022;40: TPS9605.
[9] Blank CU, Lucas MW, Scolyer RA, et al. Neoadjuvant nivolumab plus ipilimumab versus adjuvant nivolumab in macroscopic, resectable stage III melanoma: the phase 3 NADINA trial. J Clin Oncol 2024;42:LBA2.
[10] Moschos SJ, Edington HD, Land SR, et al. Neoadjuvant treatment of regional stage IIIB Melanoma with high-dose interferon Alfa-2b induces objective tumor regression in Association with modulation of tumor infiltrating host cellular immune responses. J Clin Oncol 2006;24: 3164–71.
[11] Tarhini A, Lin Y, Lin H, et al. Neoadjuvant ipilimumab (3 mg/kg or 10 mg/kg) and high dose IFN-α2b in locally/regionally advanced melanoma: safety, efficacy and impact on T-cell repertoire. J Immunother Cancer 2018;6(112):PMC6199801.
[12] Huang AC, Orlowski RJ, Xu X, et al. A single dose of neoadjuvant PD-1 blockade predicts clinical outcomes in resectable melanoma. Nat Med 2019;25:454–61.
[13] Amaria RN, Postow M, Burton EM, et al. Neoadjuvant relatlimab and nivolumab in resectable melanoma. Nature 2022;611:155–60.
[14] Mooradian M, Karunamurthy A, Wang H, et al. Randomized phase II study of neoadjuvant (neoadj) anti-PD-1 dostarlimab (D) vs. D + anti-TIM-3 cobolimab (C) in high-risk resectable melanoma (mel) (NEO-MEL-T): primary analysis. J Clin Oncol 2025;43:LBA9504-LBA9504.
[15] Miura J, Farooq MS, Gimotty PA, et al. Neoadjuvant-adjuvant pembrolizumab in clinical stage IIB/C melanoma. J Clin Oncol 2025;43:9502.
[16] Mao L, Li C, Dai J, et al. Neoadjuvant camrelizumab plus apatinib and temozolomide for resectable stage II/III acral melanoma: the CAP 03-NEO trial. J Clin Oncol 2025;43: 9512.

[17] Amaria RN, Prieto PA, Tetzlaff MT, et al. Neoadjuvant plus adjuvant dabrafenib and trametinib versus standard of care in patients with high-risk, surgically resectable melanoma: a single-centre, open-label, randomised, phase 2 trial. Lancet Oncol 2018;19: 181–93.
[18] Long GV, Saw RPM, Lo S, et al. Neoadjuvant dabrafenib combined with trametinib for resectable, stage IIIB-C, BRAF(V600) mutation-positive melanoma (NeoCombi): a single-arm, open-label, single-centre, phase 2 trial. Lancet Oncol 2019;20:961–71.
[19] Hieken TJ, Nelson GD, Flotte TJ, et al. Neoadjuvant cobimetinib and atezolizumab with or without vemurafenib for high-risk operable stage III melanoma: the phase II NeoACTIVATE trial. Nat Commun 2024;15:1430.
[20] Dummer R, Gyorki DE, Hyngstrom J, et al. Neoadjuvant talimogene laherparepvec plus surgery versus surgery alone for resectable stage IIIB–IVM1a melanoma: a randomized, open-label, phase 2 trial. Nat Med 2021;27:1789–96.
[21] Zijlker LP, Houdt WJV, Stahlie EHA, et al. Neoadjuvant T-VEC + nivolumab combination therapy for resectable early metastatic (stage IIIB/C/D-IV M1a) melanoma with injectable disease: NIVEC trial. J Clin Oncol 2023;41:9546.
[22] Network CGA. Genomic classification of cutaneous melanoma. Cell 2015;161:1681–96, PMC4580370.
[23] Long GV, Stroyakovskiy D, Gogas H, et al. Dabrafenib and trametinib versus dabrafenib and placebo for Val600 BRAF-mutant melanoma: a multicentre, double-blind, phase 3 randomised controlled trial. Lancet 2015;386:444–51.
[24] Robert C, Grob JJ, Stroyakovskiy D, et al. Long GV: five-year outcomes with dabrafenib plus trametinib in metastatic melanoma. N Engl J Med 2019;381:626–36.
[25] Saad M, Tarhini AA. Neoadjuvant therapy in Melanoma: where are we now? Curr Oncol Rep 2023;25:325–39.
[26] Ollila DW, Lopez NE, Hsueh EC. Metastasectomy for stage IV melanoma in the era of effective systemic agents. Crit Rev Oncog 2016;21:37–55.
[27] Menzies AM, Amaria RN, Rozeman EA, et al. Pathological response and survival with neoadjuvant therapy in melanoma: a pooled analysis from the International Neoadjuvant Melanoma Consortium (INMC). Nat Med 2021;27:301–9.
[28] Amaria RN, Menzies AM, Burton EM, et al, International Neoadjuvant Melanoma Consortium Members. Neoadjuvant systemic therapy in melanoma: recommendations of the International neoadjuvant Melanoma Consortium. Lancet Oncol 2019;20:e378–89.
[29] Health NIo. Adjuvant nivolumab or ipilimumab + nivolumab determined by pathological response to A single dose of neoadjvuant nivolumab. Bethesda, MD: Abramson Cancer Center at Penn Medicine; 2020.
[30] Willsmore ZN, Coumbe BGT, Crescioli S, et al. Karagiannis SN: combined anti-PD-1 and anti-CTLA-4 checkpoint blockade: treatment of melanoma and immune mechanisms of action. Eur J Immunol 2021;51:544–56.
[31] Amaria RN, Reddy SM, Tawbi HA, et al. Neoadjuvant immune checkpoint blockade in high-risk resectable melanoma. Nat Med 2018;24:1649–54, PMC6481682.
[32] Friedman JF, Sunkara B, Jehnsen JS, et al. Risk factors associated with lymphedema after lymph node dissection in melanoma patients. Am J Surg 2015;210:1178–84 [discussion: 1184].
[33] Rhodin KE, Gaughan EM, Raman V, et al. Multicenter experience with neoadjuvant therapy in melanoma highlights heterogeneity in contemporary practice. Ann Surg 2023;277: e1306–12, PMC9823148.

Advances in Surgery 60 (2026) 99–113

ADVANCES IN SURGERY

Myths and Science: Understanding the Current Landscape of Lymphatic Surgery

Min-Jeong Cho, MD[a,*], Kevin C. Chung, MD, MS[b]

[a]Department of Plastic and Reconstructive Surgery, The Ohio State University, Columbus, OH, USA; [b]Plastic Surgery and Orthopaedic Surgery, Section of Plastic Surgery, University of Michigan Medical School, Ann Arbor, MI, USA

Keywords

• Lymphedema • Lymphovenous bypass • Lymphovenous anastomosis
• Vascularized lymph node transfer • Immediate lymphatic reconstruction
• LYMPHA

Key points

- Lymphedema is a chronic, debilitating condition that leads to functional impairment and disfiguring swelling of the impacted body area.
- Microsurgical procedures such as lymphovenous bypass and vascularized lymph node transfer are effective in treating lymphedema by re-establishing the lymphatic system and restoring lymphatic fluid drainage.
- Preventive lymphatic surgery significantly decreases the risk of developing lymphedema after high-risk surgeries such as lymph node dissections.

INTRODUCTION

Lymphedema is a chronic, debilitating condition that impacts over 250 million patients worldwide and up to 10 million patients in the United States [1]. Due to impaired lymph transport, these patients experience chronic heaviness, paresthesia, and swelling, which ultimately lead to significant physical, financial, and emotional burdens [2]. Although there are multiple etiologies of lymphedema, the majority of patients in the United States are afflicted with lymphedema caused by the disruption of normal lymphatic pathways from oncologic resection, radiation, or trauma. It is estimated that patients are at

*Corresponding author. *E-mail address:* Min-Jeong.Cho@osumc.edu

https://doi.org/10.1016/j.yasu.2026.03.006

Abbreviations

BCRL	breast cancer-related lymphedema
ICG	indocyanine green
ILR	immediate lymphatic reconstruction
INOS	inducible nitric oxidase synthase
ISL	International Society of Lymphology
LVB	lymphovenous bypass
MDACC	MD Anderson Cancer Center
VLNT	vascularized lymph node transfer

4% to 65% risk of developing lymphedema after axillary node dissection, and up to 66% for inguinal node dissection for their oncologic treatment [3].

Historically, treatment of lymphedema was limited to conservative treatment such as decongestive therapy to overcome fluid excess and to debulking procedures such as liposuction for fat hypertrophy [4,5]. Though the former is effective in alleviating edema and removing excess fluid via external compression, it requires constant use of compression garments, leading to discomfort, fitting difficulties, and economic strain and time commitment for physical therapy visits [6]. Similarly, debulking procedures such as liposuction aim to decrease the size and volume of the affected limb without correcting the disrupted lymphatic system [7]. It too requires lifelong constant compression postoperatively. Therefore, microsurgical procedures such as lymphovenous bypass (LVB) and vascularized lymph node transfer (VLNT) were developed to re-establish the lymphatic system and restore lymphatic fluid drainage in preventive and therapeutic manners [8–11].

Despite the popularity, the understanding and awareness of microsurgical physiologic treatments of lymphedema are riddled with controversy. As patient survival after cancer treatment continues to increase with pharmacologic and technical advances, it is crucial to understand the current landscape of lymphedema surgery to increase access, to promote early surgical intervention, and to offer guidance to patients beyond myths regarding lymphedema surgery [12].

PATHOPHYSIOLOGY OF LYMPHEDEMA

The lymphatic system is a complex network of circulating lymphocytes, lymphatic vessels, lymph nodes, and lymphoid organs. It serves a critical role in fluid homeostasis, immune responses, and absorption of dietary fats by reabsorbing interstitial fluid from the periphery and transporting them to lymphoid organs via its network (Fig. 1) [13]. The function of lymphatic vessels is carefully regulated by a myriad of growth factors, cytokines, and lymphocytes. Lymphatic flow is unidirectional, and it is maintained by pressure gradients between the interstitial space and the lymphatic capillaries. Lymphatic vessels are lined with lymphatic endothelial cells, which possess button-like junctions to allow for the influx of fluid. Due to the pressure difference, about

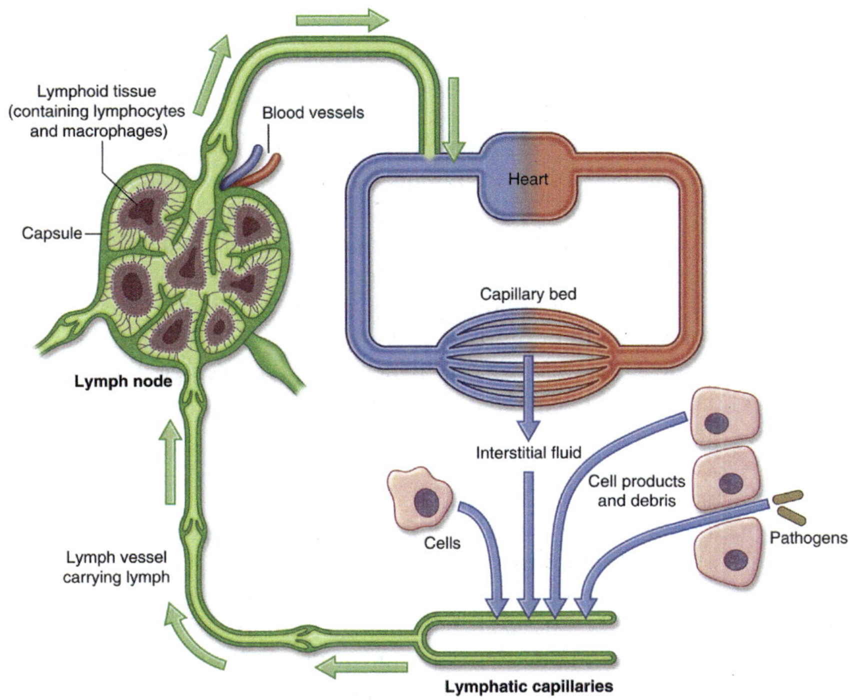

Fig. 1. Normal lymphatic circulation demonstrating the hierarchy of lymphatic structures: lymphatic capillaries, pre-collectors, collecting lymphatic vessels with valves, and lymph nodes (Richard L. Drake, A. Wayne Vogl, Adam W.M. Mitchell, Gray's Anatomy for Students, 5th Edition, 2023, Elsevier.)

10% of the interstitial fluid drains into the lymphatic capillaries to the collecting lymphatic vessels, and the lymph fluid travels to the lymph nodes with the assistance of the intrinsic muscle pump and valves [14].

In patients with a disrupted lymphatic systems such as after lymph node dissection, lymphatic stasis occurs secondary to mechanical occlusion of the drainage pathways and upregulation of cytokines and various growth factors that impair lymphatic drainage and development. Dysregulation of growth factors such as VEGF-C leads to lymphatic hyperplasia, leading to less efficient lymphatic drainage [13]. In addition, it prevents the formation of functional lymphatic vessels and development of immature lymphatic vessels. Similarly, naïve $CD4^+$ T cells promote impaired lymphangiogenesis and fibrosis in the area of lymphatic stasis and decrease lymphatic pumping by activating inducible nitric oxidase synthase (iNOS) [14,15]. As a result, patients are in a constant proinflammatory state with a collection of cytokines and immune cells that ultimately lead to lymphatic valve failure, sclerosis of lymphatics, impaired contractility, and backflow of lymph.

CLINICAL CONSIDERATIONS

Patients at risk for developing lymphedema

Although patients with primary lymphedema are born with a dysfunctional lymphatic system, patients with secondary lymphedema experience disruption or obstruction of a normal lymphatic system due to surgery, radiation, trauma or infection [1]. Of these, lymphatic filariasis is the most common cause, affecting 120 million people worldwide [16]. In nontropical countries, cancer-related etiologies such as lymph node dissection and radiation are the leading cause: (1) axillary lymph node dissection–4% to 65% of patients may develop lymphedema following surgery and radiation therapy; (2) inguinal lymph node dissection–up to 66% of patients; and for sentinel lymph node biopsy of the axilla–5% to 7% of patients [3]. On average, the presentation of secondary lymphedema may take months to years to present after the surgical intervention and/or radiation.

Staging of lymphedema

It is essential to stage the severity of lymphedema as the treatment options vary based on the status of lymphedema. Of the various types of staging systems, the International Society of Lymphology (ISL) staging system is the most commonly used [17]. The ISL staging system characterizes the severity of lymphedema according to volume changes and firmness before and after limb elevation. There are four ISL stages of lymphedema: (1) Stage 0–subclinical stage with no visible swelling but the lymphatic system has been disrupted; (2) Stage 1–early stage with mild pitting edema that resolves with limb elevation; (3) Stage 2–stage with early soft tissue fibrosis and limb swelling that does not resolve with elevation; and (4) Stage 3–late stage with severe skin fibrosis and nonpitting edema [17].

Despite the wide use of the ISL stage, it is highly subjective and there is a weak correlation between the ISL staging and indocyanine green (ICG) staging [18,19]. Therefore, ICG fluorescent lymphography has become the mainstay tool for staging of lymphedema and surgical decision-making [20]. In ICG lymphography, functionality and lymphatic flow of superficial lymphatic vessels are visualized in real-time using a near-infrared camera. Functional lymphatic vessels are characterized as linear lines whereas the obstructed vessels demonstrate reflux of ICG dye into lymphatic capillaries, which is called dermal back flow [18]. In the MD Anderson Cancer Center (MDACC) ICG lymphedema staging system (Fig. 2), the distribution and patterns of the dermal backflow are used to determine the severity of lymphedema: (1) Stage 0–normal lymphatics with no dermal backflow; (2) Stage 1–many patent lymphatic vessels with minimal patchy dermal backflow; (3) Stage 2–moderate number of patent lymphatic vessels with segmental dermal backflow; (4) Stage 3–few patent lymphatic vessels with extensive dermal backflow involving the entire extremity; (5) Stage 4–no patent lymphatic vessels seen with dermal backflow involving the entire extremity; and (6) Stage 5–ICG does not move from injection sites.

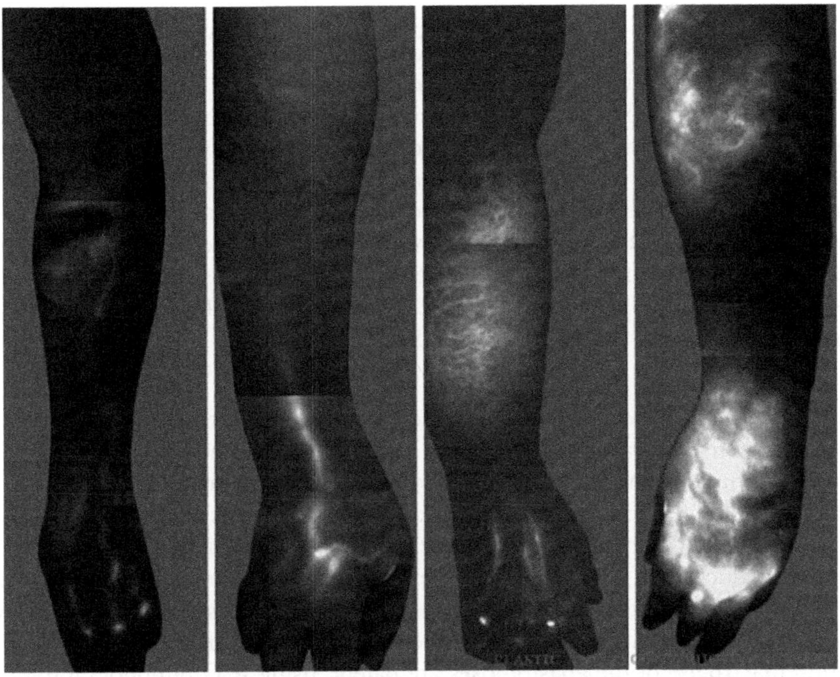

Fig. 2. Left to right. M.D. Anderson Cancer Center lymphedema staging based on indocyanine green lymphangiography. (*From* Chang DW, Suami H, Skoracki R. A prospective analysis of 100 consecutive lymphovenous bypass cases for treatment of extremity lymphedema. Plastic and reconstructive surgery. Nov 2013;132(5):1305–1314. https://doi.org/10.1097/PRS.0b013e3182a4d626; with permission.)

MICROSURGICAL TREATMENT OF LYMPHEDEMA

With the evolution of microsurgery and supermicrosurgery (defined as microsurgery on vessels that are <0.8 mm in diameter), surgical options for lymphedema have drastically changed from addressing fat hypertrophy to re-establishing functional lymphatic flow via supermicrosurgery. The main goals of the treatment are to create additional new outflow pathways for lymph fluid, decrease the dependency on compression therapy, to minimize the risk of cellulitis, to improve the quality of life, and to enhance the overall patient well-being.

Lymphovenous bypass

Surgical technique

First described in the 1960s, LVB or lymphovenous anastomosis was developed to augment lymphatic drainage by performing anastomosis between obstructed lymphatic vessels and neighboring veins [8,11]. Due to the lack of specialized microscopes, instruments, and sutures that enable surgeons to operate on vessels that are smaller than 0.8 mm, this technique was not popularized until the 2000s. The goal of this procedure is to identify functional lymphatic channels that are proximally sclerotic and shunt the flow into a neighboring vein to re-establish functional lymphatic pathway.

Traditionally, LVB is indicated in patients with earlier stages of lymphedema (MDDACC ICG lymphedema stage 1 or 2). First, 0.1 to 0.2 mL of ICG is injected intradermally into each webspace of the hand or the foot. Then, near-infrared fluorescence imaging is used to identify functional lymphatic vessels and areas of dermal backflows. LVBs are typically performed at the areas distal to the region of dermal reflux and supermicrosurgical anastomosis performed using an 11-0 or 12-0 nylon suture (Fig. 3). The patency of the lymphovenous bypass is confirmed using blue dye and/or ICG dye.

Outcomes

Since Koshima *and colleagues* have demonstrated the success of LVB with an average decrease in arm circumference by more than 4 cm, additional studies have continued to show the beneficial role of LVB in the treatment of lymphedema [8,10,21]. In a recent systematic review on the efficacy of LVB for breast cancer-related lymphedema (BCRL), 26 studies (914 patients) demonstrated volume reduction of 27.6%±30.9% in excessive arm volume, and 5 studies reported a significant improvement in total functional score after surgery (19.7±6.8 points using quality of life questionnaires) [22]. In addition, 4 studies found that 76.5% of the anastomoses are patent, using ICG lymphography. In addition, 3 studies (102 patients) reported that circumference reduction in patients who underwent LVB was greater than those who received compression alone in both upper and lower extremity lymphedema. Lastly, it was shown to

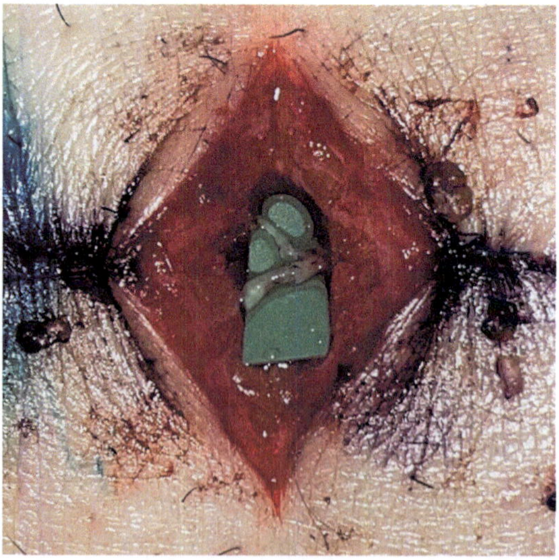

Fig. 3. A Y-shaped vein was used to perform lymphovenous bypass with 2 lymphatic vessels: end to end anastomosis into each vein branch.

be effective in reducing the number of cellulitis episodes in 3 studies (141 upper or lower extremity lymphedema patients) [22].

Despite the evidence of effectiveness and role of LVB in treating patients with lymphedema, there are heterogeneous data on its efficacy due to the following: (1) variation in anastomotic techniques; (2) assessment of patency; (3) different protocols in preoperative and postoperative compression therapy; and (4) lack of reference-standard measurements to assess the success of the surgery. Due to the limitations in identifying functional lymphatic vessels, early results on the success of LVB were variable. However, advances in imaging such as ICG lymphography, high-frequency ultrasound, and magnetic resonance lymphography enhanced the sophistication and accuracy of LVB and increased its success rate [19,23]. Nevertheless, the debate on the ideal type of anastomosis, whether it is end-to-end, end-to-side, side-to-side, or side-to-end is still being investigated [24,25].

Currently, 2 perioperative factors are emerging as the key considerations that can minimize variability in outcomes. According to a consensus study on lymphedema surgery by a panel of lymphedema surgery experts using a Delphi method, recommendations are given to maximize preoperative physiotherapy because placing patients in physiotherapy only after the surgery leads to difficulty with identifying the true treatment effect of lymphedema surgery [26]. In addition, they recommended obtaining continuous limb volume and circumference measurements for standardization of objective outcomes. While there is lack of literature on the superiority of outcome measures, multi-modal outcome assessments including limb measurements, volumetric analysis, rate of infections, and patient reported outcomes should be ascertained because the volume reduction may not be readily apparent in patients in very early stage, that may be symptomatic with limited volume change, or severe stages of lymphedema due to a fatty/fibrotic tissue [27].

Vascularized lymph node transfer

Surgical technique

Historically, vascularized lymph node transfer is the treatment of choice for patients with moderate and advanced stages of lymphedema [9]. In this procedure, lymph nodes are harvested and transferred to the affected area reconnecting their vascular supply using microsurgical anastomosis (Fig. 4). The options for donor sites include inguinal, lateral thoracic, submental, supraclavicular, omental, and jejunal lymph nodes. Although the exact mechanism and treatment effects of VLNT are unknown, many studies have theorized that proposed mechanism of VLNT is inducing lymphangiogenesis of local lymphatic channels toward the transplant node(s) via growth factors and having the transferred lymph nodes act as a *pump*, by collecting lymph fluid from the surrounding tissue and draining it into the efferent venous circulation [28,29]. Due to these mechanisms and in contrast to LVB (which results in immediate outflow augmentation), it is estimated that VLNT has a treatment delay of 6 to 12 months to be effective.

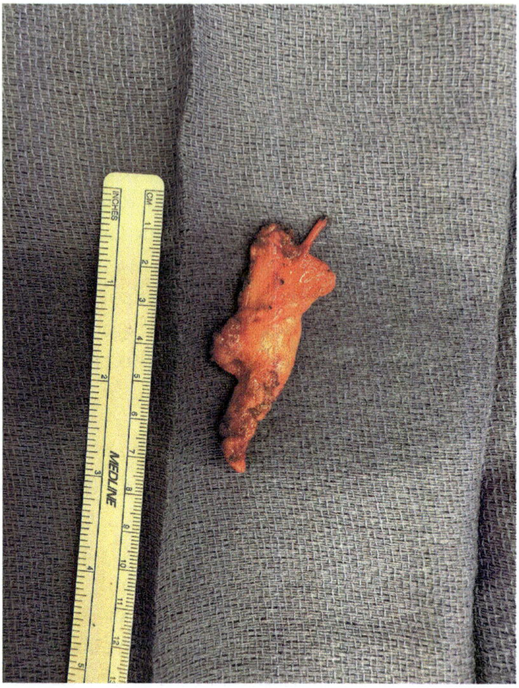

Fig. 4. Jejunal mesenteric vascularized lymph node flap.

Outcomes

VLNT has shown to be efficacious in the treatment of lymphedema, leading to a mean relative volume reduction of 43.6% in 972 patients with BCRL, and overall improvement of a total quality of life including their lymphedema symptoms, body appearance, mood, and arm function in 14 studies using LYMQOL (Lymphedema quality of life questionnaire) survey [22]. Similar to LVB, VLNT has been shown to provide a significant improvement in both circumference reduction of 24.3% and circumferential differentiation 3.9 cm in patients who underwent VLNT and rehabilitation compared to physiotherapy alone [30].

Though the efficacy of VLNT in treating lymphedema has been demonstrated, there remain questions due to the limited number of centers performing VLNTs and the relative paucity of large prospective studies with long-term outcomes: (1) ideal location of the donor site from which to harvest the lymph nodes; (2) variabilities in the recipient location (proximal vs distal); and (3) need to perform combined procedures to circumvent outcome delays. Currently, the literature includes the combined results of VLNTs from multiple donor sites due to the variability in surgeon experience, patient preference for scar location and morbidity, and risks for iatrogenic lymphedema [31]. Hence, it is difficult to identify the ideal donor site due to confounding factors. However, studies have shown that VLNT is efficacious, regardless of its recipient location (proximal: 76.9% vs distal: 80.4%) [32]. Similarly, Senger *and colleagues* found that mean volume/circumference reductions, patient satisfaction rates, and compression garment discontinuation were observed among placement strategies in their meta-analysis of 1440 patients [33].

Interestingly, the treatment effects of VLNT are delayed due to the proposed mechanisms of its action. To combat this phenomenon, microsurgeons now perform simultaneous LVB and VLNT, to promote early volume reduction in patients with functional lymphatic vessels using LVB. Garza *and colleagues* demonstrated that these patients demonstrated significant objective and subjective improvements with volume reduction of the affected limb at all time points postoperatively [34].

Preventive lymphatic surgery

Surgical technique

Similar to the introduction of de-escalation of axillary surgery to minimize lymphedema-related patient morbidity, particularly for those with advanced disease, there has been a paradigm shift in lymphedema surgery. Using techniques such as prophylactic lymphovenous bypass (pLVB), lymphatic microsurgical preventative healing approach or immediate lymphatic reconstruction (ILR), surgeons now offer procedures to prevent the development of lymphedema [12]. In this procedure, reverse axillary mapping is performed first by injecting 0.1 mL aliquots of alternating isosulfan blue and ICG dye in the hand and foot and/or circumferentially in the upper arm or the proximal thigh, respectively. After the lymph node dissection, the divided lymphatic vessels are identified using either signs of dye extravasation form the cut ends of lymphatics from the extremity or identifying dye filed ligated ends of lymphatics themselves and the tributary of the axillary or femoral veins are identified as potential recipients (Fig. 5). Based on the location and number of channels available, the damaged lymphatic system is restored by performing anastomosis between the lymphatic vessels and veins using supermicrosurgical techniques at the time of nodal resection.

Outcomes

Described in 2009, Boccardo *and colleagues* introduced preventive lymphatic surgery at the time of axillary lymph node dissection (ALND) to prevent the development of BCRL [35]. Since then, several studies have described the efficacy of this procedure. In a systematic review and meta-analysis of preventive lymphatic surgeries (18 studies; 47,465 patients), it has been reported that this procedure effectively reduces the risk of developing BCRL with a risk ratio of 0.35 [36]. In this study, 9.6% (98 of 1026 patients) developed BCRL whereas 41.6% (584 of 1405 patients) did in the group that did not receive BCRL, demonstrating the protective effect of the procedure. Similarly, Ciudad *and colleagues* demonstrated preventive lymphatic surgery is effective in reducing the incidence of both upper and lower extremity lymphedema by 18.7 per 100 patients treated and 30.3 by per 100 patients treated, respectively [37]. Lastly, Coriddi *and colleagues* found that patients who undergo preventive lymphatic

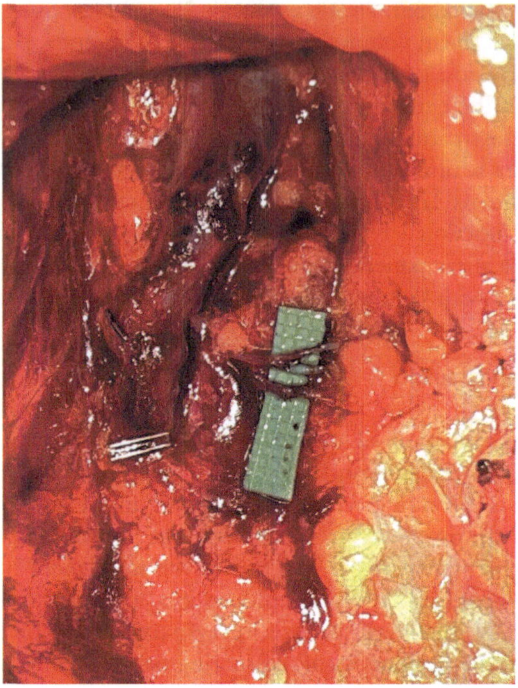

Fig. 5. pLVB was performed between the lateral thoracic vein and ligated lymphatic vessels.

surgeries have decreased need for compression, better quality of life, and better lymphatic function on ICG lymphography [38].

Because lymphedema is a chronic and noncurable disease, preventive lymphatic surgery has become increasingly popular. While many studies have demonstrated the efficacy of these procedures in preventing lymphedema, there is limited literature on directly comparing long-term outcomes of ALND with and without intervention. The data are not conclusive owing to small patient cohorts attributed to the novelty of the procedure and delay in manifestation of BCRL, which can take up to 24 months to develop. To date, there are 20 outcome-based studies published, of which only 9 include a control group with a small-size patient population (median of 41 patients in intervention group) [3]. Similar LVB studies, there is an unresolved matter on the ideal number of anastomoses and the surgical technique for anastomosis (end-to-end, side-to-end, intussusception). Previously, Sputova *and colleagues* suggested that intussusception technique (telescoping of lymphatic vessels into a vein) has inferior patency rates than supermicrosurgical anastomosis but Cho *and colleagues* found that there is no significant difference between the 2 techniques in 370 patients [3,39]. It should be noted that the evidence that does exist is compelling and all points to a significant beneficial effect of ILR at the time of nodal basin clearance.

DISCUSSION

Current consensus and recommendations on lymphedema surgery

With the advent of supermicrosurgical treatment of lymphedema, it is crucial to understand the current landscape on lymphedema surgery. Previously believed to be a novel concept, microsurgical treatment of lymphedema now offers evidence-based consensus statements and recommendations stemming from a meta-analysis of randomized and nonrandomized clinical trials. Chang *and colleagues* concluded that there is evidence to support LVB (grade 1C) and VLNT (grade 1B) in reducing the severity of lymphedema [30]. In addition, they recommend that preventive lymphatic surgery may reduce the incidence of lymphedema (grade 1B).

Importance of referring patients to lymphedema centers of excellence

It is crucial for patients to be treated at high-volume centers with the necessary technical expertise and a multidisciplinary team to receive comprehensive lymphedema treatment in addition to their comprehensive cancer care. Currently, only 22 centers around the world are recognized as Lymphatic Education & Research Network Comprehensive Center of Excellence, a designation that is given to institutions with at least 3 certified lymphedema therapists on-site and a minimum of 3 surgeons performing lymphatic surgeries. In addition, these centers must demonstrate proficiency in diagnosis, imaging, conservative management, assessment tools, interventional therapies, genetics, and consultative services. Studies revealed that it is important to perform early surgical intervention to maintain lymphatic function and prevent the progression of lymphedema with concurrent preoperative and postoperative rehabilitation to maximize prognosis [6,30]. Therefore, it is essential for surgeons and therapists to identify patients who would benefit from lymphatic surgeries early and refer them to a high-volume lymphatic center.

Secondly, lymphatic procedures are highly technically demanding and complex with evolving treatment algorithms [10]. Lymphovenous bypass surgery is considered supermicrosurgery, a technique that requires manipulating vessels ranging from 0.3 to 0.8 mm. Specialized equipment and magnification (specialized operating microscopes) are necessary to perform these procedures. These are not available in most microsurgery departments. In most plastic surgery residency programs, residents are not exposed to supermicrosurgical skills nor have experience in taking care of lymphedema patients. While there are no designated requirements to be a lymphatic surgeon, lymphedema surgeons should undergo rigorous microsurgical training. Many lymphedema patients, by the time they visit a dedicated lymphedema center, have exhausted nonsurgical management strategies, and present with advanced stage and a limited number of functional lymphatic pathways that are candidates for surgical intervention by LVB. Therefore, lymphatic procedures allow little to no room for error, and it is imperative that these patients have access to the most technically competent surgical reconstruction.

Future of lymphedema surgery

The field of lymphedema surgery continues to evolve with technological advancements and an increased understanding of pathophysiological changes. Historically, LVB was reserved for patients with early-stage lymphedema but the indications for LVB expanded with the introduction of ultrahigh-frequency ultrasound, allowing surgeons to overcome the depth of penetration limitations of ICG lymphogram and to visualize functional lymphatic vessels even in patients with advanced-stage lymphedema [40]. In addition, novel procedures such as lymph node-to-vein connection procedures, in which a healthy vein is anastomosed to a functional lymph node to augment the outflow, have shown to be effective in small series of the studies and can be integrated into the treatment algorithm [41]. In addition, robotic-assisted lymphatic surgery is being introduced to assist with precision in this technically-demanding field by facilitating promising advances in this field.

SUMMARY

Surgical treatment of lymphedema has evolved in the past several decades with technological advancements in microsurgical techniques and research on pathophysiology of lymphedema. Many studies have demonstrated that microsurgical physiologic treatment and prevention of lymphedema via restoration of the lymphatic system is effective in improving volume and functional outcomes. However, as in any active area of investigation, questions remain as lymphedema is a complex disease with a combination of fat hypertrophy, fluid excess, and tissue fibrosis. Therefore, it is critical to elevate the care of lymphedema patients by increasing access to multidisciplinary teams, by achieving consensus on the treatment algorithms for specific presentations of lymphedema, establishing rigorous surveillance programs for patients at risk of developing lymphedema and minimizing variabilities in the assessment of treatment outcomes.

CLINICS CARE POINTS

- Microsurgical physiologic treatment and prevention of lymphedema via the surgical restoration of the lymphatic system is effective in improving volume and functional outcomes.
- As lymphedema is a chronic and noncurative disease, preventive lymphatic surgery has become increasingly popular and proven to be effective in preventing the development of cancer-related lymphedema
- Lymphatic procedures are highly complex and it is crucial for patients to go to high-volume centers with a multidisciplinary team, specialized equipment and expertise to receive comprehensive lymphedema treatment
- Surveillance of patients at risk of developing lymphedema is a key component of early diagnosis and intervention, which has been shown to have greater treatment success rates.

Disclosure

M-J. Cho serves as a consultant for Fujifilm Sonosite. Neither author has a financial interest in any of the drugs, products, or devices mentioned in this article. No financial or material support was received for this research.

References

[1] Rockson SG, Rivera KK. Estimating the population burden of lymphedema. Ann N Y Acad Sci 2008;1131:147–54.
[2] Fu MR, Ridner SH, Hu SH, et al. Psychosocial impact of lymphedema: a systematic review of literature from 2004 to 2011. Psychooncology 2013;22(7):1466–84.
[3] Cho MJ, Senger JL, Park KU, et al. Preventing breast cancer-related lymphedema: a comprehensive analysis of a 9-Year single-center experience of prophylactic lymphovenous bypass. Ann Surg Oncol 2025;32(3):2007–15.
[4] Maclellan RA, Couto RA, Sullivan JE, et al. Management of primary and secondary lymphedema: analysis of 225 referrals to a center. Ann Plast Surg 2015;75(2):197–200.
[5] Moseley AL, Carati CJ, Piller NB. A systematic review of common conservative therapies for arm lymphoedema secondary to breast cancer treatment. Ann Oncol 2007;18(4):639–46.
[6] Schaverien MV, Moeller JA, Cleveland SD. Nonoperative treatment of lymphedema. Semin Plast Surg 2018;32(1):17–21.
[7] Brorson H. Liposuction in lymphedema treatment. J Reconstr Microsurg 2016;32(1):56–65.
[8] Chang DW, Suami H, Skoracki R. A prospective analysis of 100 consecutive lymphovenous bypass cases for treatment of extremity lymphedema. Plast Reconstr Surg 2013;132(5):1305–14.
[9] Cheng MH, Huang JJ, Nguyen DH, et al. A novel approach to the treatment of lower extremity lymphedema by transferring a vascularized submental lymph node flap to the ankle. Gynecol Oncol 2012;126(1):93–8.
[10] Koshima I, Inagawa K, Urushibara K, et al. Supermicrosurgical lymphaticovenular anastomosis for the treatment of lymphedema in the upper extremities. J Reconstr Microsurg 2000;16(06):437–42.
[11] Koshima I, Nanba Y, Tsutsui T, et al. Long-term Follow-Up after lymphaticovenular anastomosis for lymphedema in the leg. J Reconstr Microsurg 2003;19:209–15.
[12] Cho MJ, Flores Garcia J, Myung Y, et al. Evolving role of lymphedema surgery on breast reconstruction: a systematic review and multi-institutional algorithmic approach. J Clin Med 2024;13(21); https://doi.org/10.3390/jcm13216518.
[13] Grada AA, Phillips TJ. Lymphedema: pathophysiology and clinical manifestations. J Am Acad Dermatol 2017;77(6):1009–20.
[14] Azhar SH, Lim HY, Tan BK, et al. The unresolved pathophysiology of lymphedema. Front Physiol 2020;11:137.
[15] Aschen S, Zampell JC, Elhadad S, et al. Regulation of adipogenesis by lymphatic fluid stasis: part II. Expression of adipose differentiation genes. Plast Reconstr Surg 2012;129(4):838–47.
[16] Wynd S, Melrose WD, Durrheim DN, et al. Understanding the community impact of lymphatic filariasis: a review of the sociocultural literature. Bull World Health Organ 2007;85(6):493–8.
[17] The diagnosis and treatment of peripheral lymphedema: 2016 consensus document of the international society of lymphology. Lymphology 2016;49(4):170–84.
[18] Yamamoto T, Yamamoto N, Doi K, et al. Indocyanine green-enhanced lymphography for upper extremity lymphedema: a novel severity staging system using dermal backflow patterns. Plast Reconstr Surg 2011;128(4):941–7.

[19] Kim HB, Jung SS, Cho MJ, et al. Comparative analysis of preoperative high frequency color doppler ultrasound versus MR lymphangiography versus ICG lymphography of lymphatic vessels in lymphovenous anastomosis. J Reconstr Microsurg 2023;39(2):92–101.
[20] Suami H, Chang DW, Yamada K, et al. Use of indocyanine green fluorescent lymphography for evaluating dynamic lymphatic status. Plast Reconstr Surg 2011;127(3):74e–6e.
[21] Garza RM, Wong D, Chang DW. Optimizing outcomes in lymphedema reconstruction. Plast Reconstr Surg 2023;152(6):1131e–42e.
[22] Lilja C, Madsen CB, Damsgaard TE, et al. Surgical treatment algorithm for breast cancer lymphedema-a systematic review. Gland Surg 2024;13(5):722–48.
[23] Cho MJ, Chratian S, Visconti G, et al. Ultra high-frequency ultrasound in lymphatic surgery: the next frontier. Expet Rev Med Dev 2024;21(11):995–8.
[24] AlJindan FK, Lin CY, Cheng MH. Comparison of outcomes between side-to-end and end-to-end lymphovenous anastomoses for early-grade extremity lymphedema. Plast Reconstr Surg 2019;144(2):486–96.
[25] Yamamoto T, Yoshimatsu H, Yamamoto N, et al. Side-to-end lymphaticovenular anastomosis through temporary lymphatic expansion. PLoS One 2013;8(3):e59523.
[26] Masià J, Al Sakkaf AM, Hong JP, et al. Barcelona consensus paper on reconstructive lymphedema surgery: a Delphi study. Plast Reconstr Surg 2025; https://doi.org/10.1097/prs.0000000000012201.
[27] Morgan PA, Franks PJ, Moffatt CJ. Health-related quality of life with lymphoedema: a review of the literature. Int Wound J 2005;2(1):47–62.
[28] Patel KM, Lin CY, Cheng MH. From theory to evidence: long-term evaluation of the mechanism of action and flap integration of distal vascularized lymph node transfers. J Reconstr Microsurg 2015;31(1):26–30.
[29] Suami H, Scaglioni MF, Dixon KA, et al. Interaction between vascularized lymph node transfer and recipient lymphatics after lymph node dissection-a pilot study in a canine model. J Surg Res 2016;204(2):418–27.
[30] Chang DW, Dayan J, Greene AK, et al. Surgical treatment of lymphedema: a systematic review and meta-analysis of controlled trials. Results of a consensus conference. Plast Reconstr Surg 2021;147(4):975–93.
[31] Chang DW, Masia J, Garza R 3rd, et al. Lymphedema: surgical and medical therapy. Plast Reconstr Surg 2016;138(3 Suppl):209s–18s.
[32] Scaglioni MF, Arvanitakis M, Chen YC, et al. Comprehensive review of vascularized lymph node transfers for lymphedema: outcomes and complications. Microsurgery 2018;38(2):222–9.
[33] Senger J-LB, Rajaii R, Slater C, et al. Proximal vs. recipient site for vascular lymph node transfers for breast cancer-related lymphedema: a meta-analysis and systematic review. J Clin Med 2025;14(20); https://doi.org/10.3390/jcm14207281.
[34] Garza RM, Beederman M, Chang DW. Physical and functional outcomes of simultaneous vascularized lymph node transplant and lymphovenous bypass in the treatment of lymphedema. Plast Reconstr Surg 2022;150(1):169–80.
[35] Boccardo F, Casabona F, De Cian F, et al. Lymphedema microsurgical preventive healing approach: a new technique for primary prevention of arm lymphedema after mastectomy. Ann Surg Oncol 2009;16(3):703–8.
[36] Silva AC, Franco-Mesa C, Vieira ACP, et al. Immediate lymphovenous anastomosis is effective in preventing breast cancer-related lymphedema: a systematic review and meta-analysis. J Plast Reconstr Aesthetic Surg 2025;106:114–24.
[37] Ciudad P, Escandón JM, Bustos VP, et al. Primary prevention of cancer-related lymphedema using preventive lymphatic surgery: systematic review and meta-analysis. Indian J Plast Surg 2022;55(1):18–25.
[38] Coriddi M, Dayan J, Bloomfield E, et al. Efficacy of immediate lymphatic reconstruction to decrease incidence of breast cancer-related lymphedema: preliminary results of randomized controlled trial. Ann Surg 2023;278(4):630–7.

[39] Sputova K, Kim LM, Francis AM. Surgical prevention of lymphedema. Current Surgery Reports 2023;11(8):188–95.
[40] Cha HG, Oh TM, Cho M-J, et al. Changing the paradigm: lymphovenous anastomosis in advanced stage lower extremity lymphedema. Plast Reconstr Surg 2021;147(1):199–207.
[41] Alshomer F, Cho J, Noh H, et al. Lymphaticovenous and lymph node–to-vein anastomosis to improve milroy disease–related chylothorax and lymphedema. Plast Reconstr Surg 2025;155(3):610e–7e.

Advances in Surgery 60 (2026) 115–126
ADVANCES IN SURGERY

Active Surveillance Versus Surgery for Low-risk Well-differentiated Thyroid Cancer

Anthony T. Saxton, MD[a], Randall P. Scheri, MD[b,*]

[a]Department of Surgery, Duke University, Durham, NC, USA; [b]Duke University, Durham, NC, USA

Keywords

- Active surveillance • Thyroid lobectomy • Total thyroidectomy
- Differentiated thyroid cancer

Key points

- Attention to overdiagnosis and overtreatment of indolent thyroid cancers has brought active surveillance strategies to the forefront of modern thyroid oncology.
- Active surveillance entails structured follow-up with ultrasound by experienced groups with clear thresholds for intervention and reliable patient engagement.
- Ideal candidates for active surveillance of thyroid cancer are adults with small (<1 cm), intrathyroidal, unifocal papillary cancers without evidence of nodal disease or aggressive histology and are willing to comply with follow-up.
- Triggers for conversion from active surveillance to surgery include growth ≥ 3 mm in any dimension, new extrathyroidal extension, metastasis, patient preference, intolerable anxiety, or inability to comply with follow-up.
- When surgery is indicated or desired, a lobectomy-first strategy for most low-risk disease balances oncologic control with the lowest complication burden.

INTRODUCTION

The global incidence of thyroid cancer has risen steadily over the past three decades, largely due to the detection of small papillary thyroid carcinomas (PTCs) through increased imaging and screening. While the disease-specific mortality of differentiated thyroid cancer (DTC) remains exceedingly

*Corresponding author. DUMC 2945, Durham, NC 27110. *E-mail address:* r.scheri@duke.edu

https://doi.org/10.1016/j.yasu.2026.03.007

Abbreviations

ATA	American Thyroid Association
CT	computed tomography
DTC	differentiated thyroid cancer
PTC	papillary thyroid carcinoma
RAI	radioactive iodine
RLN	recurrent laryngeal nerve
Tg	thyroglobulin
TSH	thyroid-stimulating hormone

low, its management has historically involved thyroidectomy followed by radioactive iodine (RAI) and lifelong hormone suppression therapy. This approach, though curative in most cases, exposes patients to risk of complications and requires lifelong thyroid hormone replacement.

Recent years have brought a paradigm shift in the management of low-risk well-differentiated thyroid cancer. Evidence from Japan, Korea, and now Western centers demonstrates that selected patients with small, intrathyroidal papillary cancers can be safely managed with observation, a strategy now termed *active surveillance.* The 2025 American Thyroid Association (ATA) Guidelines formally recognize this approach, stating that "active surveillance may be offered as an appropriate management option for some patients with cT1aN0M0 PTCs," with shared clinical decision-making at its core [1].

This article examines the evolution of active surveillance versus surgical treatment for low-risk DTC, reviewing epidemiology, evidence, patient selection, and the integration of active surveillance into modern thyroid oncology.

EVOLUTION TOWARD ACTIVE SURVEILLANCE: LANDMARK STUDIES AND LONG-TERM DATA

The incidence of thyroid cancer has nearly tripled since the 1980s, yet mortality has remained stable [2,3]. The most striking example is South Korea, where the launch of a nationwide cancer screening campaign in 1999 was followed by a more than 15-fold rise in thyroid cancer incidence by 2011(4). The dramatic rise in incidence was directly and strongly correlated with the degree of screening penetration across regions, while mortality from thyroid cancer remained unchanged [4]. Similar, though less pronounced, patterns have been observed globally among developed health systems [5]. Advances in ultrasonography, fine-needle aspiration (FNA), and cytologic classification have enabled increased detection of thyroid cancers. Most of the rise in thyroid cancer incidence reflects detection of sub-2 cm tumors, whereas the rate of larger tumors has remained essentially unchanged [6]. These data strongly suggest that the observed rise in incidence reflects increased detection rather than a true surge in clinically meaningful disease.

This concept is reinforced by autopsy studies that have found stable prevalence of thyroid cancer over the past six decades [7]. In a landmark Finnish series of 101 consecutive autopsies, Harach and colleagues reported papillary thyroid carcinoma in 35.6% of individuals, two-thirds of which measured less than 1 cm [8]. Similar findings have been demonstrated in the United States [9]. Together, these studies highlight the enormous reservoir of indolent papillary microcarcinomas that have existed silently within the population long before modern imaging. This illustrates that in effect, the medical community has been "observing" a substantial volume of clinically insignificant thyroid cancer for decades.

The indolent biology of well-differentiated thyroid cancers, particularly PTCs, accounts for 10-year disease-specific survival exceeding 99% for localized tumors [10]. This natural history forms the foundation for less aggressive management strategies. However, a small subset of patients with PTC develop clinically meaningful regional and/or distant metastases, and identification of patients that will progress from the larger indolent population is a major challenge [11–13]. As such, for decades total thyroidectomy followed by RAI ablation and thyroid-stimulating hormone (TSH) suppression represented the standard of care for nearly all papillary and follicular thyroid cancers greater than 1 cm. The rationale was multifold: complete resection to minimize recurrence, facilitation of RAI uptake, and simplification of serum thyroglobulin (Tg) surveillance. Although thyroid surgery is highly effective and generally safe, it still carries meaningful risks and potential morbidity. Complication rates for total thyroidectomy, including hypocalcemia, recurrent laryngeal nerve injury, and hemorrhage/hematoma, range from 5% to 15% in population studies [14,15]. Permanent hypoparathyroidism and vocal cord paralysis may occur in 1% to 3% of cases, with increased complication rates in low-volume centers [14,15]. Furthermore, total thyroidectomy mandates lifelong levothyroxine replacement, with attendant quality-of-life impacts. In the 2010s, attention turned toward overdiagnosis and overtreatment of indolent thyroid cancers. Epidemiologic modeling increasingly suggested that although a small subset of DTC patients may develop clinically meaningful regional or distant metastases, most are unlikely ever to cause harm [5]. The potential risks of surgical management prompted reappraisal of management paradigms.

The first structured program of nonoperative management for papillary microcarcinoma was established by Ito and colleagues at Kuma Hospital in Japan in the 1990s [16]. In this cohort of 1395 patients undergoing immediate surgery or active surveillance for PTC measuring 1.0 cm or less, 15.9% of 340 patients in the active surveillance group had tumor growth $\geq$ 3 mm over 10 years of follow-up, and 3.4% had new lymph node metastasis. [16]. Updated long-term outcomes reported 20-year disease progression rates from an expanded cohort of 3222 patients, with 1.7% of patients in the active surveillance group that developed new lymph node metastasis, and a 6.6% tumor enlargement $\geq$3 mm [17]. Outcomes for delayed surgery after documented progression were equivalent to those for initial thyroidectomy [16–18].

The favorable outcomes from the early Japanese studies led to subsequent prospective studies on active surveillance in other parts of the world and expanded the criteria for patients considered for active surveillance [19]. In the United States, Ho and colleagues included patients with Bethesda V-VI thyroid nodules up to 2 cm in size in their prospective nonrandomized trial of 222 patients treated with either active surveillance or immediate surgery at Cedars-Sinai Medical Center between 2014-21 [20]. The authors reported no patients developed lymph node metastases at 7 years of follow-up, a cumulative incidence of growth $\geq$5 mm of 10.8% at 5 years, and equivalent disease-specific and overall survival between the two groups [20]. Comparable results have emerged from other cohorts from Korea [21,22], Canada [23], Colombia [24], Brazil [25], Argentina [26], Italy [27], and Memorial Sloan Kettering Cancer Center in the United States [28]. A systematic review and analysis by Chou and colleagues found similar low risk of all-cause and thyroid cancer-specific mortality, distant metastasis, and recurrence in younger adults (mean age 50s-low 60s) treated with active surveillance or immediate surgery, reinforcing that oncologic outcomes were comparable in appropriately selected low-risk tumors [29]. Collectively, these studies formed the basis for a fundamental evolution in thyroid cancer guidelines. The 2015 ATA Guidelines strongly recommended surgical treatment for cytology-confirmed thyroid malignancies, with an exception that active surveillance can be considered as an alternative to immediate surgery for patients with very low risk tumors [30]. The 2025 ATA update expanded this recommendation, with active surveillance conditionally endorsed for select cT1aN0M0 PTCs.

DEFINING THE POPULATION: WHO QUALIFIES AS "LOW RISK"?

Low-risk well-differentiated thyroid cancer generally refers to papillary or follicular carcinomas confined to the thyroid without evidence of nodal or distant spread. The 2025 ATA Guidelines define the primary candidates for active surveillance as those with cT1aN0M0 ($\leq$1 cm) papillary thyroid carcinomas [1]. No formal recommendations were made for T1b tumors between 1-2 cm given limited data on the role of active surveillance in these cancers. Ideal tumors for surveillance are unifocal, intrathyroidal, and lack sonographic evidence of extrathyroidal extension. The absence of aggressive histologic variants (tall cell, hobnail, diffuse sclerosing) and the presence of a smooth, well-circumscribed nodule on high-resolution ultrasound favor consideration of active surveillance.

Patient selection is central to safety. Candidates should be adults capable of adhering to long-term follow-up, ideally in centers with endocrine surgery and ultrasound expertise. Active surveillance may be a more appropriate strategy for older adults. A systematic review and meta-analysis by Koshkina and colleagues found that risk of PTC growth decreases with age, with older age (>60 years) associated with lower risk of tumor progression, while younger age (<40 years) predicts higher likelihood of growth or nodal involvement over time [31]. Comorbidities that increase operative risk, life expectancy considerations, and patient preference for nonsurgical management may also favor surveillance. Conversely, high anxiety about "living with cancer" may necessitate surgery despite low biologic risk.

Active surveillance is inappropriate for patients less than 18 year old, for tumors demonstrating invasion of the trachea, esophagus, or recurrent laryngeal nerve, those with gross extrathyroidal extension, or for radiographic/biopsy-proven nodal or distant metastases. Cancers abutting the posterior capsule, trachea, or recurrent laryngeal nerve pose unacceptable risk for local invasion if growth occurs and are inappropriate for active surveillance. Inability to comply with serial imaging also invalidates the safety of this approach. The 2025 ATA guidelines explicitly warn that "non-compliance with such follow-up invalidates claims for safety of this approach," underscoring the ethical duty of physicians to ensure robust surveillance infrastructure and the patient's understanding of this follow-up [1].

WHAT DOES ACTIVE SURVEILLANCE ENTAIL?

Active surveillance is a proactive, structured management pathway. Its safety depends on expert ultrasound, clear thresholds for intervention, and reliable patient engagement. Prior to enrollment, patients should undergo baseline assessment including comprehensive high-resolution neck ultrasound by an experienced sonographer surveying the thyroid and all cervical nodal basins, with documentation of maximal tumor diameter and three-dimensional measurements, its relation to the capsule, trachea/esophagus, and recurrent laryngeal nerve (RLN) groove, and characterization of any additional nodules. Cytologic confirmation with FNA is typical for nodules in which malignancy is suspected. FNA is not routinely recommended for $\leq$1 cm nodules with low-risk features unless diagnostic confirmation is necessary to support surveillance [1]. Molecular testing is not routinely required in classic low-risk scenarios and has not been shown to improve outcomes or cost-effectiveness in this population, with conflicting results reported from retrospective studies on the utility of molecular testing to risk-stratify patients for active surveillance [32,33].

Follow-up with neck ultrasound is the cornerstone of monitoring protocols and should be performed at 6-month intervals for the first 1 to 2 years, then annually if stable [16,28]. Ultrasound evaluation should be performed by clinicians experienced in thyroid cancer imaging. Routine use of other imaging modalities, such as computed tomography (CT), is not utilized for follow-up. Biochemical workup with serum thyroglobulin and anti-Tg antibodies are not recommended for routine monitoring during active surveillance because values are nonspecific in the presence of an intact thyroid and have not been shown to influence management decisions [1]. The 2025 ATA Guidelines discuss TSH targets for different clinical contexts (Recommendation 46) [1]. In most patients under active surveillance, stringent suppression is not required. Avoidance of overt hypothyroidism is sensible both for symptoms and potential effects on tumor growth, but aggressive suppression may not be necessary, particularly in older or comorbid patients [1].

Successful surveillance programs formalize scheduling, reminders, and no-show mitigation, and they document informed consent conversations emphasizing the *active* nature of surveillance and the non-negotiable requirement for long-term imaging. Clear messaging about uncertainty (eg, the small but real risk of growth, and that surveillance does not preclude later cure) can alleviate anxiety and build trust.

Clear criteria for converting from active surveillance to surgery have emerged. The 2025 ATA Guidelines designate surgery as indicated for new biopsy-proven nodal metastases, growth $\geq$ 3 mm in any dimension, new extrathyroidal extension, or patient preference [1]. Other triggers include inability to comply with follow-up or emerging anxiety intolerable to the patient. Importantly, delayed surgery in these contexts remains safe. Outcomes after conversion mirror those of immediate surgery, with no decrement in disease-specific survival or increased complication rate [28,34,35].

SURGICAL STRATEGY

Although an increasing proportion of appropriately selected patients can be managed without an operation, surgery remains the cornerstone of therapy for those with higher-risk features at presentation, for individuals who progress during surveillance, and for patients who prefer definitive excision. Accurate preoperative ultrasound mapping and biopsy of suspicious nodules can guide the extent of initial surgery and potentially reduce secondary operations [36–40]. The 2025 ATA guidelines (Recommendation 15) provide a contemporary framework for the extent of thyroidectomy and lymph-node management, reflecting a large body of comparative-effectiveness literature and real-world outcomes [1]. For unilateral cT1 tumors $\leq$2 cm without gross extrathyroidal extension or nodal/distant metastases (cN0M0), lobectomy is recommended as the initial operation, unless there are bilateral cancers or other clear indications to remove the contralateral lobe [1]. For cT2 (2–4 cm) low-risk unilateral disease, lobectomy is favored given lower complication rates and similar disease-specific outcomes in properly selected patients; total thyroidectomy may be chosen to facilitate RAI or follow-up based on disease features or patient preference [1]. In contrast, total thyroidectomy is recommended for cT3a tumors greater than 4 cm, any gross extrathyroidal extension (cT3b–cT4), clinically apparent nodal disease (cN1), or distant metastases (cM1) when there are no contraindications [1]. These statements synthesize multiple meta-analyses showing comparable survival and (for many patients) recurrence after lobectomy versus total thyroidectomy, with lower risks of complications [1,14,15,41–43].

The main potential benefits of total thyroidectomy include enabling RAI therapy when indicated, simplifying serum thyroglobulin surveillance, and possibly reducing ipsilateral/contralateral locoregional recurrence in selected intermediate-risk settings [1,44–47]. Conversely, total thyroidectomy is associated with higher rates of transient and permanent hypoparathyroidism, transient and permanent RLN injury, and hemorrhage/hematoma, with complication risks magnified in low-volume centers [14,15,48]. Even among high-volume surgeons, complication rates remain higher with total thyroidectomy than with lobectomy. These trade-offs should be discussed explicitly with patients during shared decision-making, with clarity that salvage completion thyroidectomy for contralateral recurrence after lobectomy is usually effective and rarely compromises survival [45,46,49]. High-volume endocrine surgery practice, standardized pathways, and postoperative calcium/voice protocols further minimize adverse events [50–54].

Prophylactic central compartment dissection is generally not recommended in low-risk, clinically node-negative disease [1]. Therapeutic dissection is reserved for clinically/radiographically involved nodes. Avoiding prophylactic dissection in cN0 low-risk patients reduces hypocalcemia and RLN morbidity without clear survival benefit, while thorough preoperative and intraoperative evaluation is essential to identify those with cN1 disease who do benefit from compartment-oriented clearance [55,56].

DECISION-MAKING FRAMEWORK: THE PATIENT-CENTERED APPROACH

The central philosophy in modern thyroid oncology has shifted from "which operation?" to "is any operation necessary now?" This reframing places patient values, risk tolerance, and life circumstances alongside tumor biology. Shared decision-making aligns the best available evidence with individual preferences to assist patients making complex treatment decisions [57]. For many patients with cT1aN0M0 DTC, both active surveillance and lobectomy are reasonable options with excellent disease-specific survival. The dialogue with patients should transparently address [1]: the very low disease-specific mortality regardless of initial choice [2]; the comparative morbidities of surgery (especially total thyroidectomy) versus the surveillance burden [3]; triggers for conversion to surgery; and [4] the feasibility of reliable follow-up. Counseling tools such as plain-language handouts and visual risk displays and documented preference-sensitive discussions help patients make informed choices and support medicolegal robustness.

Patient age, comorbidities, and psychosocial considerations should also play a role in treatment decisions. Older patients (>60 years) are less likely to progress on surveillance and may particularly benefit from avoiding anesthesia and surgical complications, while young adults (<40 years) have slightly higher progression rates and may prefer early excision for peace of mind [31]. Occupational voice users or those with high public-facing demands may prioritize avoidance of even small RLN risk. The psychological impact of observation varies by individual. Some patients experience reassurance from avoiding surgery; others report persistent anxiety about disease progression. Longitudinal surveys show that, with adequate counseling and structured follow-up, quality of life and cancer-related anxiety are comparable to post-surgical patients [58]. However, individuals with pronounced cancer anxiety may not tolerate surveillance despite low biologic risk, and their preference for surgery should be respected after counseling.

Although active surveillance presupposes experienced ultrasonography and reliable longitudinal care, access to these resources is not uniformly distributed. Programs should anticipate transportation barriers, language needs, and financial constraints. Embedding surveillance within health-system registries and navigation services can narrow disparities [59]. Active surveillance markedly reduces upfront costs associated with hospital stay, anesthesia, and surgical complications, with economic models suggesting that active surveillance is generally more cost-effective for patients diagnosed at an older age [60,61]. For healthcare systems facing rising rates of thyroid cancer, the policy implications are substantial.

FUTURE DIRECTIONS AND RESEARCH GAPS

While randomized trials remain challenging, multicenter prospective registries with standardized imaging thresholds, core sonographic reporting, and patient-reported outcomes can further validate safety and identify rare adverse trajectories. Pragmatic trials comparing surveillance to lobectomy in Western populations, particularly for tumors 1 to 2 cm, would refine boundaries of candidacy for active surveillance [19]. Further research is needed to determine whether specific genomic alterations (eg, BRAF and TERT) or transcriptomic signatures predict progression in cT1 tumors and could individualize surveillance intensity [62]. At present, routine molecular testing is not recommended for classic small intrathyroidal DTC because clinical risk stratification suffices and cost-effectiveness is unproven [1]. Finally, more granular understanding of anxiety trajectories, decisional regret, quality of life including voice and swallowing outcomes, endocrine symptoms, and financial toxicity across strategies will help tailor counseling and personalized treatment decisions.

SUMMARY

Low-risk well-differentiated thyroid cancer has an excellent prognosis, and management is increasingly preference-sensitive. The accumulated evidence from Japan, Korea, and Western centers demonstrates that active surveillance is a safe and effective initial option for carefully selected patients with small PTC if expert ultrasound and structured follow-up are available. The 2025 ATA Guidelines endorse this approach as a conditional recommendation with low-certainty evidence, emphasizing shared decision-making and explicit thresholds for conversion to surgery [1]. Routine measurement of thyroglobulin during surveillance is not recommended, and ultrasound at 6-month intervals for 1 to 2 years, then annually if stable, is advised [1].

When surgery is chosen up-front or required after progression, the operation should be risk-adapted. Lobectomy is the preferred initial procedure for most unilateral cT1–T2N0M0 tumors, offering excellent oncologic control with lower rates of hypocalcemia and RLN injury than total thyroidectomy [1,63]. Total thyroidectomy is reserved for larger primary tumors (>4 cm), gross extrathyroidal extension, clinically apparent nodal disease, distant metastasis, or when required to enable adjuvant RAI and facilitate biomarker surveillance [1].

Prophylactic central compartment dissection is not recommended for low risk cN0 disease, as therapeutic dissection is performed for clinically involved nodes.

CLINICS CARE POINTS

- Consensus guidelines have addressed overdiagnosis and overtreatment of indolent thyroid cancers by including active surveillance as an alternative treatment option for low-risk cT1aN0M0 PTC.
- Candidates for active surveillance include patients with small (<1 cm), intrathyroidal, unifocal papillary cancers without evidence of nodal disease or aggressive histology.
- Growth $\geq$ 3 mm in any dimension, new extrathyroidal extension, metastasis, patient preference, intolerable anxiety, or inability to comply with follow-up should trigger conversion to surgical management.
- Further research evaluating active surveillance in tumors greater than 1 cm and incorporation of molecular profiling may meaningfully broaden the population of patients who can be safely offered active surveillance.

Disclosures

The authors have no disclosures.

References

[1] Ringel MD, Sosa JA, Baloch Z, et al. American Thyroid Association Management guidelines for adult patients with differentiated thyroid cancer. Thyroid 2025;35(8):841–985.
[2] Siegel RL, Kratzer TB, Giaquinto AN, et al. Cancer statistics. CA Cancer J Clin 2025;75(1): 10–45.
[3] Davies L, Welch HG. Current thyroid cancer trends in the United States. JAMA Otolaryngol Head Neck Surg 2014;140(4):317–22.
[4] Ahn HS, Kim HJ, Welch HG. Korea's thyroid-cancer "epidemic"–screening and overdiagnosis. N Engl J Med 2014;371(19):1765–7.
[5] Brito JP, Morris JC, Montori VM. Thyroid cancer: zealous imaging has increased detection and treatment of low risk tumours. Br Med J 2013;347:f4706.
[6] Davies L, Welch HG. Increasing incidence of thyroid cancer in the United States, 1973-2002. JAMA 2006;295(18):2164–7.
[7] Furuya-Kanamori L, Bell KJL, Clark J, et al. Prevalence of differentiated thyroid cancer in autopsy studies over six decades: a meta-analysis. J Clin Oncol 2016;34(30): 3672–9.
[8] Harach HR, Franssila KO, Wasenius VM. Occult papillary carcinoma of the thyroid. A "normal" finding in Finland. A systematic autopsy study. Cancer 1985;56(3):531–8.
[9] Fukunaga FH, Yatani R. Geographic pathology of occult thyroid carcinomas. Cancer 1975;36(3):1095–9.
[10] Surveillance Research Program NCI. SEER*Explorer: an interactive website for SEER cancer statistics. 2025. Available at: https://seer.cancer.gov/statistics-network/explorer/.
[11] Mazzaferri EL. Management of low-risk differentiated thyroid cancer. Endocr Pract 2007;13(5):498–512.
[12] Hay ID. Management of patients with low-risk papillary thyroid carcinoma. Endocr Pract 2007;13(5):521–33.

[13] Yu XM, Wan Y, Sippel RS, et al. Should all papillary thyroid microcarcinomas be aggressively treated? An analysis of 18,445 cases. Ann Surg 2011;254(4):653–60.
[14] Weiss A, Parina RP, Tang JA, et al. Outcomes of thyroidectomy from a large California state database. Am J Surg 2015;210(6):1170–6 [discussion: 6-7].
[15] Hsiao V, Light TJ, Adil AA, et al. Complication rates of total thyroidectomy vs hemithyroidectomy for treatment of papillary thyroid microcarcinoma: a systematic review and meta-analysis. JAMA Otolaryngol Head Neck Surg 2022;148(6):531–9.
[16] Ito Y, Miyauchi A, Inoue H, et al. An observational trial for papillary thyroid microcarcinoma in Japanese patients. World J Surg 2010;34(1):28–35.
[17] Miyauchi A, Ito Y, Fujishima M, et al. Long-term outcomes of active surveillance and immediate surgery for adult patients with low-risk papillary thyroid microcarcinoma: 30-year experience. Thyroid 2023;33(7):817–25.
[18] Ito Y, Miyauchi A, Kihara M, et al. Patient age is significantly related to the progression of papillary microcarcinoma of the thyroid under observation. Thyroid 2014;24(1):27–34.
[19] Kim MJ, Moon JH, Lee EK, et al. Active surveillance for low-risk thyroid cancers: a review of current practice guidelines. Endocrinol Metab 2024;39(1):47–60.
[20] Ho AS, Kim S, Zalt C, et al. Expanded parameters in active surveillance for low-risk papillary thyroid carcinoma: a nonrandomized controlled trial. JAMA Oncol 2022;8(11):1588–96.
[21] Lee EK, Moon JH, Hwangbo Y, et al. Progression of low-risk papillary thyroid microcarcinoma during active surveillance: interim analysis of a multicenter prospective cohort study of active surveillance on papillary thyroid microcarcinoma in Korea. Thyroid 2022;32(11):1328–36.
[22] Jeon MJ, Kang YE, Moon JH, et al. Protocol for a Korean multicenter prospective cohort study of active surveillance or surgery (KoMPASS) in papillary thyroid microcarcinoma. Endocrinol Metab 2021;36(2):359–64.
[23] Sawka AM, Ghai S, Rotstein L, et al, Canadian Active Surveillance Study Group Greater Toronto Area. A quantitative analysis examining patients' choice of active surveillance or surgery for managing low-risk papillary thyroid cancer. Thyroid 2022;32(3):255–62.
[24] Sanabria A. Experience with active surveillance of thyroid low-risk carcinoma in a developing country. Thyroid 2020;30(7):985–91.
[25] Rosario PW, Mourão GF, Calsolari MR. Active surveillance in adults with low-risk papillary thyroid microcarcinomas: a prospective study. Horm Metab Res 2019;51(11):703–8.
[26] Smulever A, Pitoia F. Active surveillance in papillary thyroid carcinoma: not easily accepted but possible in Latin America. Arch Endocrinol Metab 2019;63(5):462–9.
[27] Molinaro E, Campopiano MC, Pieruzzi L, et al. Active surveillance in papillary thyroid microcarcinomas is feasible and safe: experience at a single Italian center. J Clin Endocrinol Metab 2020;105(3):e172–80.
[28] Tuttle RM, Fagin JA, Minkowitz G, et al. Natural history and tumor volume kinetics of papillary thyroid cancers during active surveillance. JAMA Otolaryngol Head Neck Surg 2017;143(10):1015–20.
[29] Chou R, Dana T, Haymart M, et al. Active surveillance versus thyroid surgery for differentiated thyroid cancer: a systematic review. Thyroid 2022;32(4):351–67.
[30] Haugen BR, Alexander EK, Bible KC, et al. 2015 American thyroid association management guidelines for adult patients with thyroid nodules and differentiated thyroid cancer: the American thyroid association guidelines task force on thyroid nodules and differentiated thyroid cancer. Thyroid 2016;26(1):1–133.
[31] Koshkina A, Fazelzad R, Sugitani I, et al. Association of patient age with progression of low-risk papillary thyroid carcinoma under active surveillance: a systematic review and meta-analysis. JAMA Otolaryngol Head Neck Surg 2020;146(6):552–60.
[32] Kim KJ, Kim SG, Tan J, et al. BRAF V600E status may facilitate decision-making on active surveillance of low-risk papillary thyroid microcarcinoma. Eur J Cancer 2020;124:161–9.

[33] Lee J, Ha EJ, Roh J, et al. Presence of TERT ± BRAF V600E mutation is not a risk factor for the clinical management of patients with papillary thyroid microcarcinoma. Surgery 2021;170(3):743–7.
[34] Ito Y, Miyauchi A, Fujishima M, et al. Active surveillance for adult low-risk papillary thyroid microcarcinoma-a review focused on the 30-year experience of Kuma Hospital. Endocr J 2024;71(1):7–21.
[35] Oh HS, Ha J, Kim HI, et al. Active surveillance of low-risk papillary thyroid microcarcinoma: a multi-center cohort study in Korea. Thyroid 2018;28(12):1587–94.
[36] Lamartina L, Bidault S, Hadoux J, et al. Can preoperative ultrasound predict extrathyroidal extension of differentiated thyroid cancer? Eur J Endocrinol 2021;185(1):13–22.
[37] Leong D, Ng K, Nguyen H, et al. Preoperative ultrasound characteristics in determining the likelihood of requiring completion thyroidectomy for cytologically confirmed (bethesda VI) papillary thyroid tumors with 1 - 4 Cm in diameter. Asian J Surg 2022;45(1):197–201.
[38] Raffaelli M, Sessa L, De Crea C, et al. Is it possible to intraoperatively modulate the extent of thyroidectomy in small papillary thyroid carcinoma? Surgery 2021;169(1):77–81.
[39] Marshall R, Alexander D, Fleming J, et al. Utility of intraoperative frozen sections of thyroid tissue in the age of molecular testing. Clin Otolaryngol 2021;46(5):991–7.
[40] Staubitz JI, Elmrich I, Musholt PB, et al, Prospective Evaluation Study Thyroid Surgery PETS 2 Study Group. Targeted use of intraoperative frozen-section analysis lowers the frequency of completion thyroidectomy. BJS Open 2021;5(2).
[41] Bojoga A, Koot A, Bonenkamp J, et al. The impact of the extent of surgery on the long-term outcomes of patients with low-risk differentiated non-medullary thyroid cancer: a systematic meta-analysis. J Clin Med 2020;9(7).
[42] Gartland RM, Lubitz CC. Impact of extent of surgery on tumor recurrence and survival for papillary thyroid cancer patients. Ann Surg Oncol 2018;25(9):2520–5.
[43] Rodriguez Schaap PM, Botti M, Otten RHJ, et al. Hemithyroidectomy versus total thyroidectomy for well differentiated T1-2 N0 thyroid cancer: systematic review and meta-analysis. BJS Open 2020;4(6):987–94.
[44] Chan S, Karamali K, Kolodziejczyk A, et al. Systematic review of recurrence rate after hemithyroidectomy for low-risk well-differentiated thyroid cancer. Eur Thyroid J 2020;9(2):73–84.
[45] Vargas-Pinto S, Romero Arenas MA. Lobectomy compared to total thyroidectomy for low-risk papillary thyroid cancer: a systematic review. J Surg Res 2019;242:244–51.
[46] Zhang C, Li Y, Li J, et al. Total thyroidectomy versus lobectomy for papillary thyroid cancer: a systematic review and meta-analysis. Medicine (Baltim) 2020;99(6):e19073.
[47] Barbaro D, Basili G, Materazzi G. Total thyroidectomy vs. lobectomy in differentiated thyroid cancer: is there a reasonable size cut-off for decision? A narrative review. Gland Surg 2021;10(7):2275–83.
[48] Kandil E, Krishnan B, Noureldine SI, et al. Hemithyroidectomy: a meta-analysis of postoperative need for hormone replacement and complications. ORL J Otorhinolaryngol Relat Spec 2013;75(1):6–17.
[49] Rajjoub SR, Yan H, Calcatera NA, et al. Thyroid lobectomy is not sufficient for T2 papillary thyroid cancers. Surgery 2018;163(5):1134–43.
[50] Sosa JA, Bowman HM, Tielsch JM, et al. The importance of surgeon experience for clinical and economic outcomes from thyroidectomy. Ann Surg 1998;228(3):320–30.
[51] Loyo M, Tufano RP, Gourin CG. National trends in thyroid surgery and the effect of volume on short-term outcomes. Laryngoscope 2013;123(8):2056–63.
[52] Tuggle CT, Roman S, Udelsman R, et al. Same-day thyroidectomy: a review of practice patterns and outcomes for 1,168 procedures in New York State. Ann Surg Oncol 2011;18(4):1035–40.
[53] Kandil E, Noureldine SI, Abbas A, et al. The impact of surgical volume on patient outcomes following thyroid surgery. Surgery 2013;154(6):1346–52, ; discussion 52-3.

[54] Duclos A, Peix JL, Colin C, et al, CATHY Study Group. Influence of experience on performance of individual surgeons in thyroid surgery: prospective cross sectional multicentre study. Br Med J 2012;344:d8041.
[55] Chen L, Wu YH, Lee CH, et al. Prophylactic central neck dissection for papillary thyroid carcinoma with clinically uninvolved central neck lymph nodes: a systematic review and meta-analysis. World J Surg 2018;42(9):2846–57.
[56] Hughes DT, Rosen JE, Evans DB, et al. Prophylactic central compartment neck dissection in papillary thyroid cancer and effect on locoregional recurrence. Ann Surg Oncol 2018;25(9):2526–34.
[57] Schumm MA, Shu ML, Leung AM, et al. Patient preference in physician decision-making for patients with Low- to intermediate-risk differentiated thyroid cancer. JAMA Surg 2023;158(8):886–8.
[58] Jeon MJ, Lee YM, Sung TY, et al. Quality of life in patients with papillary thyroid microcarcinoma managed by active surveillance or lobectomy: a cross-sectional study. Thyroid 2019;29(7):956–62.
[59] Lamartina L, Grani G, Durante C, et al. Follow-up of differentiated thyroid cancer - what should (and what should not) be done. Nat Rev Endocrinol 2018;14(9):538–51.
[60] Youssef MR, Attia AS, Omar M, et al. Thyroid lobectomy as a cost-effective approach in low-risk papillary thyroid cancer versus active surveillance. Surgery 2022;171(1):190–6.
[61] Baek HS, Jeong CH, Ha J, et al. Cost-effectiveness analysis of active surveillance compared to early surgery in small papillary thyroid cancer: a systemic review. Cancer Manag Res 2021;13:6721–30.
[62] Silaghi H, Lozovanu V, Georgescu CE, et al. State of the art in the current management and future directions of targeted therapy for differentiated thyroid cancer. Int J Mol Sci 2022;23(7).
[63] Mazzaferri EL. Long-term outcome of patients with differentiated thyroid carcinoma: effect of therapy. Endocr Pract 2000;6(6):469–76.

Advances in Surgery 60 (2026) 127–148

ADVANCES IN SURGERY

Sarcoma of the Breast

A Rare and Heterogeneous Entity

Shoshana T. Levi, MD[a], Heather A. Lillemoe, MD[a,b,*]

[a]Department of Surgical Oncology, The University of Texas MD Anderson Cancer Center, Houston, TX, USA; [b]Department of Breast Surgical Oncology, The University of Texas MD Anderson Cancer Center, Houston, TX, USA

Keywords

• Breast sarcoma • Angiosarcoma of the breast • Soft-tissue sarcoma
• Radiation associated malignancy

Key points

- Breast sarcomas comprise a heterogeneous group of malignancies and are extremely rare.
- Radiation therapy (RT) to the breast confers a slight risk of developing secondary sarcoma, most commonly angiosarcoma.
- Diagnosis and management of breast sarcoma should be determined by expert sarcoma pathologists and multidisciplinary teams.
- Treatment guidelines and histology specific considerations for soft tissue sarcoma of the extremity and trunk can inform decision making for breast sarcoma.
- Surgical resection is the primary treatment of breast sarcomas. The use of adjuvant chemotherapy and RT should be individualized and discussed in a multidisciplinary setting.

INTRODUCTION

Background

Breast sarcomas are extremely rare malignancies accounting for less than 0.01% of all breast cancers with an estimated incidence of 4.5 cases per million women per year [1–3]. In addition to their rarity, breast sarcomas are composed of a heterogenous group of histologies, making them difficult to study. In this article, we review the clinicopathologic features and management

*Corresponding author. Department of Breast Surgical Oncology, UT MD Anderson, 1400 Pressler Street, Unit 1434, Houston, TX 77030. *E-mail address:* halillemoe@mdanderson.org

https://doi.org/10.1016/j.yasu.2026.03.008

Abbreviations

AJCC	American Joint Committee on Cancer
BCT	breast-conserving therapy
CNB	core needle biopsy
CNS	central nervous system
FNA	fine needle aspiration
LNM	lymph node metastases
MDACC	MD Anderson Cancer Center
NCCN	National Comprehensive Cancer Network
OS	overall survival
PD	progressive disease
PT	phyllodes tumor
RAAS	radiation-associated angiosarcomas
RT	radiation therapy
SEER	Surveillance, Epidemiology and End Results
STS	soft tissue sarcoma
WLE	wide local excision

approaches for the rare and diverse group of malignancies that make up breast sarcomas.

Etiology and predisposing factors

Like breast carcinomas derived from epithelial tissues, breast sarcomas largely affect women, with only 1.5% to 3.8% of cases occurring in men [1,4]. While this is more frequent than the less than 1% of male breast cancers that account for invasive epithelial breast cancers, female sex is clearly a predisposing factor for breast sarcoma. Additionally, radiation exposure and lymphedema–which predominantly affect females who have undergone prior treatment for breast cancer–are well-known risk factors for the development of secondary breast sarcoma.

Radiation

Radiation-associated sarcomas have been recognized since the 1940s, approximately 20 years after peak utilization of radium for neoplastic diseases [5]. The diagnostic criteria are generally as follows: (1) the malignancy must be histopathologically confirmed to be a sarcoma and must be different from the primary malignancy; (2) the sarcoma must arise within the irradiated field; and (3) there must be a latency period of approximately 3 to 4 years after receipt of radiation therapy (RT). While radiation for breast-conserving therapy (BCT) is known to be associated with the development of secondary sarcomas, the risk-benefit ratio still greatly favors receipt of RT. In a study evaluating the incidence of secondary breast sarcomas using the Surveillance, Epidemiology and End Results (SEER) Cancer Incidence database (1973–1997), 274,572 cases of primary invasive breast cancer were reported with an associated 263 cases of subsequent sarcomas [6]. Of the sarcoma cases identified, 87 had received RT (0.1% of patients who had received radiation) and 176 had not (0.09% of patients who had not received radiation). The cumulative incidence of sarcoma 15 years after initial breast cancer diagnosis differed only slightly between the groups with 3.2 per 1000 (standard error = 0.4) versus 2.3 per 1000 (standard error = 0.2) (P=.001) in radiated versus non-radiated cases, respectively. Interestingly, angiosarcoma accounted for 56.8% of cases in the radiated group versus only 5.7% in the non-radiated group [6].

Lymphedema

The development of upper extremity angiosarcoma in the setting of post-mastectomy chronic lymphedema was initially described by Stewart and Treves in 1948 [7]. While there is a clear association between chronic lymphedema and secondary sarcoma of the extremity in this eponymous disease (Stewart-Treves Syndrome), the association between chronic lymphedema and secondary sarcoma of the breast remains unclear. Post-mastectomy lymphedema and post-radiation status are frequently seen concomitantly so it is difficult to attribute risk to lymphedema alone.

Interestingly, in an updated SEER-based study evaluating the risk of sarcoma after treatment for breast cancer (1973–2003), the authors found partial mastectomy (HR, 7.12; 95% CI, 3.2–16.0) and lymph node dissections (HR, 2.57; 95% CI, 1.3–5.0) to be independent risk factors for development of breast angiosarcoma [8]. Such findings support the notion that lymphedema may be a contributing risk factor to the formation of secondary angiosarcoma.

Genetic predispositions

Several cancer predisposition syndromes, such as Li-Fraumeni and retinoblastoma, are known to be associated with a moderate-to-high lifetime risk of developing soft tissue sarcoma (STS) [9]. With the recent widespread use of genetic sequencing, additional germline pathogenic or likely pathogenic variants (GPVs) have been identified and implicated in causing susceptibility to sarcoma formation. One study evaluated germline DNA from 177 children, adolescents, and young adults with soft tissue or bone sarcoma and found GPVs in 21.5% of the patients [10]. These findings highlight the importance of comprehensive genetic testing, particularly in young patients without other identifiable risk factors.

CLINICAL PRESENTATION AND DIAGNOSTIC WORK-UP

Clinical presentation

Breast sarcomas are most often diagnosed in the 5th or 6th decades of life with a median age of diagnosis of 50 years [11,12]. Patients with radiation-associated sarcomas tend to present at an older age, given they typically develop after a latency period following the treatment of a primary cancer. Several studies focusing on radiation-associated angiosarcomas (RAAS) reported median age of presentation to be 62 to 72 years [13–15]. Similarly, 2 retrospective case series reported an approximately 30 year difference in age of presentation between primary and radiation-associated breast sarcoma (39.4–45.5 years vs 70.6–75.8 years) [16,17].

Breast sarcomas tend to be large, with a median size greater than 5 cm and sizes up to 30 cm documented in the literature [11]. Primary breast sarcomas typically present as firm, rapidly expanding, unilateral masses without palpable lymphadenopathy, given their propensity to disseminate via hematogenous, rather than lymphangitic spread. In contrast, RAAS typically present with skin changes such as skin nodules, violaceous skin lesions, or ulceration, rather than a discreet mass (Fig. 1A–D) [13,14,16]. The lack of a distinct mass in such cases can lead to diagnostic delay, thus the recognition of such skin changes as characteristic of RAAS is imperative.

Diagnostic workup

Imaging of primary tumor

Initial imaging with diagnostic mammography and ultrasound can reveal non-specific findings, and these modalities may be insufficient for determining the extent of disease. Mammographic abnormalities are typically reported as an isodense (14%–50%) or hyperdense (50%–86%) mass with indistinct (23%–73%) or microlobulated (7%–70%) borders. Spiculations (3%) and calcifications (3%–21%) are less frequently reported [18–20]. On ultrasound imaging, the

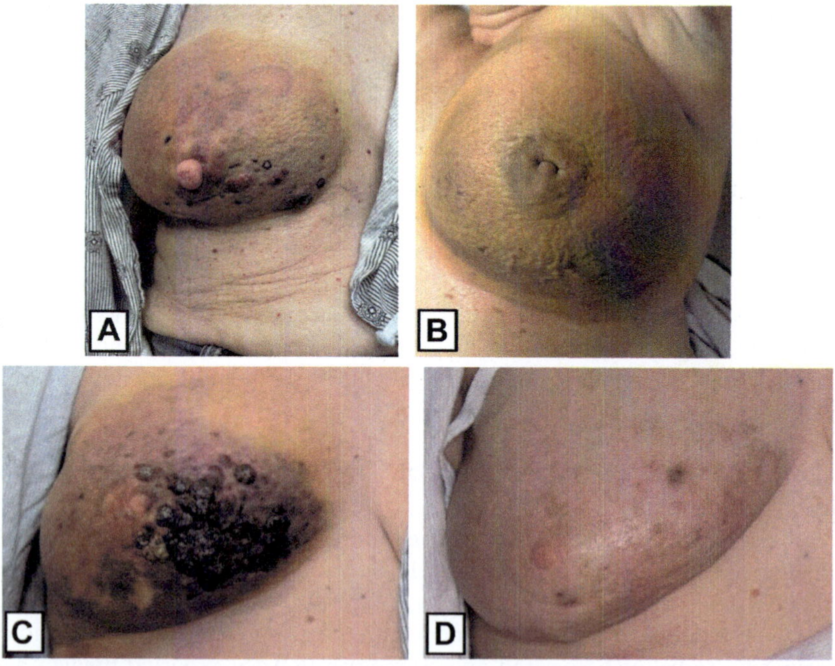

Fig. 1. Radiation-associated angiosarcoma of the breast. (*A* and *B*) Pre-treatment photographs of patients presenting with radiation-associated angiosarcoma of the breast after prior treatment for breast carcinoma. (*C* and *D*) Radiation-associated angiosarcoma of the breast pre-treatment (*C*) and post-treatment (*D*) with neoadjuvant chemotherapy.

majority of primary breast sarcomas are reported as hypoechoic (63%–82%) with posterior acoustic shadowing (50%–79%) [18–20].

While MRI characteristics are similarly variable, rapid contrast enhancement was a universal finding in the small sample of patients for whom kinetics were evaluated (12 of 12 patients) [18–20]. Importantly, MRI can provide resolution in patients with mammographically or sonographically occult lesions or in patients with dense breasts. Additionally, MRI yields a comprehensive assessment of a tumor's relationship to surrounding structures such as skin and chest wall, which can be critical for surgical planning (Fig. 2). For tumors with more extensive chest wall involvement, dedicated chest wall imaging may also be required for surgical planning.

In RAAS, radiologic findings mirror clinical findings with cutaneous nodularity and thickening noted on mammography, ultrasonography, and MRI [16].

The variability in imaging characteristics likely reflects the heterogeneity in sarcoma histologies and is further limited by the nature of small case series from which these data are derived. This highlights the importance of communication between radiologists and clinicians when there is a high suspicion for non-carcinoma breast mass.

Biopsy

Diagnosis of breast sarcoma follows the same principles as diagnosis of STS of the extremity and trunk and is based on tissue biopsy. Core needle biopsy (CNB) is preferred as it allows for determination of grade and histologic subtype, as compared with fine needle aspiration (FNA), and is less invasive compared with open, surgical biopsy. If CNB does not yield adequate tissue for diagnosis, an incisional biopsy can be considered. Importantly, the location of any open biopsy site should be carefully oriented within the future definitive oncologic resection field. Image guidance for biopsy is particularly useful for

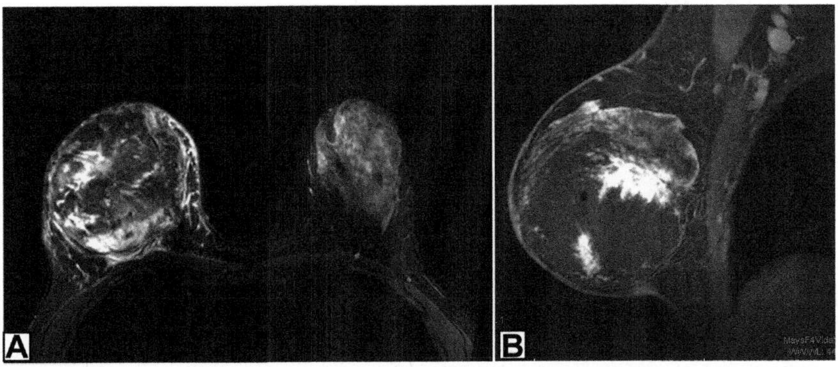

Fig. 2. Bilateral breast contrast-enhanced MRI in a patient with primary breast angiosarcoma showing a large, irregularly shaped mass with circumscribed margins and heterogeneous internal enhancement in the (*A*) axial and (*B*) sagittal views. There is global skin thickening without evidence of nipple or chest wall invasion.

deeper lesions or lesions with large necrotic components to target non-necrotic regions for improved diagnostic accuracy. For RAAS, a punch biopsy of involved skin is often used for tissue diagnosis, particularly if there is minimal subcutaneous extension.

Clinical staging

For initial clinical staging, the University of Texas MD Anderson Cancer Center (MDACC) Algorithm for Breast Sarcoma (Fig. 3) recommends CT

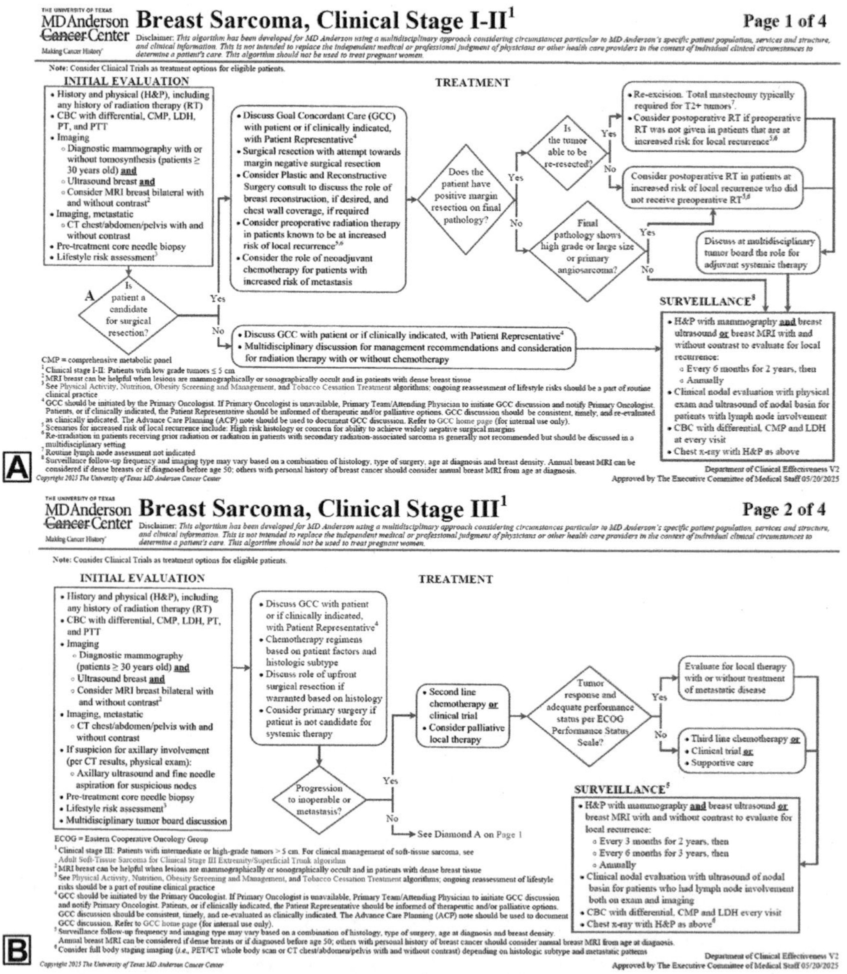

Fig. 3. The University of Texas MD Anderson Cancer Center Breast Sarcoma Clinical Practice Algorithm for (*A*) Clinical Stage I-II and (*B*) Clinical Stage III Disease. Previously published materials are unchanged from the source, used with permission from the University of Texas MD Anderson Cancer Center. [Copyright held by, and used with permission of, The Board of Regents of the University of Texas System through The University of Texas MD Anderson Cancer Center.]

chest/abdomen/pelvis with and without contrast to evaluate for metastatic disease. If there is clinical concern for regional lymph node involvement, axillary ultrasound with FNA is recommended. Histology specific considerations based on unique metastatic patterns can be extrapolated from National Comprehensive Cancer Network (NCCN) Clinical Practice Guidelines in Oncology for extremity and trunk sarcomas [21]. For example, central nervous system (CNS) MRI may be indicated for angiosarcoma, and PET/CT or bone scan may be indicated for leiomyosarcoma given the propensity for CNS and bone metastases, respectively.

PATHOLOGY AND STAGING

Pathology

Assessment of grade and histologic subtype is paramount in determining the optimal treatment of each individual sarcoma. Furthermore, given the rarity and diversity of sarcomas, expert review by a sarcoma pathologist is critical for establishing the correct diagnosis. A study by the Hellenic Group of Sarcoma and Rare Cancers found that expert pathologist review of sarcoma cases in Greece led to modifications in histologic diagnosis in 31% of cases with a resulting change in management in 14% of cases [22]. Similarly, a recent retrospective, single-institution study in the United States found major discordance rates (benign/malignant, histologic subtype, nondiagnostic/diagnostic, and major grading discrepancies) of 44% in sarcoma pathology reports between high and low volume centers [23]. These studies highlight the importance of expert pathologic review for sarcomas to determine optimal treatment of patients.

It is worth noting that metaplastic carcinomas of epithelial origin can have large sarcomatoid components, making it difficult to distinguish them from breast sarcomas. Differentiation between the 2 entities is important for prognostic and treatment planning purposes and can largely be accomplished with the use of wide spectrum screening keratin staining [2,24].

Staging

Breast sarcomas

Breast sarcomas are staged according to the staging system for STS of the extremity and trunk as published in The Cancer Staging Manual of the American Joint Committee on Cancer (AJCC) [25]. The 8th edition was published in 2017 with several notable updates including (1) separation of STS by location (extremity and trunk, retroperitoneum, head and neck, and visceral); (2) transition from a four-grade classification to a 3 grade classification; (3) upstaging of extremity and trunk sarcomas with lymph node metastases (LNM) to stage IV; and (4) expanding T factor classification to four categories with elimination of depth of tumor as a prognostic factor [26]. Notably, upstaging for LNM is unique to sarcomas of the extremities and trunk and is not reflected in the 8th edition of the Union for International Cancer Control TNM Classification of Malignant Tumors [26,27].

Subsequent studies have disputed the validity of grouping patients with distant metastases and loco-regional LNM within the same prognostic stage. A SEER-based analysis of 21,396 patients and a single-center retrospective review of 2689 patients with sarcoma of the extremity and trunk demonstrated significant differences in survival between distant and nodal metastasis [28,29]. Additionally, several histologic subtypes denoted by the "CARE" acronym (clear cell sarcoma, angiosarcoma, rhabdomyosarcoma, and epithelioid sarcoma) have higher propensities for regional LNM [30], further arguing against universal upstaging of LNM to stage IV disease.

Phyllodes tumors

Phyllodes tumors (PTs) are distinct fibroepithelial tumors of the breast that account for less than 1% of all breast tumors. They are classified by the World Health Organization as benign, borderline, or malignant based on the degree of stromal cellularity (mild, moderate, marked or diffuse), stromal cell atypia (mild, moderate, marked), mitotic activity (<5, 5–9, >9 per 10 HPF), tumor margin (well-defined, well-defined but may be focally infiltrative, infiltrative), and stromal overgrowth (absent, focal, present). Additionally, the presence of heterologous elements, other than well-differentiated liposarcoma, leads to automatic classification as malignant PT [31]. In the absence of heterologous elements, a PT needs to exhibit all malignant criteria in order to be classified as malignant. This can lead to challenges in assigning a classification when most, but not all, of these subjective criteria are met [32]. Malignant phyllodes tumors are managed along similar guiding principles as primary breast sarcomas.

TREATMENT APPROACH—GENERAL CONSIDERATIONS

Surgical resection

Primary tumor

Surgical resection with widely negative margins is the cornerstone of treatment for breast sarcomas. Most authors recommend a margin of at least 1 cm with several retrospective studies showing no difference in outcomes with more extensive mastectomy compared with wide local excision (WLE) [33–37]. Thus, partial mastectomy is considered safe and adequate, particularly for smaller tumors where good cosmetic outcomes can be achieved. Special considerations are important to note for RAAS, which are discussed in further detail below.

Lymph nodes

Routine axillary lymph node sampling is not recommended for breast sarcoma, given the low rates of LNM and the lack of associated clinical benefit. In 6 retrospective case series, there were a cumulative 158 cases of breast sarcoma with axillary lymph node sampling and only 5 cases (3.2%) with positive lymph nodes (excluding cases of carcinosarcoma) [33–35,37–39]. Additionally, a SEER-based study evaluating the role of lymph node evaluation in breast sarcoma from 1988 to 2002 found that examination of nodes had no impact on survival and out of 129 patients with documented assessment of their regional lymphatics, only 6 (4.6%) were found to have positive nodes [40]. Instead, directed surgical management of confirmed LNM should be utilized. In a retrospective study looking at patients with extremity soft-tissue sarcoma, 76 patients who underwent surgical resection of isolated LNM were found to have similar 5 year overall survival (OS) rates to patients with localized AJCC stage III sarcomas (52.9% [95% CI, 40.9%–64.9%] vs 49.3% [95% CI, 45.7%–53.5%]) [29]. These findings illustrate that isolated LNM, in the absence of distant disease, can be managed surgically with favorable outcomes.

Reconstruction

Oncoplastic reconstruction is an important pillar in the multidisciplinary treatment of breast sarcoma. Considerations for the type of reconstruction include patient preference, previous exposure to RT or plans for adjuvant RT, and extent of the sarcoma resection. Two reviews of the breast sarcoma reconstruction experience at the University of Texas MDACC highlight the diversity of reconstructive options after breast sarcoma resection, which included immediate, delayed, and staged approaches. The following techniques were utilized: local tissue rearrangement, local flap, pedicled flap, free flap, tissue expander placement, permanent implant placement, and skin grafting [41,42]. Coordination with and engagement of reconstructive teams, along with possible thoracic surgeon collaboration, is particularly important in cases with extensive local tissue or chest wall involvement as illustrated in Fig. 4.

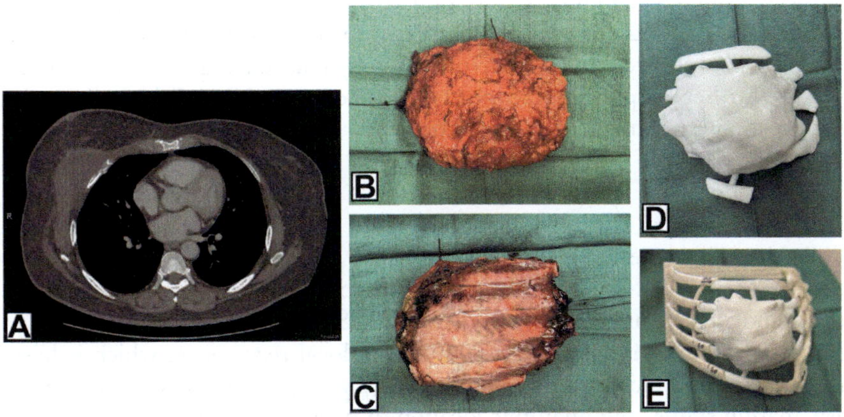

Fig. 4. Radiation-associated breast and chest wall pleomorphic and spindle cell sarcoma. (*A*) Cross-sectional computed tomography (CT) imaging showing right anterior chest wall mass with pectoralis musculature and rib involvement. (*B* and *C*) Post-resection specimen anterior (*B*) and posterior (*C*) views after wide-margin surgical resection via inframammary breast conserving approach. (*D* and *E*) 3-Dimensional reconstructed tumor model based on CT-imaging and used for pre-operative planning of chest wall reconstruction.

Systemic therapy

The nuanced use of chemotherapy for the treatment of breast sarcoma again emphasizes the heterogeneity of the disease and the importance of multidisciplinary discussion. The use of chemotherapy is individualized and informed by data from STS of the extremity and trunk. A common limitation of much of these data are the heterogeneous patient populations within studies in terms of tumor location, histology, grade, and chemotherapy dosing. Nonetheless, a meta-analysis of 18 randomized controlled trials representing 1953 patients with STS demonstrated marginal benefit of chemotherapy for localized resectable disease in terms of local recurrence, distant recurrence, overall recurrence, and OS [43]. Notably, the benefit to OS was only seen with combination doxorubicin and ifosfamide and not with doxorubicin alone [43].

The preferred regimen for resectable STS is doxorubicin, ifosfamide, and mesna (AIM) and its use can be considered to facilitate surgical resection or for patients with a high risk of developing metastatic disease, which is based on histology, grade, size, and recurrent versus primary disease. These factors should be weighed against the risks of a highly toxic chemotherapy regimen. A special consideration for radiation-associated sarcomas is that many patients may have prior exposure to anthracyclines from treatment of primary breast carcinoma. Given the cumulative dose risk of cardiotoxicity, additional treatment with doxorubicin may be limited. Alternative treatment regimens such as gemcitabine plus docetaxel [44,45] or dacarbazine (DTIC) [46] have been shown to have activity against advanced or metastatic STS and may be utilized. Furthermore, histology specific agents such as paclitaxel for angiosarcoma [47,48] or trabectedin for myxoid liposarcoma [49] or leiomyosarcoma [50] can be considered. Notably, a randomized trial evaluating histology-tailored neoadjuvant chemotherapy to standard epirubicin plus ifosfamide in localized high-risk STS showed no benefit of histology-tailored regimens [51]. These findings further emphasize the need for expert multidisciplinary discussion when planning treatments for this patient population.

Radiation therapy

Like chemotherapy, RT for breast sarcoma is utilized on a case-by-case basis. While there is some conflicting retrospective data specifically for breast sarcoma [1,33,34,36,52–54], recommendations for the use of RT can similarly be extrapolated from extremity and trunk STS guidelines [21,55]. RT is typically reserved for patients with a high risk of local recurrence, which is based on several factors including histology, grade, size, recurrent versus primary disease, margin status, and anatomic location or proximity to vital structures [55]. Pre-operative administration is recommended to minimize late toxicities such as fibrosis and edema and for tumor downstaging [21,55]. Post-operative RT may be favored if there are specific wound healing concerns, as wound complications are more common with pre-operative RT, or if formal pathology is needed for final recommendations. Re-irradiation for radiation-associated breast sarcoma is a controversial topic, given the concerns for cumulative toxicity; however, some studies have shown benefits in local recurrence with the administration of radiation in these patients [56]. Multidisciplinary input is recommended to strongly consider both risks and benefits of this approach.

A comprehensive treatment schema for patients with breast sarcoma that encompasses the above recommendations is illustrated in Fig. 3.

TREATMENT APPROACH—TUMOR-SPECIFIC CONSIDERATIONS

Radiation associated angiosarcoma

RAAS arise from the overlying dermis rather than the underlying breast parenchyma and are therefore considered cutaneous sarcomas. They are diffusely infiltrative within the dermis and can range from well to poorly differentiated with varying degrees of cytologic atypia, necrosis, and mitotic index [57]. Multifocal disease is commonly identified with reported incidences between 42% and 70% in retrospective series [13,14,58,59]. The multifocal nature of RAAS can lead to false negative resection margins and partially explains the historically high rates of local recurrence seen after mastectomies or WLE. Additionally, all skin within the irradiated field is considered at risk from a radiation damage perspective. Two retrospective series compared mastectomy alone to mastectomy with excision of all overlying irradiated skin and found marked improvements in local recurrence (median local recurrence free survival: 80.8 vs 10.0 months, P=.065 and 5-year local recurrence rate: 23 vs 76%, P<.01), distant metastasis (median recurrence free survival: 72.6 vs 10.0 months, P=.098 and 5-year distant metastasis rate: 18 vs 47%, P=.02) and survival (OS: not achieved vs 29 months, P=.054 and 5-year disease-specific survival: 86 vs 46%, P<.01) for patients who underwent radical excision of all irradiated skin [13,58]. Thus, a more radical resection of irradiated field is preferred over standard mastectomy or WLE. If the prior radiation treatment plan cannot be accessed, standard anatomic landmarks can be used to guide extent of skin excision (superior: clavicle, medial: mid-sternum, inferior: rectus sheath, lateral: anterior border of latissimus dorsi).

Phyllodes tumors

Like breast sarcoma, the mainstay of treatment of PT is surgical resection without axillary staging. The required extent of negative margins remains controversial due to conflicting data. For instance, a meta-analysis from 2019 showed that a positive surgical margin was associated with a higher rate of local recurrence (LR) only for malignant PT [60], whereas another meta-analysis from 2020 observed decreased LR for benign, borderline, and malignant PT when margins were ≥10 mm [61]. Subsequent large cohort studies have shown positive margin status, but not margin width, as a risk factor for LR for all PT [62,63]. Current NCCN guidelines suggest grossly negative margins for benign PT and WLE with intention of obtaining ≥1 cm for borderline and malignant PT. It is noted that narrow surgical margins are not an absolute indication for mastectomy when BCT does not achieve 1 cm or greater margins [64].

Importantly, the entire clinical picture including tumor histopathologic details and size should be considered when making this recommendation.

While there are no prospective randomized trials evaluating the role of RT for PT, a meta-analysis has demonstrated decreased risk of LR in patients with borderline or malignant PT who received RT following BCT. The decreased LR was not seen in patients who had undergone mastectomy and there was no observed difference in survival [65]. Thus, RT may be considered for patients whose risk of recurrence poses significant morbidity, such as within the chest wall [64]. While its use is more limited in borderline PT, RT should be considered for patients with malignant PT who are intermediate or high-risk for local recurrence. This includes patients with tumor size greater than 5 cm who undergo mastectomy (intermediate risk) and patients with any tumor size who undergo BCT or have nodal positivity (high risk) [66].

Desmoid tumor

Desmoid tumors are rare, locally destructive tumors characterized by fibroblastic proliferation. While they do not have metastatic potential, they can confer significant morbidity to patients. They have widely variable and unpredictable clinical courses with nearly 30% of patients experiencing spontaneous regression [67]. Thus, the initial treatment approach for desmoid is active surveillance [68]. For patients with progressive disease (PD), medical therapy has supplanted surgical resection as the next line of therapy, given the high morbidity and LR risk associated with surgical resection [68]. Nirogacestat, the only FDA-approved medication for the treatment of desmoid [69], and sorafenib [70] have both been shown to have improved progression-free survival and objective response rates compared with placebo in phase 3 clinical trials. There is no evidence to support the use of NSAIDs (beyond pain control) or antihormonal therapy, but cytotoxic chemotherapy remains a treatment option based on nonrandomized studies [71]. Surgical resection is an option for PD or for tumors that do not pose a significant risk of surgical morbidity, particularly when weighed against the side effects of medical therapy. MRI is useful for delineating extent of disease to accurately assess surgical risk.

Recurrent and metastatic disease

Locally recurrent STS should be managed with surgical re-resection with negative margins if feasible. An R0 resection should be attempted as margin status remains an important risk factor for additional LR [72]. In a retrospective study, re-irradiation for patients with locally recurrent STS who were initially treated with resection and RT did not improve subsequent local control and was associated with higher complication rates [73].

Patients with limited metastatic disease who are good surgical candidates should be offered resection. Retrospective series have reported 5 year OS rates as high as 50% after pulmonary metastasectomy [74]. These favorable outcomes depend on careful patient selection with consideration of tumor burden, location of metastatic disease, status of the primary tumor, ability to achieve R0 resection, and patient fitness for surgery.

Table 1
Clinical outcomes of breast sarcoma

Publication, year	N	Median follow-up in months (range)	Histologic subtypes (n)	Risk factors	LR rate Median time to LR in months (range)	DM rate	Clinical outcomes
Adem et al [2], 2004	25	6.4 (7–492)	Primary breast sarcomas: FS (6), AS (6), UPS (6), LMS (2), MFS (3), HPC (1), OGS (1)	OS: tumor size	44% 15 (2–36)	40%	5 y OS: 66% 5 y CSS: 70% 5y OS for tumors ≤5 cm vs >5 cm: 91% vs 50%
Barrow et al [52], 1999	59	40 (3–399)	MFH, FS, or stromal sarcoma (32), AS (17), OGS (3), other (7)	LR: margin status OS: tumor size, histology	36% NR	47%	Median DFS: 18 mo Median OS for tumors 0-2 cm vs 21.-4.9 cm vs >5 cm: 80 vs 37 vs 20 mo Median OS for AS vs OGS vs MFH vs other: 237 vs 169 vs 40 vs 20 mo
Billings et al [59], 2004	27	44 (12–91)	RAAS	N/A	64% NR	41%	Median survival: 33.5 mo (range 4–91)
Bousquet et al [34], 2007	103	64 (12–309)	AS (42), MFH (14), FS (12), LS (7), LMS (6), OGS (2), other (20)	LR: residual tumor[a], cellular pleomorphism, angiosarcoma DFS: premenopausal status, angiosarcoma, cellular pleomorphism, histologic grade 3, residual tumor	55% 10.5 (2–113)	36%	5y DFS: 44% 10 y DFS: 36% 5 y OS: 55% 10 y OS: 51%

(continued on next page)

Table 1
(continued)

Publication, year	N	Median follow-up in months (range)	Histologic subtypes (n)	Risk factors	LR rate Median time to LR in months (range)	DM rate	Clinical outcomes
Confavreux et al [36], 2006	70	31.7 (NR)	Primary breast sarcomas: AS (17), SCC (6), LS (3), FS (3), OGS (2), LMS (2), RMS (1), other (10) Phyllodes: Grade I (5), Grade II (5), Grade III (16)	OS: histology, age, R0 vs R1 + R2	50% 8.4 (1.3–85.3)	NR	Median DFS: 1.15 y 3 y OS for age >60 vs ≤60: 27% vs 61% 3 y OS for R0 vs R1 + R2: 72% vs 38.5% 3 y OS for AS vs non-AS[b]: 23% vs 57.6%
Fields et al [39], 2008	13	5.3 (1–14) years	Primary breast sarcomas: LMS (3), MFH (3), FS (3), CS (1), AS (1), ECS (1), RMS (1)	OS: tumor size	54% NR	54%	5 y OS for tumors <5 cm vs >5 cm: 83% vs 42%
Li et al [58], 2017	76	27 (11–60)	RAAS	DSS: age, radicality of surgery[c], margin	Radical: 16% 15 (NR) Conservative: 68% 5 (NR)	R: 13% C: 37%	5 y DSS for radical vs conservative resection: 86% vs 46% Radical 5 y DSS for negative vs positive margin: 63% vs 14%

McGowan et al [33], 2000	78	9.5 (0.9–31) years	Malignant phyllodes (32), stromal sarcoma (14), AS (8), FS (7), CS (5), LS (4), other (8)	LRFR: margin status CSS: tumor grade, radiation dose			5 y LRFR for positive vs negative margins: 33% vs 80% 5 y CSS for grade I or II tumors vs grade III or IV tumors: 84% vs 55% 5 y CSS for >48 Gy vs ≤48 Gy vs no RT: 91% vs 50% vs 50% 10 y CSS: 48%
Mergancová et al [15], 2022	53	30 (5–186)	RAAS	N/A[d]	43%[e] 7.5 (3–66)	17%	3-y survival: 56% 5 y survival: 33%
Morgan et al [13], 2012	33	23.8 (1–199)	RAAS	Radicality of surgery	52% NR	27%	Median LRFS for radical vs conservative resection: 80.8 vs 10.0 mo Median RFS for radical vs conservative resection: 72.6 vs 10.0 mo Median OS for radical vs conservative resection: not reached vs 29 mo
Pandey et al [75], 2004	19	25 (NR)	Primary breast sarcomas: AS (8), SSC (4), UPS (2), stromal sarcoma (2), MFH (1), RMS (1), other (1)	DFS: margin status	37% NR	10%	3 y DFS: 39%

(continued on next page)

Table 1
(*continued*)

Publication, year	N	Median follow-up in months (range)	Histologic subtypes (n)	Risk factors	LR rate Median time to LR in months (range)	DM rate	Clinical outcomes
Torres et al [14], 2016	95	10.3 (2.4–31.8) years	RAAS	LR: receipt of chemotherapy	48% 1.8 (0.1–15.8) years	27%	1 y DSS: 93.5% 5 y DSS: 62.5%
Zelek et al [76], 2003	83	7.8 (0.25–24) years	Primary breast sarcomas: MFH (57), AS (8), LS (7), SSC (2), OGS (2), RMS (2), LMS (2), neurosarcoma (2)	OS: tumor size, histologic grade DFS: tumor size, histologic grade	30% NR	35%	10 y OS for tumors grade 1 vs 2 vs 3: 82% vs 62% vs 36% 10 y OS for tumors 5 cm vs 5–10 cm vs >10 cm: 76% vs 68% vs 28% 10 y DFS for tumors grade 1 vs 2 vs 3: 61% vs 51% vs 25% 10 y DFS for tumors <5 cm vs 5–10 cm vs >10 cm: 66% vs 55% vs 15%

Histologic subtypes: Angiosarcoma (AS), carcinosarcoma (CS), dermatofibrosarcoma protuberans (DFP), epithelioid cell sarcoma (ECS), fibrosarcoma (FS), hemangiopericytoma (HPC), leiomyosarcoma (LMS), liposarcoma (LS), malignant fibrous histiocytoma (MFH), myxofibrosarcoma (MFS), osteosarcoma or osteogenic sarcoma (OGS) rhabdomyosarcoma (RMS), spindle cell sarcoma (SCC), undifferentiated pleomorphic sarcoma (UPS).

Abbreviations: CSS, cause-specific survival; DFS, Disease-free survival; DM, distant metastasis rate; DSS, Disease-specific survival; LR, local recurrence; LRFR, local relapse-free rate; NR, not reported; OS, Overall survival; RFS, Recurrence-free survival.

[a]Residual tumor defined as margin <1 cm, microscopically involved margin, incomplete initial surgery, or gross residual tumor.

[b]Excluding Grade I and II phyllodes that had an OS of 100%.

[c]Radical resection: mastectomy plus all irradiated skin, Conservative resection: mastectomy/wide excision.

[d]Surgical management did not include resection of all irradiated skin.

[e]9 patients excluded from LR rate due to progression within 3 mo after surgery.

OUTCOMES AND FOLLOW-UP

Breast sarcomas, like other STS, have high rates of both local and distant recurrence with survival influenced by several risk factors including tumor size, grade, histology, and quality of surgical resection [75] (Table 1). While 2 studies showed worse prognosis for primary angiosarcoma compared with other histologies [36,76], another study showed improved survival for primary angiosarcoma [52]. Two studies comparing radiation-associated sarcomas to radiation-naïve sarcomas found no difference in OS between the 2 groups [6,17]. Because of the rarity of these tumors, the heterogeneity of the histologies, and the limitations of existing staging systems as previously discussed, it can be difficult to provide accurate prognoses to patients. Several nomograms for STS [77], and even a phyllodes-specific nomogram [78], have been validated and are available for use. Additional breast sarcoma-specific nomograms have been constructed and studied [79]. The use of these nomograms may provide providers and patients with more reliable and individualized risk assessments.

Most local recurrence events occur within 2 years, but late recurrences have been reported as far out as 15 years (see Table 1). Thus, long-term surveillance is critical. Fig. 3 provides institutional consensus guidelines for surveillance of patients after treatment of their breast sarcoma.

SUMMARY

Breast sarcomas are rare and histologically diverse. They can arise spontaneously, or in association with prior RT. They are aggressive in nature and frequently recur or disseminate. Surgery remains the mainstay of treatment, and BCT can be safely pursued, except in the case of RAAS, where radical excision is recommended. The use of chemotherapy and RT should be individualized based on a patient's risk of distant metastasis and local recurrence, respectively. Optimal treatment requires expert consensus in a multidisciplinary team.

CLINICS CARE POINTS

- FNA does not allow for accurate assessment of sarcoma. Core needle or incisional biopsies are required for the comprehensive evaluation of a sarcoma to create optimal treatment plans.
- Expert pathologic review and referral to a high-volume tertiary care center with expertise in sarcoma is recommended for improved patient outcomes.
- Multidisciplinary review and discussion are crucial for the management of these patients.
- Primary breast sarcomas and non-angiosarcoma radiation associated sarcomas can be managed surgically with wide margins. RAAS should be managed with mastectomy and radical resection of irradiated skin for improved outcomes.

Disclosure

The authors have nothing to disclose.

Funding

This work was supported by National Institutes Health T32 CA 009599 and the MD Anderson Cancer Center support grant P30 CA016672.

References

[1] Lee JS, Yoon K, Onyshchenko M. Sarcoma of the breast: clinical characteristics and outcomes of 991 patients from the National Cancer Database. Sarcoma 2021;2021; https://doi.org/10.1155/2021/8828158.

[2] Adem C, Reynolds C, Ingle JN, et al. Primary breast sarcoma: clinicopathologic series from the Mayo Clinic and review of the literature. Br J Cancer 2004;91(2); https://doi.org/10.1038/sj.bjc.6601920.

[3] May DS, Stroup NE. The incidence of sarcomas of the breast among women in the United States, 1973–1986. Plast Reconstr Surg 1991;87(1); https://doi.org/10.1097/00006534-199101000-00045.

[4] Li GZ, Raut CP, Hunt KK, et al. Breast sarcomas, phyllodes tumors, and desmoid tumors: epidemiology, diagnosis, staging, and histology-specific management considerations. Am Soc Clin Oncol Edu Book 2021;(41); https://doi.org/10.1200/edbk_321341.

[5] Cahan WG, Woodard HQ, Higinbotham NL, et al. Sarcoma arising in irradiated bone. Cancer 1948;82(1); https://doi.org/10.1002/(sici)1097-0142(19980101)82:1<8::aid-cncr3>3.0.co;2-w.

[6] Yap J, Chuba PJ, Thomas R, et al. Sarcoma as a second malignancy after treatment for breast cancer. Int J Radiat Oncol Biol Phys 2002;52(5); https://doi.org/10.1016/S0360-3016(01)02799-7.

[7] Stewart FW, Treves N. Lymphangiosarcoma in postmastectomy lymphedema. A report of six cases in elephantiasis chirurgica. Cancer 1948;1(1); https://doi.org/10.1002/1097-0142(194805)1:1<64::AID-CNCR2820010105>3.0.CO;2-W.

[8] Mery CM, George S, Bertagnolli MM, et al. Secondary sarcomas after radiotherapy for breast cancer: sustained risk and poor survival. Cancer 2009;115(18); https://doi.org/10.1002/cncr.24462.

[9] Connolly EA, Boye K, Bonvalot S, et al. Genetic predisposition in sarcomas: clinical implications and management. eClinicalMedicine 2025;83:103203; https://doi.org/10.1016/j.eclinm.2025.103203.

[10] Carvalho NDA, Santiago KM, Maia JML, et al. Prevalence and clinical implications of germline pathogenic variants in cancer predisposing genes in young patients across sarcoma subtypes. J Med Genet 2023;61(1); https://doi.org/10.1136/jmg-2023-109269.

[11] Lim SZ, Ong KW, Tan BKT, et al. Sarcoma of the breast: an update on a rare entity. J Clin Pathol 2016;69(5); https://doi.org/10.1136/jclinpath-2015-203545.

[12] Al-Benna S, Poggemann K, Steinau HU, et al. Diagnosis and management of primary breast sarcoma. Breast Cancer Res Treat 2010;122(3); https://doi.org/10.1007/s10549-010-0915-y.

[13] Morgan EA, Kozono DE, Wang Q, et al. Cutaneous radiation-associated angiosarcoma of the breast: poor prognosis in a rare secondary malignancy. Ann Surg Oncol 2012;19(12); https://doi.org/10.1245/s10434-012-2563-4.

[14] Torres KE, Ravi V, Kin K, et al. Long-term outcomes in patients with radiation-associated angiosarcomas of the breast following surgery and radiotherapy for breast cancer. Ann Surg Oncol 2013;20; https://doi.org/10.1245/s10434-012-2755-y.

[15] Mergancová J, Lierová A, Coufal O, et al. Radiation-associated angiosarcoma of the breast: an international multicenter analysis. Surg Oncol 2022;41; https://doi.org/10.1016/j.suronc.2022.101726.

[16] Bentley H, Roberts J, Hayes M, et al. The role of imaging in the diagnosis of primary and secondary breast angiosarcoma: twenty-five-year experience of a provincial cancer Institution. Clin Breast Cancer 2023;23(2); https://doi.org/10.1016/j.clbc.2022.11.003.
[17] Vorburger SA, Xing Y, Hunt KK, et al. Angiosarcoma of the breast. Cancer 2005;104(12): 2682–8.
[18] Wienbeck S, Meyer HJ, Herzog A, et al. Imaging findings of primary breast sarcoma: results of a first multicenter study. Eur J Radiol 2017;88; https://doi.org/10.1016/j.ejrad.2016.12.020.
[19] Surov A, Holzhausen HJ, Ruschke K, et al. Primary breast sarcoma: prevalence, clinical signs, and radiological features. Acta radiol 2011;52(6); https://doi.org/10.1258/ar.2011.100468.
[20] Smith TB, Gilcrease MZ, Santiago L, et al. Imaging features of primary breast sarcoma. Am J Roentgenol 2012;198(4); https://doi.org/10.2214/AJR.11.7341.
[21] National Comprehensive Cancer Network. Soft Tissue Sarcoma (Version 1.2025). Available at: https://www.nccn.org/professionals/physician_gls/pdf/sarcoma.pdf. Accessed October 28, 2025.
[22] Kokkali S, Boukovinas I, de Bree E, et al. The impact of expert pathology review and molecular diagnostics on the management of sarcoma patients: a prospective study of the hellenic group of sarcomas and rare cancers. Cancers (Basel) 2024;16(13):2314.
[23] Eckardt MA, Siena NM, Copeland AR, et al. Dedicated review of sarcoma pathology is necessary for corroborative diagnosis in nearly one half of referred patients. Surgery 2025;188:109610; https://doi.org/10.1016/j.surg.2025.109610.
[24] Adem C, Reynolds C, Adlakha H, et al. Wide spectrum screening keratin as a marker of metaplastic spindle cell carcinoma of the breast: an immunohistochemical study of 24 patients. Histopathology 2002;40(6); https://doi.org/10.1046/j.1365-2559.2002.01417.x.
[25] Amin M, Edge S, Greene F. Chapter 41: AJCC cancer staging manual. 8th edition. New York (NY): Springer Cham; 2017. p. 507–16.
[26] Tanaka K, Ozaki T. New TNM classification (AJCC eighth edition) of bone and soft tissue sarcomas: JCOG bone and soft tissue tumor study group. Jpn J Clin Oncol 2019;49(2); https://doi.org/10.1093/jjco/hyy157.
[27] Brierley J, Gospodarowicz MD, Wittekind CT. TNM classification of malignant tumors International Union against cancer. 8th. Oxford, England: Wiley; 2017.
[28] Cates JMM. The AJCC 8th edition staging system for soft tissue sarcoma of the extremities or trunk: a cohort study of the SEER database. JNCCN Journal of the National Comprehensive Cancer Network 2018;16(2); https://doi.org/10.6004/jnccn.2017.7042.
[29] Basile G, Mattei JC, Alshaygy I, et al. Curability of patients with lymph node metastases from extremity soft-tissue sarcoma. Cancer 2020;126(23); https://doi.org/10.1002/cncr.33189.
[30] Ashamalla M, Guirguis A, Mokhtar BE, et al. Clinical presentation and patterns of care in SCARE soft tissue sarcoma. Int J Radiat Oncol Biol Phys 2017;99(2); https://doi.org/10.1016/j.ijrobp.2017.06.2403.
[31] WHO Classification of Tumours. Chapter 3: Breast Tumours. 5th EditionVol 2. Lyon, France: IARC Publications; 2019. p. 172–6.
[32] Tan PH, Ellis IO, Allison KH, et al. Malignant phyllodes tumours of the breast: the case for revising WHO's 'full house' diagnostic criteria. Histopathology 2025;87(2):169–82.
[33] McGowan TS, Cummings BJ, O'Sullivan B, et al. An analysis of 78 breast sarcoma patients without distant metastases at presentation. Int J Radiat Oncol Biol Phys 2000;46(2); https://doi.org/10.1016/S0360-3016(99)00444-7.
[34] Bousquet G, Confavreux C, Magné N, et al. Outcome and prognostic factors in breast sarcoma: a multicenter study from the rare cancer network. Radiother Oncol 2007;85(3); https://doi.org/10.1016/j.radonc.2007.10.015.

[35] McGregor GI, Knowling MA, Este FA. Sarcoma and cystosarcoma phyllodes tumors of the breast-A retrospective review of 58 cases. Am J Surg 1994;167(5); https://doi.org/10.1016/0002-9610(94)90238-0.
[36] Confavreux C, Lurkin A, Mitton N, et al. Sarcomas and malignant phyllodes tumours of the breast - a retrospective study. Eur J Cancer 2006;42(16); https://doi.org/10.1016/j.ejca.2006.05.040.
[37] Gutman H, Pollock RE, Ross MI, et al. Sarcoma of the breast: implications for extent of therapy. The M. D. Anderson experience. Surgery 1994;116(3).
[38] Christensen L, Schiodt T, Blichert-Toft M, et al. Sarcomas of the breast: a clinico-pathological study of 67 patients with long term follow-up. Eur J Surg Oncol 1988;14(3).
[39] Fields RC, Aft RL, Gillanders WE, et al. Treatment and outcomes of patients with primary breast sarcoma. Am J Surg 2008;196(4); https://doi.org/10.1016/j.amjsurg.2008.06.010.
[40] Gullett NP, Delman K, Folpe AL, et al. National surgical patterns of care: regional lymphadenectomy of breast sarcomas. Am J Clin Oncol: Cancer Clin Trials 2007;30(5); https://doi.org/10.1097/COC.0b013e31804b40f4.
[41] Crosby MA, Chike-Obi CJ, Baumann DP, et al. Reconstructive outcomes in patients with sarcoma of the breast. Plast Reconstr Surg 2010;126(6); https://doi.org/10.1097/PRS.0b013e3181f5276f.
[42] Kiefer J, Paidisetty P, Elmorsi RAI, et al. Contemporary trends in reconstruction for patients with sarcoma of the breast. J Surg Oncol 2025;131(6):1013–23.
[43] Pervaiz N, Colterjohn N, Farrokhyar F, et al. A systematic meta-analysis of randomized controlled trials of adjuvant chemotherapy for localized resectable soft-tissue sarcoma. Cancer 2008;113(3); https://doi.org/10.1002/cncr.23592.
[44] Maki RG, Wathen JK, Patel SR, et al. Randomized phase II study of gemcitabine and docetaxel compared with gemcitabine alone in patients with metastatic soft tissue sarcomas: results of sarcoma alliance for research through collaboration study 002. J Clin Oncol 2007;25(19); https://doi.org/10.1200/jco.2006.10.4117.
[45] Seddon B, Strauss SJ, Whelan J, et al. Gemcitabine and docetaxel versus doxorubicin as first-line treatment in previously untreated advanced unresectable or metastatic soft-tissue sarcomas (GeDDiS): a randomised controlled phase 3 trial. Lancet Oncol 2017;18(10); https://doi.org/10.1016/S1470-2045(17)30622-8.
[46] García-del-Muro X, López-Pousa A, Maurel J, et al. Randomized phase II study comparing gemcitabine plus dacarbazine versus dacarbazine alone in patients with previously treated soft tissue sarcoma: a Spanish group for research on sarcomas study. J Clin Oncol 2011;29(18); https://doi.org/10.1200/JCO.2010.33.6107.
[47] Penel N, Bui BN, Bay JO, et al. Phase II trial of weekly paclitaxel for unresectable angiosarcoma: the ANGIOTAX study. J Clin Oncol 2008;26(32); https://doi.org/10.1200/JCO.2008.17.3146.
[48] Fury MG, Antonescu CR, Van Zee K, et al. A 14-year retrospective review of angiosarcoma: clinical characteristics, prognostic factors, and treatment outcomes with surgery and chemotherapy. Cancer J 2005;11(3); https://doi.org/10.1097/00130404-200505000-00011.
[49] Sanfilippo R, Hindi N, Cruz Jurado J, et al. Effectiveness and safety of trabectedin and radiotherapy for patients with myxoid liposarcoma: a nonrandomized clinical trial. JAMA Oncol 2023;9(5); https://doi.org/10.1001/jamaoncol.2023.0056.
[50] Pautier P, Italiano A, Piperno-Neumann S, et al. Doxorubicin alone versus doxorubicin with trabectedin followed by trabectedin alone as first-line therapy for metastatic or unresectable leiomyosarcoma (LMS-04): a randomised, multicentre, open-label phase 3 trial. Lancet Oncol 2022;23(8); https://doi.org/10.1016/S1470-2045(22)00380-1.
[51] Gronchi A, Ferrari S, Quagliuolo V, et al. Histotype-tailored neoadjuvant chemotherapy versus standard chemotherapy in patients with high-risk soft-tissue sarcomas (ISG-STS 1001): an international, open-label, randomised, controlled, phase 3, multicentre trial. Lancet Oncol 2017;18(6); https://doi.org/10.1016/S1470-2045(17)30334-0.

[52] Barrow BJ, Janjan NA, Gutman H, et al. Role of radiotherapy in sarcoma of the breast - a retrospective review of the M.D. Anderson experience. Radiother Oncol 1999;52(2); https://doi.org/10.1016/S0167-8140(99)00070-5.
[53] Blanchard DK, Reynolds CA, Grant CS, et al. Primary nonphylloides breast sarcomas. Am J Surg 2003;186(4); https://doi.org/10.1016/S0002-9610(03)00269-1.
[54] Johnstone PAS, Pierce LJ, Merino MJ, et al. Primary soft tissue sarcomas of the breast: local-regional control with post-operative radiotherapy. Int J Radiat Oncol Biol Phys 1993;27(3); https://doi.org/10.1016/0360-3016(93)90395-C.
[55] Salerno KE, Alektiar KM, Baldini EH, et al. Radiation therapy for treatment of soft tissue sarcoma in adults: executive Summary of an ASTRO clinical practice guideline. Pract Radiat Oncol 2021;11(5); https://doi.org/10.1016/j.prro.2021.04.005.
[56] Depla AL, Scharloo-Karels CH, De Jong MAA, et al. Treatment and prognostic factors of radiation-associated angiosarcoma (RAAS) after primary breast cancer: a systematic review. Eur J Cancer 2014;50(10); https://doi.org/10.1016/j.ejca.2014.03.002.
[57] Brenn T, Fletcher CDM. Postradiation vascular proliferations: an increasing problem. Histopathology 2006;48(1); https://doi.org/10.1111/j.1365-2559.2005.02293.x.
[58] Li GZ, Fairweather M, Wang J, et al. Cutaneous radiation-associated breast angiosarcoma: radicality of surgery impacts survival. Ann Surg 2017;265(4).
[59] Billings SD, McKenney JK, Folpe AL, et al. Cutaneous angiosarcoma following breast-conserving surgery and radiation: an analysis of 27 cases. Am J Surg Pathol 2004;28(6); https://doi.org/10.1097/01.pas.0000126055.33916.0b.
[60] Lu Y, Chen Y, Zhu L, et al. Local recurrence of benign, borderline, and malignant phyllodes tumors of the breast: a systematic review and meta-analysis. Ann Surg Oncol 2019;26(5); https://doi.org/10.1245/s10434-018-07134-5.
[61] Toussaint A, Piaget-Rossel R, Stormacq C, et al. Width of margins in phyllodes tumors of the breast: the controversy drags on?—a systematic review and meta-analysis. Breast Cancer Res Treat 2021;185(1); https://doi.org/10.1007/s10549-020-05924-8.
[62] Van Olmen J, Beerthuizen A, Bekers E, et al. Management of benign phyllodes tumors: a Dutch population-based retrospective cohort between 1989 and 2022. Eur J Surg Oncol 2024;50(2); https://doi.org/10.1016/j.ejso.2023.107601.
[63] Bartels SAL, van Olmen JP, Scholten AN, et al. Real-world data on malignant and borderline phyllodes tumors of the breast: a population-based study of all 921 cases in the Netherlands (1989 –2020). Eur J Cancer 2024;201; https://doi.org/10.1016/j.ejca.2024.113924.
[64] National Comprehensive Cancer Network. Breast cancer. Phyllodes tumor (Version 5.2025). Available at: https://www.nccn.org/professionals/physician_gls/pdf/breast.pdf. Accessed November 11, 2025.
[65] Zeng S, Zhang X, Yang D, et al. Effects of adjuvant radiotherapy on borderline and malignant phyllodes tumors: a systematic review and meta-analysis. Mol Clin Oncol 2015;3(3); https://doi.org/10.3892/mco.2015.503.
[66] Zheng WH, Long ZQ, Kou J, et al. Postoperative radiation therapy in localized breast malignant phyllodes tumors: RPA-derived risk model identifies high-benefit subgroups with local control improvement. Breast 2025;84:104617; https://doi.org/10.1016/j.breast.2025.104617.
[67] Bonvalot S, Ternes N, Fiore M, et al. Spontaneous regression of primary abdominal wall desmoid tumors: more common than previously thought. Ann Surg Oncol 2013;20(13); https://doi.org/10.1245/s10434-013-3197-x.
[68] Kasper B, Baldini EH, Bonvalot S, et al. Current management of desmoid tumors. JAMA Oncol 2024;10(8):1121.
[69] Gounder M, Ratan R, Alcindor T, et al. Nirogacestat, a γ-secretase inhibitor for desmoid tumors. N Engl J Med 2023;388(10); https://doi.org/10.1056/nejmoa2210140.
[70] Gounder MM, Mahoney MR, Van Tine BA, et al. Sorafenib for advanced and refractory desmoid tumors. N Engl J Med 2018;379(25); https://doi.org/10.1056/nejmoa1805052.

[71] Alman B, Attia S, Baumgarten C, et al. The management of desmoid tumours: a joint global consensus-based guideline approach for adult and paediatric patients. Eur J Cancer 2020;127; https://doi.org/10.1016/j.ejca.2019.11.013.
[72] Sugiura H, Tsukushi S, Yoshida M, et al. What is the success of repeat surgical treatment of a local recurrence after initial wide resection of soft tissue sarcomas? Clin Orthop Relat Res 2018;476(9); https://doi.org/10.1007/s11999.0000000000000158.
[73] Torres MA, Ballo MT, Butler CE, et al. Management of locally recurrent soft-tissue sarcoma after prior surgery and radiation therapy. Int J Radiat Oncol Biol Phys 2007;67(4); https://doi.org/10.1016/j.ijrobp.2006.10.036.
[74] Gonzalez MR, Inchaustegui ML, Ruiz-Arellanos K, et al. Management of oligometastatic disease in soft tissue sarcomas. J Cancer Metastasis Treat 2023;9; https://doi.org/10.20517/2394-4722.2022.132.
[75] Pandey M, Mathew A, Abraham EK, et al. Primary sarcoma of the breast. J Surg Oncol 2004;87(3):121–5.
[76] Zelek L, Llombart-Cussac A, Terrier P, et al. Prognostic factors in primary breast sarcomas: a series of patients with long-term follow-up. J Clin Oncol 2003;21(13):2583–8.
[77] Danieli M, Gronchi A. Staging systems and nomograms for soft tissue sarcoma. Curr Oncol 2023;30(4); https://doi.org/10.3390/curroncol30040278.
[78] Tan PH, Thike AA, Tan WJ, et al. Predicting clinical behaviour of breast phyllodes tumours: a nomogram based on histological criteria and surgical margins. J Clin Pathol 2012;65(1); https://doi.org/10.1136/jclinpath-2011-200368.
[79] Ding P, Zhang L, Pei S, et al. Nomogram construction for overall survival in breast angiosarcoma based on clinicopathological features: a population-based cohort study. Discov Oncol 2025;16(1):351.

Advances in Surgery 60 (2026) 149–167

ADVANCES IN SURGERY

What Do Population-based Studies Tell Us about the Ideal Timing of Surgical Resection for Colorectal Cancer?

Adom Bondzi-Simpson, MD, MSc[a,*], Julie Hallet, MD, MSc[b]

[a]Department of Surgery, University of Toronto, Toronto, Ontario, Canada; [b]Division of General Surgery, Department of Surgery, University of Toronto, Toronto, Ontario, Canada

Keywords

• Wait time • Surgical delay • Treatment delay • Colorectal cancer • Health services research • Health systems • Quality monitoring • Quality indicator

Key points

- Population-based studies provide the strongest evidence on wait times for colorectal cancer surgery, offering robust, generalizable estimates that challenge long-standing assumptions about timging of surgery.
- For stage I to III colon cancer, wait times of 30 to 45 days from the decision to treat are safe and do not compromise survival.
- Rectal cancer requires individualized timing after neoadjuvant therapy; surgery at 6 to 12 weeks, balances tumor regression, technical feasibility, and opportunities for organ preservation.
- Wait-time targets should function as flexible, evidence-informed quality indicators. Rigid historical benchmarks, often policy-driven rather than biologically grounded, may distort system behavior without improving outcomes.
- The waiting period itself is an opportunity for intervention. Prehabilitation, optimized nutrition, psychosocial support, and patient navigation can improve readiness, experience, and outcomes.

*Corresponding author. Department of Surgery, University of Toronto, Stewart Building, 139 College Street, 5th Floor, Toronto, Ontario, M5T 1P5, Canada. *E-mail address:* adom.bondzisimpson@mail.utoronto.ca

https://doi.org/10.1016/j.yasu.2026.03.014

Abbreviations

COVID-19	coronavirus disease 2019
CRC	colorectal cancer
GP	general practitioner
MDT	multidisciplinary tumor board
NCDB	National Cancer Database
NOM	nonoperative management
OR	operating room
OS	overall survival
SEER	Surveillance, Epidemiology, and End Results
TNT	total neoadjuvant therapy
UK	United Kingdom
US	United States of America
WTs	wait times

INTRODUCTION

Importance of wait times

At the turn of the twenty-first century, the Institute of Medicine outlined a framework that would shape contemporary health care quality monitoring systems [1,2]. Its 6 pillars–safe, effective, patient-centered, efficient, equitable, and timely care–established timeliness not merely as a matter of system efficiency, but also as a core dimension of quality. Since then, health systems have increasingly prioritized the measurement, reporting, and improvement of wait times (WTs), particularly for elective and time-sensitive cancer surgery.

For patients, surgeons, and health systems globally, WTs for elective cancer surgery represent a critical component of health care performance [3–5]. Timely surgery is valued not only to mitigate concerns about disease progression and survival but also to reduce anxiety for patients and families navigating the uncertainty between diagnosis and treatment [6,7]. As a result, a range of WT targets have been implemented across health systems, with public reporting at the level of surgeons, hospitals, networks, and national authorities [8].

Globally, colorectal cancer (CRC) is the third most common malignancy worldwide [9]. Given the high burden of disease and well-defined treatment pathways, CRC is often one of the first cancer sites targeted by health care systems globally for quality improvement strategies [10,11]. Surgical resection is a mainstay of curative-intent therapy [12,13]. Therefore, the analysis of WTs in CRC surgery is an effective model for exploring the construct of delivery of timely care. Gaining clarity on how we conceptualize, validate, and report WTs for elective surgery will aid surgeons and health systems to ensure high-quality care for patients and their families.

Historical context: the "Two-Week Wait" referral pathway in the National Health Services

In 2000, the United Kingdom implemented the National Health Service Cancer Plan, which included the introduction of the "Two-Week Wait" referral pathway [14]. Designed to expedite evaluation of patients with alarm symptoms, the policy sought to ensure rapid diagnosis and timely initiation of therapy. The plan formally introduced 2 additional targets: (1) definitive treatment within 31 days of the decision to treat, and (2) treatment within 62 days of referral from primary care [14,15]. These intervals were justified by the assumptions that faster diagnosis would lead to earlier stage disease and that shorter waits might alleviate anxiety.

These policy-driven targets–rather than biologically informed evidence–were subsequently adopted or adapted across health systems in Europe (United Kingdom, Denmark, the Netherlands, Switzerland, and New Zealand) and North America (Canada and the United States of America). More than 2 decades later, key questions remain: How has the evidence evolved since these standards were introduced? Do current WT targets meaningfully influence oncologic or patient-centered outcomes? And how should targets be refined to optimize the quality of care?

Why population-based studies are vital

Population-based studies leverage comprehensive health administrative datasets that capture health care encounters, treatments, outcomes, and long-term follow-up for residents within a defined jurisdiction (local, regional, and national levels). These datasets offer unique strengths for evaluating WTs: they reflect real-world practice, minimize selection bias, and provide sufficiently large sample sizes to detect clinically meaningful associations. As such, population-level analyses represent the most robust method for examining whether delays to curative-intent CRC surgery influence survival or other outcomes.

This article explores the question: What do population-based studies tell us about the ideal timing of surgical resection for CRC? To establish this, we first examine how WTs are conceptualized and defined (Table 1).

FRAMEWORK FOR CONCEPTUALIZING WAIT TIMES IN COLORECTAL CANCER SURGERY

Conceptualizing and Defining Wait Times

Understanding WT for curative-intent CRC surgery requires mapping the patient journey from symptom onset (or screening detection) to operative intervention. Numerous intervals exist along this continuum, including the diagnostic phase, referral processes, multidisciplinary assessments, staging investigations, and surgical planning.

The Aarhus statement classifies WT into 3 broad intervals [16,17].

1. *Primary care interval*: from first cancer-related contact with a general practitioner to referral to secondary care.
2. *Referral interval*: from referral to histologic diagnosis.
3. *Treatment interval:* from diagnosis to initiation of treatment.

Fig. 1 outlines WT intervals with reference to those typically and not-typically captured within health administrative databases. Population-based

Table 1
Conceptual definitions and commonly used wait time intervals in colorectal cancer care

Wait time interval	Definition	Typical anchor dates	Commonly captured in administrative data?	Primary system lever
Primary care interval	Time from first cancer-related symptom or screening abnormality to referral to secondary care	Symptom onset → GP referral	Rarely	Primary care access and screening programs
Referral interval	Time from referral to endoscopic/histologic diagnosis	GP referral → biopsy/pathology	Inconsistently	Diagnostic capacity and endoscopy access
Treatment interval	Time from diagnosis to initiation of treatment	Diagnosis → surgery or neoadjuvant therapy	Commonly	Surgical capacity and system throughput
Decision-to-treat interval	Time from formal decision to treat to surgery	Consent/MDT decision → surgery	Commonly (Canada, UK)	OR availability and scheduling efficiency
Diagnosis-to-surgery interval	Time from pathologic diagnosis to surgical resection	Pathology date → surgery	Common in research	Composite system performance

Abbreviations: GP, general practitioner; MDT, multidisciplinary tumor board; OR, operating room; UK, United Kingdom.

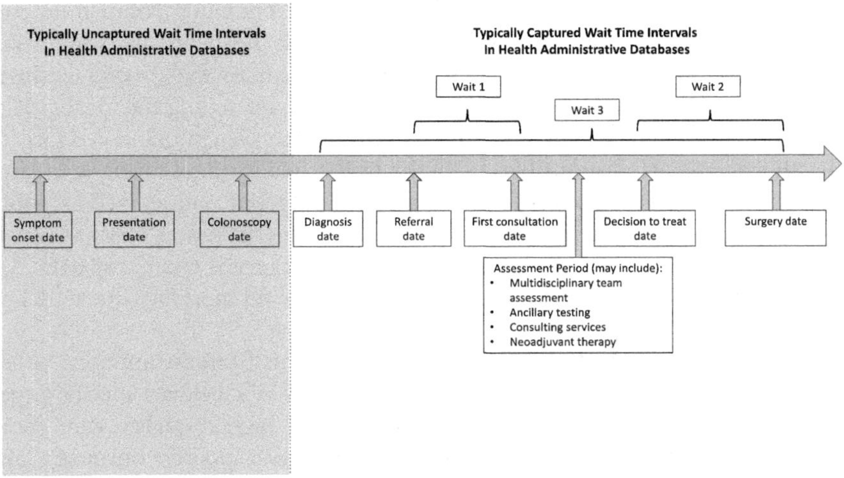

Fig. 1. Key wait-time intervals along the colorectal cancer care continuum and their capture within health administrative databases. This schematic illustrates the major time points along the patient journey from symptom onset (or screening detection) to definitive surgical treatment. The continuum includes symptom onset (variably captured), first presentation to a primary care provider, referral to specialist care, diagnostic testing and histologic confirmation, decision-to-treat date (formal consent and surgical planning), and date of surgery. Health administrative datasets typically capture only portions of these intervals—most reliably the diagnostic and treatment intervals (eg, diagnosis-to-surgery and decision-to-treat-to-surgery). "Wait 1" and "Wait 2" represent commonly monitored intervals within quality-reporting systems in Canada and in many countries in Western Europe. "Wait 3" reflects intervals typically examined in observational research using administrative data. Some dates may overlap depending on clinical scenario.

datasets traditionally capture only some of these intervals–typically the treatment interval and portions of the diagnostic trajectory. These captured intervals represent the segments most directly influenced by health-system performance and resource allocation.

WT metrics are, thus, not simply measures of elapsed time; they represent actionable windows through which surgeons, hospitals, and health systems understand and optimize performance. Achieving or failing to meet WT targets drives quality improvement efforts, shapes resource distribution, and influences patient and provider expectations in systems globally [18–25]. Therefore, what constitutes an *appropriate* WT target has profound implications for system design, policy-making, and patient outcomes.

What Constitutes "Ideal Timing" for Surgery

The ideal timing of elective surgery is dependent on several factors that consider the patient, the surgeon, and the health care system. Patients who experience disease and its associated quality-of-life impacts have both (1) expectations of timeliness as a health services user and (2) the desire to have the best possible outcomes. Surgeon must balance possible tensions between patient expectations of timely and high-quality care with operating room time constraints, and case volume/surgical backlogs. While hospitals are responsible for building and distributing operating room resources that maximize high-quality care. Furthermore, hospitals are responsible for setting the local quality improvement agenda to improve adherence to health system mandated targets. Health systems are responsible for building the quality monitoring standards including setting WT targets for hospitals and surgeons and as well as public reporting and accountability (Fig. 2). Therefore, the definition of what constitutes "ideal" or "appropriate" WTs for elective surgery is context-specific. Ultimately, this process balances the risk of morbidity and mortality due to delays to surgery with system capacity.

In cancer surgery, WT in quality monitoring stems from assumptions of better cancer control and access to care. Shorter WT, or WT below a specific target, is assumed to provide better cancer control and higher quality care [3–5]. Conversely delays in care may be associated with poorer oncologic and patient-centered outcomes. Therefore, our current knowledge of ideal WTs for elective CRC surgery stems from studies exploring associations of delays to surgery with outcomes of interest to patients, surgeons, and health systems.

Current Knowledge

The strongest evidence exploring the appropriate timing for curative-intent CRC surgery comes from population-based studies, multiinstitutional

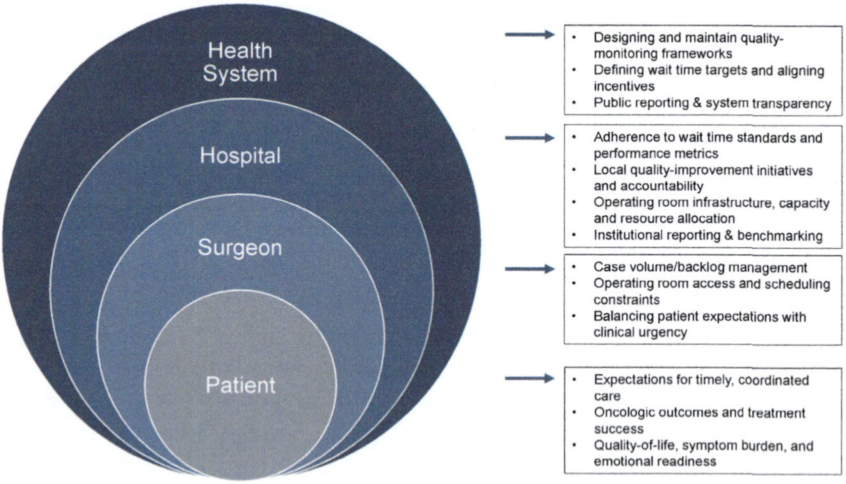

Fig. 2. Multilevel considerations influencing wait times for curative-intent colorectal cancer surgery across patients, surgeons, hospitals, and health systems. This figure depicts the distinct but interrelated factors shaping timely access to CRC surgery across 4 levels including the patient, surgeon, hospital, and health system. Together, these domains illustrate how "ideal timing" for elective cancer surgery is shaped not only by clinical urgency but also by broader structural and operational factors across the cancer care system.

observational studies or randomized control trials [26–34]. However, the majority of studies in this field has typically relied on small single institutional studies with varying estimates. These studies have often blended colon and rectal cancer subtypes in their analysis. However, recognizing the difference in treatment paradigms, patterns of referral, and tumor biology with these distinct entities, WTs for colon and rectal cancer should be analyzed separately. With neoadjuvant therapy increasingly being considered in rectal cancer and with ever more emphasis on organ preservation, WTs for rectal cancer may be distinctly different to colon cancer as providers continue to delay surgery to assess tumor response to therapy [35,36].

Historical consensus taking in to account the genetic pathways and pathogenesis of CRC is that this disease represents a slow growing process. Through the adenoma-adenocarcinoma sequence malignancy may take up to 15 years from onset to eventual malignancy [37,38]. Therefore, traditionally, surgeons have not conceptualized WTs to elective cancer surgery (which happens in the order of weeks to months) as having a significant effect on disease progression (which happens in the order of years to decades). Extending this logic, surgeons have not traditionally conceptualized longer WT to elective CRC surgery with poorer survival. In colon cancer, studies have largely failed to demonstrate clear associations between increasing WT intervals and survival [29,34,39–41]. Despite this, health systems across North America and Europe have utilized a 14 to 30 day window for WT from either the date of diagnosis or date of "decision to treat" [22–25,42]. This decision reflects the goal to expedite surgery for curative-intent CRC as these patients may "need it most," which ultimately serves as a marker of system efficiency. The premise underpinning these decisions can likely be traced back to original conceptions of the Two-Week Wait referral pathway in the United Kingdom in the 2000s where the goal was to have quick diagnosis for earlier stage disease and reduce patient anxiety [14,15].

Unlike colon cancer, rectal cancer timing is often dictated by multimodal therapy. The interval between neoadjuvant chemoradiation and surgery influences tumor regression, downstaging, and the feasibility organ preservation. Therefore, in rectal cancer, WTs have primarily focused on appropriate timing after neoadjuvant therapy [31–33,43–47]. Traditional guidance recommended resection at 6 to 8 weeks [31,33,44,46]. Although, more contemporary studies have observed added benefit for up to 12 weeks or slightly beyond [43,45,47,48]. Given these complexities, defining a universal WT target for rectal cancer is problematic. Ideal timing is necessarily individualized and anchored in treatment sequencing and goals of care.

Why Population-Based Evidence Matters

Despite traditional dogma often relying on smaller single-institution studies, these studies may be prone to bias and may not capture the true signal for entire populations. Furthermore, less often is this question of the ideal WT to curative-intent cancer surgery solvable with a randomized control trial.

Therefore, population-based studies are a powerful tool for inferring ideal timing for elective cancer surgery (Table 2). Drawing on the large statistical power of health administrative datasets to explore associations between wait intervals and oncologic and patient-centered outcomes, allows surgeons and health systems to appraise the ideal or acceptable WTs. Next, we will discuss specifically what population-based studies tell us about the ideal timing of elective curative-intent surgical resection in CRC.

DISCUSSION

Important lessons from the coronavirus disease 2019 pandemic

The coronavirus disease 2019 (COVID-19) pandemic provided an interesting natural experiment. As health systems were strained and resources allocated toward the acute global pandemic, health systems were challenged with finding the sweet spot for WTs that balanced immediate health care needs versus acceptable oncologic outcomes. During this period, cancer surgeries were delayed beyond usual WT targets. Therefore, this context renewed interest in understanding the association between delays in cancer surgery and survival, particularly for common malignancies such as CRC.

Early in the pandemic, preliminary reports and meta-analyses suggested that treatment delays of 4 to 12 weeks could result in poorer survival [6,49,50]. However, these studies largely relayed on single-institutional retrospective studies from historical cohorts. As higher quality data accrued, a more nuanced picture emerged. Using population-based estimates from the Surveillance, Epidemiology, and End Results (SEER) database, Min and colleagues [51] found no effect of intermediate (1–2 months) or longer (3–6 months) treatment delays on overall or cancer-specific survival. Similarly, in Manitoba, Canada, Lambert and colleagues [52] used an interrupted time series to determine when observed cancer survival deviated from expected trends during the pandemic. Despite substantial disruption to surgical services during this time period, they observed no measurable impact of pandemic-related delays on 1 year overall survival for colon or rectal cancer.

Multi-institutional prospective cohorts complemented these population-based observations. Data from Italy (the COVID-Delay study) and the international COVIDSurg Collaborative showed a substantial drop in early stage CRC diagnoses but did not identify a clear association between surgical delay and short-term oncologic surrogates such as resectability or completeness of resection [53,54]. Together, these findings challenge simple assumptions that any deviation from traditional WT benchmarks necessarily translates into worse oncologic outcomes.

Taken together, 2 key lessons from the COVID-19 era emerge for CRC surgery. First, population-based studies provide more robust and generalizable estimates of the impact of surgical delay on cancer survival than small single-center series and should be prioritized when setting or revising WT standards. Second, current WT targets–many of which were designed in the early 2000s based on policy priorities rather than formal outcomes-based validation–may

Table 2
Population-based evidence linking surgical wait time and survival in colorectal cancer

Study/Region	Data source	Population	Wait time definition	Key survival finding
Grass et al, [27] 2020 (USA)	NCDB	Colon, stage I–III	Diagnosis → surgery	Worse survival beyond ~40 d
Kucejko et al, [30] 2020 (USA)	NCDB + SEER-Medicare	Colon, stage I–III	Diagnosis → surgery	Worse survival >7 wk
Bondzi-Simpson et al, [26] 2025 (Canada)	Ontario administrative data	CRC, stage I–III	Decision to treat → surgery	No survival benefit <28 d; worse survival >45 d
Castelo et al, [55] 2023 (Canada)	Ontario administrative data	CRC <50 y	Presentation → treatment	No association with OS
Iversen et al, [34] 2009 (Denmark)	National registry	Colon and rectal	First contact[a] → treatment	Delays of >60 d may affect rectal, not colon cancer survival
Strous et al, [28] 2024 (Netherlands)	Multicenter cohort	Colon	Diagnosis → surgery	Delays up to 49 d are noninferior for cancer-free survival
Yun et al, [29] 2012 (Korea)	National database	Colon and rectal	Diagnosis → surgery	Colon safe; rectal worse with delay of >28 d

Abbreviations: CRC, colorectal cancer; NCDB, National Cancer Database; OS, overall survival; SEER, Surveillance, Epidemiology, and End Results; US, United States of America.

[a]First contact defined as date of first contact with physician in health care system related to cancer diagnosis.

not represent biologically meaningful thresholds for survival. To maintain the relevance and effectiveness of WT monitoring as a quality indicator, traditional targets must be revisited and, where appropriate, recalibrated in light of contemporary population-based evidence.

Global contemporary landscape of wait time and survival in colorectal cancer

Examining population-based studies across jurisdictions provides a more complete understanding of how delays to curative-intent CRC surgery relate to survival and where there may be safe latitude for flexibility.

In the United States, population-level analyses of WTs for colon cancer surgery have primarily leveraged the National Cancer Database (NCDB), SEER-Medicare, and Veterans Affairs data. In the largest study to date (n = 118,504), Grass and colleagues [27] evaluated the association between time from diagnosis to surgery and survival in stage I to III colon cancer using NCDB data. They observed a 6% increase in the hazard of death for every 14 day delay and identified an inflection point in risk beyond approximately 40 days. Kucejko and colleagues [30] combined NCDB and SEER-Medicare data (n = 46,649) and similarly reported increased hazard of death associated with surgical delays beyond 7 weeks. These US data suggest that while some delay is tolerable, prolonged deferral of surgery may eventually impact survival.

Single-payer systems such as Canada, the United Kingdom, and several European countries offer complementary insights. In these settings, universal coverage and comprehensive cancer registries allow capture of all encounters and longitudinal follow-up, making them well suited for evaluating "real-world" WTs and outcomes at a population level.

Using health administrative data in Ontario, Canada's most populous province, we recently evaluated the association between WT to curative-intent CRC surgery and overall survival, and the relationship between meeting traditional (<28 days) versus new data-informed targets and survival [26]. Among 35,533 patients with stage I to III CRC, increasing time from decision to operate to surgery was associated with higher hazard of death, with the most pronounced increase beyond 45 days. After adjustment for confounders, undergoing surgery within the traditional 28 day target was not associated with improved overall survival. In contrast, surgery within a new, less stringent 45 day target was independently associated with a 10% reduction in the hazard of death. Put differently, missing the traditional 28 day benchmark did not translate into worse outcomes, but missing a 45 day threshold did. Castelo and colleagues [55] similarly examined time from presentation to treatment in adults aged younger than 50 years with CRC in Ontario and found that longer time to treatment was not associated with adverse overall or cause-specific survival. These findings collectively support the notion that WT targets can be made more flexible without compromising survival, at least for selected populations.

European data have further shaped our understanding of acceptable delays. In Denmark, Iversen and colleagues [34] demonstrated that provider delays (from first physician contact to treatment) and hospital delays (from referral to treatment) of at least 60 days did not adversely impact CRC survival in aggregate. In the Netherlands, a multi-institutional cohort study found that a prolonged treatment interval–even beyond 49 days–was noninferior for cancer-free survival compared with the national target of 35 days or less [28]. These findings informed a shift away from rigid benchmarks: current Dutch guidelines now recommend that 80% of patients be treated within 35 days, with a national upper limit of 49 days, reflecting a more directional, data-driven approach to targets rather than a single inflexible cutoff [40].

In Asia, Yun and colleagues examined the impact of surgical treatment delay in Korea, defining "delay" as definitive resection more than 1 month after diagnosis [29]. They found no association between delay and 5 year overall survival in colon cancer after adjustment, but identified worse 5 year survival in rectal cancer with prolonged delays. This divergence underscores important biological and treatment-pathway differences between colon and rectal cancer and supports analyzing these entities separately when defining or interpreting WT standards.

Taken together, while single-center series have reported heterogeneous associations between delay and survival and have often attributed safe outcomes to appropriate prioritization and triage [39–41], population-based studies provide a more robust and generalizable picture. They suggest that for stage I to III colon cancer, moderate delays within a 30 to 45 day window from decision to treat are unlikely to compromise survival, whereas excessive delays may carry risk. For rectal cancer, the relationship between timing, neoadjuvant therapy, and surgical outcomes is more complex and requires a tailored approach. From a health system perspective, these data support moving away from overly rigid, historically derived targets toward evidence-informed, flexible windows that remain safe for patients while allowing more pragmatic management of competing demands for operative resources (Table 3).

FUTURE CONSIDERATIONS

Key conceptual questions for wait time targets

Several conceptual questions must be addressed to refine WT targets for curative-intent cancer surgery in the future.

First, *when should the clock start?* The choice of anchor point–symptom onset, first primary care contact, date of referral, date of diagnosis, or decision to treat–has major implications for both measurement and interpretation. To date, most research has used diagnosis-to-surgery intervals, whereas many health systems, particularly in Europe and Canada, monitor WT from (1) first general practitioner presentation to specialist consultation (referral interval) and (2) decision to treat to surgery (time-to-treatment interval). Clarifying the rationale for the chosen interval is essential: different stages of the cancer care continuum reflect distinct system functions (access to primary care,

Table 3
Evidence-informed interpretation of wait time targets by disease site

Cancer site	Clinical context	Evidence-supported timing window	Key considerations
Colon cancer	Stage I–III, curative intent	~30–49 d from decision to treat	Moderate "delays" safe; excessive delays may increase mortality
Rectal cancer	Postneoadjuvant chemoradiation	~6–12 wk after completion	Tumor response, organ preservation, and technical difficulty
Rectal cancer (TNT/NOM)	Total neoadjuvant therapy or watch-and-wait	Highly individualized	Distinguish intentional delay from system failure
All CRC	Prehabilitation window	Variable within safe interval	Opportunity for fitness, nutrition, and psychosocial optimization

Abbreviations: CRC, colorectal cancer; NOM, nonoperative management; TNT, total neoadjuvant therapy.

diagnostic capacity, and surgical throughput) and will respond to different policy levers. Health administrative databases must, therefore, be designed to capture multiple key dates along the continuum to enable meaningful interval-specific analyses and policy development.

Second, *what outcome are we trying to influence?* Much of the existing literature links WTs to overall or cancer-specific survival. While survival is fundamental for evaluating oncologic safety, it does not capture the full patient experience or the broader goals of timely care. Future research should explicitly link specific intervals to other relevant outcomes, including pathologic stage migration, margin status, perioperative morbidity, quality of life, psychological distress, and patient-reported outcomes and experience. Clear articulation of which outcome a given target is intended to influence and why will be critical for interpretation and for designing interventions that are both clinically meaningful and patient-centered.

Third, *which biological and treatment factors should shape targets?* Current WT standards frequently apply a "one-size-fits-all" approach across multiple cancer types and stages. Yet CRC is heterogeneous: colon and rectal cancer differ in natural history, patterns of spread, and treatment paradigms; stage impacts urgency and potential benefit of earlier intervention; and surgical intent (curative vs palliative) further modifies priorities. Future target-setting should consider disease site, stage, and treatment pathway explicitly, with an emphasis on stage I to III curative-intent disease where surgical delay is most relevant.

Fourth, *how should neoadjuvant therapy be incorporated?* For rectal cancer in particular, the concept of WT cannot be reduced to a single interval. "Delays" after chemoradiation may reflect deliberate clinical decisions to maximize tumor response and enable organ preservation, rather than system failure [35,36]. At the same time, excessively prolonged intervals may increase technical

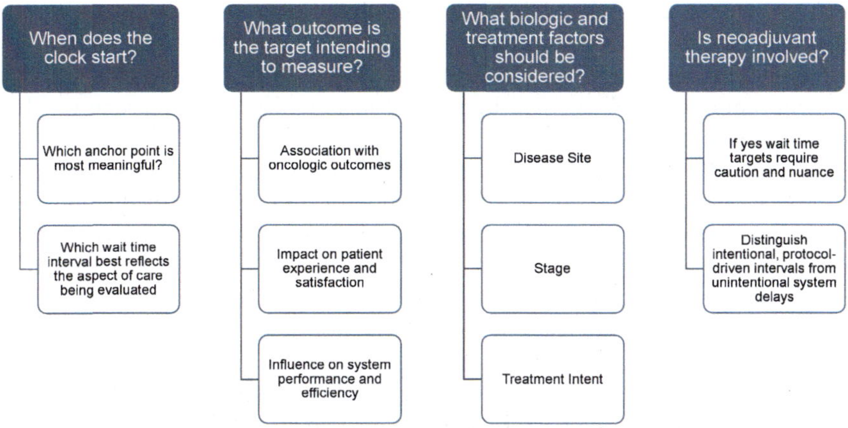

Fig. 3. Left to right. Four key conceptual questions required to refine future wait-time targets for curative-intent colorectal cancer surgery. This framework outlines the foundational questions that must be addressed to develop biologically plausible, clinically meaningful, and system-responsive wait-time standards: When should the clock start? Selecting the appropriate anchor point (example symptom onset, first primary care contact, referral, diagnosis, or decision-to-treat) determines what aspect of system performance is being measured and which policy levers apply. What outcome is the target intended to influence? Beyond survival, wait-time targets should reflect associations with stage migration, margin status, perioperative morbidity, psychological distress, patient experience, and other relevant endpoint(s). Which biological and treatment factors should shape the target? Differences in tumor biology, disease site (colon vs rectal), stage, and treatment sequencing (eg, curative vs palliative intent) require nuance rather than "one-size-fits-all" thresholds. Is neoadjuvant therapy involved? In rectal cancer, intervals after chemoradiation may reflect intentional oncologic strategy (eg, maximizing response for organ preservation) rather than system delay. Metrics must distinguish planned, protocol-driven timing from unintentional postponement. Collectively, these questions provide the conceptual scaffolding for future wait-time indicators that are evidence-informed, clinically coherent, and operationally feasible.

difficulty of surgery, complicate recovery in a radiated field, or risk tumor regrowth. As total neoadjuvant therapy becomes more common and nonoperative management strategies expand, WT metrics will need to distinguish between intentional, protocolized delays and unintended system-driven postponements (Fig. 3).

Gaps in knowledge priorities for future research

Addressing existing evidence gaps will be essential for refining WT standards and ensuring they function as useful quality indicators rather than blunt performance metrics.

First, *prediagnostic intervals remain underexplored*, despite their likely impact on stage at presentation and long-term outcomes. The period from symptom onset to first presentation, referral time to colonoscopy, and time from endoscopy to histologic diagnosis are challenging to capture in administrative data, but they reflect broader issues of access, health literacy, and primary care capacity. In many systems, these intervals likely contribute more to stage migration and survival than modest variation in postdiagnosis surgical WTs. Methodological work–potentially integrating electronic medical records, primary care data, and patient-reported timelines–will be needed to quantify and intervene on these earlier delays.

Second, *WT targets must be developed explicitly as quality indicators, not simply operational benchmarks.* Targeting is a cornerstone of performance evaluation: it allows continuous monitoring, benchmarking within and across systems, identification of unwarranted variation, and design of quality improvement strategies [56–58]. Robust indicators should be reliable, valid, and actionable at the point of care [59–61]. They should demonstrate variation among hospitals, health networks, or surgeons, and be meaningfully associated with outcomes. This has important implications for health systems. For example, if the WT targets are too strict, health care providers will be under pressure to meet them. Resources may be diverted toward achieving those WT targets, and thus not available for other activities. Conversely, if the WT targets are too permissive, patients risk getting surgery too late and their long-term outcomes may be compromised. Systems may be considered as efficient even though outcomes are not optimal, and lower quality care may be overlooked. Future research should, therefore, focus on developing and validating WT indicators using transparent methods, with explicit justification for thresholds, ranges, and performance categories.

Third, *more research is needed to understand who meets or misses targets, and why.* Once targets are appropriately defined, population-based studies can characterize patient-level, provider-level, and system-level factors associated with adherence or nonadherence [62–65]. This includes examining the influence of socioeconomic status, geography, comorbidity, hospital volume, and organizational structures on WT performance. Such analyses will not only reveal inequities in timely care but also identify modifiable levers for improvement from scheduling practices and diagnostic pathways to regional resource allocation.

Fourth, *we must reimagine what can be achieved during the waiting period itself.* Emerging evidence suggests that, within safe windows, more flexible WT targets for CRC do not compromise survival [26–28,30,55]. This creates an opportunity to reorient some system effort from relentlessly shortening waits toward enhancing what happens while patients wait. Prehabilitation and structured exercise interventions have been shown to improve outcomes for patients undergoing CRC surgery [40,66]. At the same time, patient navigation programs can provide substantial support to patients and families through education, coordination of care, and advance care planning [67]. Conceptualizing the waiting period as an active phase of preparation–physical, nutritional, psychological, and logistical–may offer greater gains in patient-centered outcomes than marginal reductions in already acceptable WTs.

Collectively, these future directions point toward a more sophisticated approach to WTs: one that integrates biologic plausibility, population-based evidence, and patient-centered priorities; distinguishes between harmful delay and intentional, protocol-driven timing; and leverages the waiting interval as a window for meaningful intervention rather than merely a metric to be compressed.

SUMMARY

The contemporary evidence from population-based studies challenges long-standing assumptions about the urgency of surgical resection for CRC and provides a more nuanced understanding of what constitutes "ideal timing." For colon cancer, whole-population analyses consistently demonstrate that moderate delays typically within a 30 to 45 day window from the decision to treat do not compromise overall survival. These findings stand in contrast to historical targets such as the 14 or 28 day benchmarks, which were largely policy-driven rather than biologically informed. By anchoring target-setting in outcomes-based evidence rather than historical convention, health systems can adopt wait-time standards that are both clinically defensible and operationally achievable.

Rectal cancer requires a more tailored approach. Here, "timing" is intimately tied to treatment sequencing and the biological effects of neoadjuvant therapy. Population-based and multi-institutional data reinforce that surgery approximately 6 to 12 weeks after chemoradiation is safe, and in some settings potentially advantageous, though excessively prolonged intervals may increase technical difficulty and risk overtreatment in patients eligible for organ-preserving strategies. Thus, ideal timing in rectal cancer is inherently individualized and must incorporate tumor response, planned treatment pathway, and the broader goals of care.

Taken together, these insights underscore that WTs should be conceptualized not as rigid thresholds but as directional, evidence-informed quality indicators that balance patient experience, oncologic safety, and system capacity. Population-based data offer unique methodological advantages for setting such targets: they reflect real-world practice, capture entire cancer populations, and provide robust estimates of the relationship between delay and outcome. As health systems evolve, WTs should be integrated with broader measures of quality including patient-centered outcomes, access to care, and opportunities for prehabilitation and leveraged to drive improvements not only in *when* surgery occurs, but *what patients experience* while they wait. Ultimately, the ideal timing of CRC surgery is both a clinical and system-level construct, best defined through rigorous evidence and applied with flexibility, nuance, and an unwavering commitment to high-quality cancer care.

CLINIC CARE POINTS

- *Define the WT interval clearly and consistently*: WT conclusions depend heavily on *where the clock starts* (diagnosis, referral, and decision to treat); misalignment leads to erroneous comparisons and misguided targets.

- *Use population-based evidence to guide expectations:* Large administrative datasets capture real-world patterns, minimize selection bias, and provide the most reliable estimates of the effect of delay on survival.
- *Distinguish colon from rectal cancer—timing considerations are fundamentally different:* Colon cancer timing is shaped by system capacity and operative prioritization, whereas rectal cancer timing is influenced by tumor biology, neoadjuvant response, organ-preservation goals, and technical considerations in a radiated field.
- *For stage I to III colon cancer, moderate WTs are safe:* Population-based studies support *30 to 45 days* from decision to treat as a clinically acceptable window that does not compromise overall survival.
- *Avoid rigid adherence to historical targets:* Traditional 14 to 28 day benchmarks were policy-driven rather than evidence-based; overly strict targets may distort system behavior without improving outcomes.
- *For rectal cancer after chemoradiation, timing should be individualized:* Most evidence supports surgery at *6 to 12 weeks,* balancing tumor regression, technical feasibility, and goals of organ preservation.
- *Recognize pitfalls of interpreting delays in isolation:* Apparent "long waits" may reflect appropriate sequencing (eg, optimization and prehabilitation) rather than system failure, and may not represent poorer-quality care.
- *Use WT data as an actionable quality indicator:* Targets should be reliable, valid, and actionable at the hospital or surgeon level, enabling benchmarking, resource allocation, and continuous quality improvement.
- *Leverage the waiting period to improve outcomes:* Prehabilitation, nutrition optimization, psychosocial support, and patient navigation can meaningfully improve patient readiness and experience, particularly when evidence supports more flexible WT windows.
- *Monitor for inequities in meeting WT targets:* Monitor for disparities in meeting WT targets by patient groups; underserved groups may systematically face longer waits and poorer outcomes despite population-level safety signals.

Funding

This work was supported by the Sunnybrook Health Sciences Centre AFP Innovation Fund.

Disclosure

The authors have nothing to disclose.

References

1 Institute of Medicine (US) Committee on Quality of Health Care in America. To err is human: building a safer health system. In: Kohn LT, Corrigan JM, Donaldson MS, editors. Washington (DC): National Academies Press (US); 2000.

2 Institute of Medicine (US) Committee on Quality of Health Care in America. Crossing the quality chasm: a new health system for the 21st century. Washington (DC): National Academies Press (US); 2001.

[3] Elkomy S, Cookson G. Performance management strategy: waiting time in the English national health services. Public Organ Rev 2020;20(1):95–112.

[4] McIntyre D, Chow CK. Waiting time as an indicator for health services under strain: a narrative review. INQUIRY: The Journal of Health Care Organization, Provision, and Financing 2020;57:0046958020910305.
[5] Stoop AP, Vrangbæk K, Berg M. Theory and practice of waiting time data as a performance indicator in health care: a case study from the Netherlands. Health Policy 2005;73(1):41–51.
[6] Whittaker TM, Abdelrazek MEG, Fitzpatrick AJ, et al. Delay to elective colorectal cancer surgery and implications for survival: a systematic review and meta-analysis. Colorectal Dis 2021;23(7):1699–711.
[7] Hanna TP, King WD, Thibodeau S, et al. Mortality due to cancer treatment delay: systematic review and meta-analysis. Br Med J 2020;371:m4087.
[8] Rechel B, McKee M, Haas M, et al. Public reporting on quality, waiting times and patient experience in 11 high-income countries. Health Policy 2016;120(4):377–83.
[9] Morgan E, Arnold M, Gini A, et al. Global burden of colorectal cancer in 2020 and 2040: incidence and mortality estimates from GLOBOCAN. Gut 2023;72(2):338–44.
[10] Xi Y, Xu P. Global colorectal cancer burden in 2020 and projections to 2040. Transl Oncol 2021;14(10):101174.
[11] Global, regional, and national burden of colorectal cancer and its risk factors, 1990-2019: a systematic analysis for the global burden of disease study 2019. Lancet Gastroenterol Hepatol 2022;7(7):627–47.
[12] Mahmoud N, Bullard Dunn K. Metastasectomy for stage IV colorectal cancer. Dis Colon Rectum 2010;53(7):1080–92.
[13] van den Berg I, Coebergh van den Braak RRJ, van Vugt JLA, et al. Actual survival after resection of primary colorectal cancer: results from a prospective multicenter study. World J Surg Oncol 2021;19(1):96.
[14] The NHS Cancer plan: a plan for investment, a plan for reform (2000).
[15] Sharpe D, Williams RN, Ubhi SS, et al. The "two-week wait" referral pathway allows prompt treatment but does not improve outcome for patients with oesophago-gastric cancer. Eur J Surg Oncol 2010;36(10):977–81.
[16] Helsper CCW, van Erp NNF, Peeters P, et al. Time to diagnosis and treatment for cancer patients in the Netherlands: room for improvement? Eur J Cancer 2017;87:113–21.
[17] Weller D, Vedsted P, Rubin G, et al. The aarhus statement: improving design and reporting of studies on early cancer diagnosis. Br J Cancer 2012;106(7):1262–7.
[18] Berwick DM, Kelley E, Kruk ME, et al. Three global health-care quality reports in 2018. Lancet 2018;392(10143):194–5.
[19] Cevasco M, Ashley SW. Quality measurement and improvement in general surgery. Perm J. Fall 2011;15(4):48–53.
[20] McGory ML, Shekelle PG, Ko CY. Development of quality indicators for patients undergoing colorectal cancer surgery. J Natl Cancer Inst 2006;98(22):1623–33.
[21] Santhirapala V, Johnson WD, Meara JG. Essential need for quality in surgical health-care systems. Lancet 2018;392(10155):1309.
[22] Ontario Go. First ever common benchmarks will allow Canadians to measure progress in reducing wait times. 2024. Available at: https://news.ontario.ca/en/release/90066/first-ever-common-benchmarks-will-allow-canadians-to-measure-progress-in-reducing-wait-times. Accessed March 17, 2024.
[23] Ontario HQ. Measuring wait times for cancer surgeries. 2025. Available at: https://www.hqontario.ca/System-Performance/Measuring-System-Performance/Measuring-Wait-Times-for-Cancer-Surgeries. Accessed January 13, 2025.
[24] Services NH. National cancer waiting times monitoring dataset guidance. 2024. Available at: https://www.england.nhs.uk/publication/national-cancer-waiting-times-monitoring-dataset-guidance/. Accessed January 1, 2024.
[25] Services NH. Changes to cancer waiting times standards from 1 October 2023. 2024. Available at: https://www.england.nhs.uk/long-read/changes-to-cancer-waiting-times-standards-from-1-october-2023/. Accessed January 7, 2024.

[26] Bondzi-Simpson A, Sutradhar R, Wright FC, et al. Association of traditional and new surgical wait time targets and survival for curative-intent colorectal cancer surgery: a population-based cohort study. Ann Surg 2025;282(4):608–19.
[27] Grass F, Behm KT, Duchalais E, et al. Impact of delay to surgery on survival in stage I-III colon cancer. Eur J Surg Oncol 2020;46(3):455–61.
[28] Strous MTA, Molenaar CJL, Franssen RFW, et al. Treatment interval in curative treatment of colon cancer, does it impact (cancer free) survival? A non-inferiority analysis. Br J Cancer 2024;130(2):251–9.
[29] Yun YH, Kim YA, Min YH, et al. The influence of hospital volume and surgical treatment delay on long-term survival after cancer surgery. Ann Oncol 2012;23(10):2731–7.
[30] Kucejko RJ, Holleran TJ, Stein DE, et al. How soon should patients with Colon cancer undergo definitive resection? Dis Colon Rectum 2020;63(2):172–82.
[31] Francois Y, Nemoz CJ, Baulieux J, et al. Influence of the interval between preoperative radiation therapy and surgery on downstaging and on the rate of sphincter-sparing surgery for rectal cancer: the Lyon R90-01 randomized trial. J Clin Oncol 1999;17(8):2396.
[32] Garcia-Aguilar J, Smith DD, Avila K, et al, Timing of Rectal Cancer Response to Chemoradiation Consortium. Optimal timing of surgery after chemoradiation for advanced rectal cancer: preliminary results of a multicenter, nonrandomized phase II prospective trial. Ann Surg 2011;254(1):97–102.
[33] Sun Z, Adam MA, Kim J, et al. Optimal timing to surgery after neoadjuvant chemoradiotherapy for locally advanced rectal cancer. J Am Coll Surg 2016;222(4):367–74.
[34] Iversen LH, Antonsen S, Laurberg S, et al. Therapeutic delay reduces survival of rectal cancer but not of colonic cancer. Br J Surg 2009;96(10):1183–9.
[35] Burger JWA, Grotenhuis BA. Neoadjuvant treatment of rectal cancer: from adjunct to surgery to primary organ sparing treatment. Br J Surg 2024;111(12):znae300.
[36] Petrelli F, Trevisan F, Cabiddu M, et al. Total neoadjuvant therapy in rectal cancer: a systematic review and meta-analysis of treatment outcomes. Ann Surg 2020;271(3):440–8.
[37] Hamilton SR. The adenoma-adenocarcinoma sequence in the large bowel: variations on a theme. J Cell Biochem Suppl 1992;16g:41–6.
[38] Muto T, Bussey HJ, Morson BC. The evolution of cancer of the colon and rectum. Cancer 1975;36(6):2251–70.
[39] Amri R, Bordeianou LG, Sylla P, et al. Treatment delay in surgically-treated colon cancer: does it affect outcomes? Ann Surg Oncol 2014;21(12):3909–16.
[40] Strous MTA, Janssen-Heijnen MLG, Vogelaar FJ. Impact of therapeutic delay in colorectal cancer on overall survival and cancer recurrence - is there a safe timeframe for prehabilitation? Eur J Surg Oncol 2019;45(12):2295–301.
[41] Trepanier M, Paradis T, Kouyoumdjian A, et al. The impact of delays to definitive surgical care on survival in colorectal cancer patients. J Gastrointest Surg 2020;24(1):115–22.
[42] Olesen F, Hansen RP, Vedsted P. Delay in diagnosis: the experience in Denmark. Br J Cancer 2009;101(Suppl 2):S5–8.
[43] Foster JD, Jones EL, Falk S, et al. Timing of surgery after long-course neoadjuvant chemoradiotherapy for rectal cancer: a systematic review of the literature. Dis Colon Rectum 2013;56(7):921–30.
[44] Habr-Gama A, Perez RO, Proscurshim I, et al. Interval between surgery and neoadjuvant chemoradiation therapy for distal rectal cancer: does delayed surgery have an impact on outcome? Int J Radiat Oncol Biol Phys 2008;71(4):1181–8.
[45] Karahan SN, Oruc M, Erozkan K, et al. Optimal timing for rectal cancer surgery after total neoadjuvant therapy: when does surgery get really challenging? Dis Colon Rectum 2025;68(12):1403–13.
[46] Lim SB, Choi HS, Jeong SY, et al. Optimal surgery time after preoperative chemoradiotherapy for locally advanced rectal cancers. Ann Surg 2008;248(2):243–51.
[47] Sloothaak DA, Geijsen DE, van Leersum NJ, et al. Optimal time interval between neoadjuvant chemoradiotherapy and surgery for rectal cancer. Br J Surg 2013;100(7):933–9.

[48] Ahmadinejad M, Parvizi A, Sheikhi S, et al. Optimal timing of surgery after neoadjuvant chemoradiotherapy in rectal cancer: a retrospective analysis. Eur J Surg Oncol 2025;51 (6):109702.
[49] Garcia-Botello S, Martín-Arevalo J, Cozar-Lozano C, et al. Does delaying curative surgery for colorectal cancer influence long-term disease-free survival? A cohort study. Langenbecks Arch Surg 2021;406(7):2383–90.
[50] Johnson BA, Waddimba AC, Ogola GO, et al. A systematic review and meta-analysis of surgery delays and survival in breast, lung and colon cancers: implication for surgical triage during the COVID-19 pandemic. Am J Surg 2021;222(2):311–8.
[51] Min Y, Liu Z, Huang R, et al. Survival outcomes following treatment delays among patients with early-stage female cancers: a nationwide study. J Transl Med 2022;20(1):560.
[52] Lambert P, Galloway K, Feely A, et al. Measuring the impact of COVID-19 on cancer survival using an interrupted time series analysis. JNCI Cancer Spectr 2024;8(1); https://doi.org/10.1093/jncics/pkae001.
[53] The impact of surgical delay on resectability of colorectal cancer: an international prospective cohort study. Colorectal Dis 2022;24(6):708–26.
[54] Mentrasti G, Cantini L, Zichi C, et al. Alarming drop in early stage colorectal cancer diagnoses after COVID-19 outbreak: a real-world analysis from the Italian COVID-DELAY Study. Oncologist 2022;27(9):e723–30.
[55] Castelo M, Paszat L, Hansen BE, et al. Analysis of time to treatment and survival among adults younger than 50 years of age with colorectal cancer in Canada. JAMA Netw Open 2023;6(8):e2327109.
[56] Ettorchi-Tardy A, Levif M, Michel P. Benchmarking: a method for continuous quality improvement in health. Healthc Policy 2012;7(4):e101–19.
[57] Nolte E. International benchmarking of healthcare quality: a review of the literature. Rand Health Q. Winter 2012;1(4):6.
[58] Willmington C, Belardi P, Murante AM, et al. The contribution of benchmarking to quality improvement in healthcare. A systematic literature review. BMC Health Serv Res 2022;22(1):139.
[59] Anema HA, van der Veer SN, Kievit J, et al. Influences of definition ambiguity on hospital performance indicator scores: examples from the Netherlands. Eur J Publ Health 2014;24(1): 73–8.
[60] Fischer C, Lingsma HF, Anema HA, et al. Testing the construct validity of hospital care quality indicators: a case study on hip replacement. BMC Health Serv Res 2016;16(1):551.
[61] Schang L, Blotenberg I, Boywitt D. What makes a good quality indicator set? A systematic review of criteria. Int J Qual Health Care 2021;33(3); https://doi.org/10.1093/intqhc/mzab107.
[62] Gillis A, Dixon M, Smith A, et al. A patient-centred approach toward surgical wait times for colon cancer: a population-based analysis. Can J Surg 2014;57(2):94–100.
[63] Merkow RP, Bilimoria KY, Sherman KL, et al. Efficiency of colorectal cancer care among veterans: analysis of treatment wait times at Veterans Affairs Medical Centers. J Oncol Pract 2013;9(4):e154–63.
[64] Porter G, Urquhart R, Kendell C, et al. Timely access and quality of care in colorectal cancer: a population-based cohort study using administrative data. BMC Res Notes 2013;6:355.
[65] Singh H, De Coster C, Shu E, et al. Wait times from presentation to treatment for colorectal cancer: a population-based study. Can J Gastroenterol 2010;24(1):33–9.
[66] Courneya KS, Vardy JL, O'Callaghan CJ, et al. Structured exercise after adjuvant chemotherapy for Colon cancer. N Engl J Med 2025;393(1):13–25.
[67] Chen M, Wu VS, Falk D, et al. Patient navigation in cancer treatment: a systematic review. Curr Oncol Rep 2024;26(5):504–37.

Advances in Surgery 60 (2026) 169–182
ADVANCES IN SURGERY

When Should Anticoagulation Be Started after Major Trauma?

Andrew J. Kerwin, MD*, Elizabeth A. Mannino, MD, Amanda Dooley Romero, MD, Dina M. Filiberto, MD

Division of Trauma & Surgical Critical Care, Department of Surgery, University of Tennessee Health Science Center, 910 Madison Avenue, Suite 220, Memphis, TN 38163, USA

Keywords

• Deep venous thrombosis • Venous thromboembolism prophylaxis • Major trauma • Pulmonary embolism

Key points

- Venous thromboembolism (VTE) is a feared complication following major trauma and use of pharmacologic prophylaxis is essential.
- Timing of initiation of venous thromboprophylaxis is debated depending on the constellation of injuries present.
- Early initiation of pharmacologic VTE prophylaxis within 24 hours of admission is safe and reduces the incidence of VTE.
- Initiation of pharmacologic VTE prophylaxis within 24 hours of admission should be a quality metric for all trauma programs.

INTRODUCTION

Nearly 100 years ago, McCartney [1] recognized a link between lower extremity fractures and fatal pulmonary embolism (PE). Using postmortem examinations, he identified that the incidence of fatal PE was 3.32% following trauma. Subsequent studies from this period sought to pinpoint the etiology of venous thrombosis and PE. Investigators hypothesized trauma, surgery, age, obesity, cardiac disease, and reduced venous return, particularly from the legs [2]. Additional studies from the 1960s recognized PE as a significant cause of mortality in injured patients [3–5]. These early investigations hypothesized that the

*Corresponding author. *E-mail address:* Akerwin1@uthsc.edu

https://doi.org/10.1016/j.yasu.2026.03.009

Abbreviations

CAMP	coumadin, aspirin, Plavix
CLOTT	Consortium of Leaders in Traumatic Thromboembolism
CT	computed tomography
DVT	deep venous thrombosis
EDH	epidural hematoma
ICH	intracranial hemorrhage
IVH	intraventricular hemorrhage
PE	pulmonary embolism
SAH	subarachnoid hemorrhage
SCIs	spinal cord injuries
SDH	subdural hematoma
TBI	traumatic brain injury
TQIP	Trauma Quality Improvement Program
VTE	venous thromboembolism
WTA	Western Trauma Association

source of these pulmonary emboli was from the deep veins of the lower extremity. These findings were subsequently confirmed in autopsy studies.

Since identifying that venous thrombosis and PE were significant causes of postoperative and posttrauma morbidity and mortality, early investigators questioned how best to prevent venous thrombosis and PE. Some suggested elevation of the lower extremities to improve venous return and decrease venous pooling, while others suggested anticoagulation [4].

Since those early studies, subsequent research has confirmed that patients with major trauma are at significant risk for developing complications secondary to venous thromboembolism (VTE), defined as both PE and deep venous thrombosis (DVT). Because of the potential for VTE to cause significant morbidity and mortality, it is a feared complication following major trauma. The incidence following major trauma is estimated to be as high as 63% without prophylaxis [4,6–8]. The Centers for Disease Control estimate that nearly 900,000 people in the United States develop VTE each year [9], and the incidence of VTE is increasing [10–12]. Of those who develop VTE, 60,000 to 100,000 people die because of it. In addition to the significant morbidity and mortality related to VTE, hospital costs are increased significantly for those who develop VTE [13].

The increased incidence of VTE is likely due to greater awareness of the disease, routine screening [8], and improved imaging technology [14–17]. Because of the significant morbidity and mortality associated with VTE, some authors have suggested routine screening with duplex ultrasonography of asymptomatic patients to diagnose a DVT. The evidence surrounding this practice is conflicting [18,19], and there is wide variability in the use of routine screening among trauma centers [20]. Routine screening for VTE will identify more DVTs [21]; however, the clinical significance of these DVTs is unclear. Limiting routine screening to patients at the highest risk of developing a

DVT may provide the best value when deciding on the utility of this resource [22]. Intensivists performing screening duplex scans in the intensive care unit have been shown to produce results similar to those of scans performed by vascular sonographers [23]. This could eliminate the need for a vascular sonographer and increase the value of routine DVT screening.

Many authors have extensively studied VTE to identify risk factors for its development [21,24,25]. Important risk factors for developing VTE include age 40 years or greater, the presence of shock (systolic blood pressure <90 mm Hg) on admission, long-bone fractures, ventilator days greater than 3, venous injury, the need for a major operative procedure, spinal cord injury with paralysis, and major injuries to the chest, abdomen, and pelvis. A comprehensive list of risk factors following trauma is shown in Box 1.

Given concerns about developing VTE after major trauma, investigators have sought ways to prevent its development. This can be challenging given concerns about bleeding after major trauma, especially for injuries involving the brain, spine, or solid organs in the abdomen. A period of observation is usually implemented to ensure there is no further bleeding from the injuries, but the length of this observation period is debated. Additionally, many patients miss doses of their pharmacologic prophylactic agent due to invasive procedures [26,27]. Early initiation of pharmacologic prophylaxis is frequently defined as starting within 48 hours of admission, but it can also be defined as less than 24 hours or less than 72 hours [28]. Delays in initiation and missed doses of pharmacologic prophylaxis will lead to an increased incidence of VTE. In 2022, the Consensus Conference to Implement Optimal VTE Prophylaxis

Box 1: Risk factors for development of venous thromboembolism following trauma

- Age ≥40 years
- Presence of shock on admission
- Need for transfusions
- Need for surgery
- Pelvic or lower extremity fracture
- Spinal cord injury
- Major traumatic brain injury
- Major injury to chest, abdomen, and pelvis
- Major venous injury
- Presence of femoral venous catheter
- Ventilator days greater than 3
- Delay in initiation of pharmacologic VTE prophylaxis
- Missed doses of pharmacologic VTE prophylaxis

in Trauma (https://www.nattrauma.org/research/research-policies-templates-guidelines/vte-conference/) was convened to define optimal use of pharmacologic prophylaxis in trauma because of the significant associated morbidity and mortality.

Venous thromboembolism in patients with blunt solid organ injury

Nonoperative management is the standard for hemodynamically stable trauma patients with blunt solid organ injuries. Pharmacologic VTE prophylaxis is frequently held for 24 to 72 hours due to concern for delayed bleeding from the injured organ requiring emergent surgery. However, trauma patients with blunt solid organ injury are known to develop a hypercoagulable phenotype as early as 12 hours of injury [29]. Studies have demonstrated hypercoagulability in patients with blunt solid organ injury using serial thromboelastography, which shows decreased time to clot formation, increased clot propagation and strength, and tissue plasminogen activator resistance [30]. Several studies have aimed to determine the optimal timing of VTE prophylaxis in patients with blunt solid organ injury. A 2014 study evaluated the timing of VTE prophylaxis initiation in patients with blunt solid organ injury managed nonoperatively [31]. Patients were divided into 3 groups based on the time of initiation of pharmacologic prophylaxis. Early group patients had initiation within less than 48 hours, intermediate group within 48 to 72 hours, and late group greater than 72 hours. In this cohort, there was no significant difference in operative intervention or postprophylaxis blood transfusion requirement by initiation time, thus demonstrating the safety of early administration of low molecular weight heparin VTE prophylaxis in patients with blunt solid organ injury.

A retrospective American College of Surgeons Trauma Quality Improvement Program (TQIP) study evaluated 36,187 patients with blunt solid organ injury who underwent nonoperative management [32]. These patients received either early (<48 hours), late (>48 hours), or no pharmacologic VTE prophylaxis. Patients receiving early VTE prophylaxis had significantly lower rates of DVT and PE compared to the other 2 groups, with no significant differences in postprophylaxis initiation transfusions, failure of nonoperative management, or mortality. A single-center prospective study of 118 patients with blunt solid organ injury managed nonoperatively demonstrated that early initiation (<48 hours) of VTE prophylaxis resulted in a lower incidence of VTE without an associated risk of bleeding [33]. Subsequently, a multicenter trial involving 19 trauma centers with 1773 patients was conducted to validate the initial single-center study [34]. Once again, early initiation (<48 hours) of pharmacologic VTE prophylaxis was associated with significantly reduced rates of VTE and no increased risk of bleeding complications. A more recent 2025 study evaluated TQIP data retrospectively to determine the effects of initiation of VTE prophylaxis early (less than 48 hours) versus late (greater than 48 hours). Among the 23,668 patients, early VTE prophylaxis was associated with lower mortality, lower rates of failure of nonoperative management, lower rates of stroke, and DVT/PE. Later administration of VTE prophylaxis was associated with higher mortality rates, failure of nonoperative management, and longer length of hospital stay [35].

Society guidelines have sought to standardize the timing of initiation of pharmacologic VTE prophylaxis to address wide variability among trauma centers. The current recommendation from the American Association for the Surgery of Trauma is early initiation of VTE prophylaxis in patients with blunt solid organ injury within 24 to 48 hours [36]. Patients with grade IV and V injuries must be assessed with caution, and initiation of VTE prophylaxis should only be initiated once bleeding has stabilized. The Western Trauma Association (WTA) recommends the initiation of VTE prophylaxis in patients with blunt solid organ injury within 24 hours [37].

Venous thromboembolism in patients with pelvic and extremity fractures

Pelvic fractures and long bone fractures are risk factors associated with a significantly higher rate of VTE in patients with trauma [19]. At the same time, there is the competing concern about bleeding from the fractures, which could be exacerbated by early initiation of pharmacologic VTE prophylaxis. This concern has led to withholding prophylaxis initiation for as long as 72 hours after admission for patients requiring interventions for pelvic and extremity fractures. Additionally, doses may be held in the perioperative period and expose the patient to an increased VTE risk. There are limited data in this area, but the data do point to early initiation of prophylaxis as safe and effective.

A 2019 retrospective TQIP study examined the effect of the timing of initiation of pharmacologic VTE prophylaxis in patients with severe blunt pelvic fractures [38]. Patients were stratified into 2 groups based on the timing of prophylaxis initiation. The study found that early initiation (<48 hours) was associated with a lower incidence of VTE and lower mortality than late initiation (>48 hours). Salottolo and colleagues [39] conducted a multicenter retrospective study to assess the effect of the timing of initiation and holding perioperative prophylaxis in patients with hip, femur, or tibia fractures requiring surgery. They divided patients into 4 groups: (1) prophylaxis initiated preoperatively and continued, (2) initiated preoperatively but held perioperative doses, (3) initiated within 12 hours of the procedure, and (4) initiated greater than 12 hours after the procedure. The incidence of VTE was similar across all 4 groups. Notably, the incidence of clinically significant hemorrhage, defined as occurring within 24 hours of the procedure and requiring action, was similar across all 4 groups. They concluded that prophylaxis should start early (<24 hours) and not be interrupted in patients with orthopedic injuries.

Findings from a 2024 TQIP study by Kobzeva-Herzog and colleagues [40] of patients requiring surgery for pelvis, hip, and femur fractures within 24 hours of admission showed similar outcomes to those in the Salottolo study. Patients who received prophylaxis greater than 12 hours after their intervention had an increased incidence of VTE compared to those who received it less than

12 hours from intervention. The need for orthopedic reinterventions was similar between the 2 groups, suggesting no increased risk of postoperative hemorrhage when prophylaxis was initiated within 12 hours of orthopedic intervention. These studies add to the recent WTA algorithm, which recommends initiating pharmacologic VTE prophylaxis within 24 hours for most patients [37].

Venous thromboembolism prophylaxis in patients with traumatic brain injury

The risk of VTE in patients who sustain a major trauma is 3% to 5%. Traumatic brain injury (TBI) has been identified as a higher risk condition with an estimated VTE risk of 8% to 10%. This risk depends on the timing of pharmacologic prophylaxis initiation, with VTE risk increasing by up to 15% when prophylaxis is delayed beyond 48 hours [41]. On the other hand, clinicians are concerned with the risk of intracranial hemorrhage (ICH) progression. A recent study by Burczak showed that ICH progression occurred in 3% of patients with TBI [42].

Given the competing priorities, researchers have attempted to define the optimal initiation time in the setting of TBI. Current recommendations for timing of initiation of VTE prophylaxis attempt to balance the risk of VTE versus the risk of ICH progression. Recommendations are stratified by hemorrhage progression risk using the modified Berne-Norwood criteria [43–46] (Table 1) and the Brain Injury Guidelines [47] (Table 2), which classify patients based on injury severity patterns and clinical factors, including history of anticoagulation, ICH progression on imaging, and operative intervention. Patients deemed to be at higher risk have typically had delays in initiation or never had prophylaxis initiated.

The recent American College of Surgeons TQIP Best Practices Guidelines for the Management of Traumatic Brain Injury are multidisciplinary recommendations on VTE prophylaxis [48]. The guidelines recommend

Table 1
Modified Berne-Norwood criteria

Low risk	Moderate risk	High risk
SDH or EDH ≤8 mm	SDH or EDH ≥8 mm	ICP monitor placement
Contusion ≤2 cm	Contusion ≥2 cm	Craniotomy
Single contusion per lobe	Multiple contusions per lobe	Evidence of progression at 72 h
Isolated SAH	Scattered SAH	
Isolated IVH	More than isolated IVH	
	Evidence of ICH progression at 24 h	

Abbreviations: EDH, epidural hematoma; ICH, intracranial hemorrhage; IVH, intraventricular hemorrhage; SAH, subarachnoid hemorrhage; SDH, subdural hematoma.

Data from Pastorek RA, Cripps MW, Bernstein IH, et al. The Parkland Protocol's modified Berne-Norwood criteria predict two tiers of risk for traumatic brain injury progression. *J Neurotrauma* 2014;31(20):1737–3.

Table 2
Brain injury guidelines

Variable	BIG 1	BIG 2	BIG 3
Loss of consciousness	Yes/No	Yes/No	Yes/No
Neurologic examination	Normal	Normal	Abnormal
Intoxication	No	No	Yes/No
CAMP[a]	No	No	Yes
SDH	≤4 mm	5–7 mm	≥8 mm
EDH	≤4 mm	5–7 mm	≥8 mm
IPH	≤4 mm, 1 location	3–7 mm, 2 locations	≥8 mm, multiple locations
SAH	Trace	Localized	Scattered
IVH	No	No	Yes

[a]CAMP, coumadin, aspirin, plavix.
Joseph, Bellal MD et al., Prospective validation of the brain injury guidelines: Managing traumatic brain injury without neurosurgical consultation. Journal of Trauma and Acute Care Surgery 77(6):p 984-988, December 2014. https://doi.org/10.1097/TA.0000000000000428.

initiating pharmacologic VTE prophylaxis within 24 hours for low-risk, nonoperative patients with TBI and within 24 to 48 hours for moderate-risk or high-risk patients, provided that follow-up computed tomography (CT) imaging demonstrates ICH stability. Additionally, it is recommended to initiate or resume prophylaxis within 24 to 48 hours after craniotomy or craniectomy if the postoperative CT is stable. Patients with intracranial pressure (ICP) monitors who do not undergo craniotomy should be treated similarly to nonoperative patients with TBI and withholding prophylaxis before ICP monitor placement is not recommended. The WTA also states that the majority of TBI patients with a stable CT may be initiated on VTE prophylaxis within 24 hours and nearly all should receive prophylaxis by 72 hours, noting that trauma centers that initiate prophylaxis within 24 hours demonstrate significantly lower VTE rates with no difference in rates of late neurosurgical intervention [37].

Several recent studies and meta-analyses have supported these recommendation guidelines. A 2025 systematic review of 30 studies found a 7% risk of ICH progression following initiation of VTE prophylaxis, with no significant difference between early (≤72 hours) and late initiation. Furthermore, this study found no increased risk of ICH progression when VTE prophylaxis groups were compared to untreated groups [49]. Additional studies suggest that initiation within 48 hours offers the optimal risk–benefit profile. A 2025 meta-analysis of 14 studies (n = 24,401) also demonstrated that early prophylaxis was associated with significantly lower VTE, and the most consistent benefit was observed at the 48 hour mark or less. Importantly, mortality was significantly lower when prophylaxis was initiated at 48 hours or less, and there was no significant increase in hemorrhage progression, neurosurgical intervention, or mortality in the early prophylaxis groups [50].

Venous thromboembolism prophylaxis in patients with spinal column and spinal cord injuries

Patients with spinal column injuries and spinal cord injuries (SCIs) are another group of patients where initiation of and interruption of pharmacologic VTE prophylaxis occurs. This is due to fear of bleeding at the site of injury, resulting in devastating neurologic deterioration. This has led to variability in prophylaxis use among spine surgeons [51,52]. Sharpe [53] reviewed 705 patients who required surgical stabilization of a spinal column fracture to determine the effect of preoperative pharmacologic VTE prophylaxis on the incidence of VTE and risk of bleeding complications. Patients who received at least 50% of their scheduled VTE prophylaxis doses were less likely to develop PE. Overall, the incidence of postoperative hemorrhage in patients who received at least 50% of their scheduled doses was low and not statistically significantly different from that in patients who received less than 50% of their scheduled doses (2.1% vs 2.9%). Additional data from Dornbush [54] demonstrated that the incidence of postoperative hemorrhage following VTE prophylaxis initiation was only 0.7%, and it did not differ between those who received prophylaxis within 48 hours and those who received it after 48 hours. Finally, a recent systematic review and meta-analysis demonstrated that initiating pharmacologic VTE prophylaxis within 48 hours of injury was associated with significantly lower odds of VTE, with no significant increase in major bleeding [55].

When should pharmacologic venous thromboembolism prophylaxis be initiated?

Given the debate regarding the timing of initiating pharmacologic VTE prophylaxis and the risks of bleeding, the Consortium of Leaders in Traumatic Thromboembolism (CLOTT) study was formed to address these questions. The CLOTT study group is 17 level 1 trauma centers that developed a multicenter, prospective observational trial of VTE management following major trauma. Enrolling centers are shown in Box 2. The trial is the most extensive study of VTE management to date with 7880 patients enrolled. Two important studies from the CLOTT study group help address the timing of initiation. In 2022, the study group examined the timing of prophylaxis initiation for patients with spinal cord injury [56]. They demonstrated that the risk of VTE was high in patients with spinal cord injury and that initiation of VTE prophylaxis in 48 hours or less was independently associated with decreased incidence of VTEs. With respect to TBI, the group showed in a 2023 study that patients receiving VTE prophylaxis 48 hours or less had lower VTE and DVT rates compared to those starting greater than 48 hours, with equivalent rates of PE, ICH progression, and other bleeding events [57]. On multivariate logistic regression analysis, initiation of pharmacologic VTE prophylaxis greater than 48 hours was an independent risk factor for VTE. It is important to note that this study demonstrated that initiation of VTE in 48 hours or less was not associated with a progression of ICH or any other risk of bleeding.

Box 2: Consortium of Leaders in Traumatic Thromboembolism Study Group Sites

- Christiana Health Care
- Denver Health
- Johns Hopkins
- Lancaster General
- Massachusetts General
- Medical College of Wisconsin
- Medical University of South Carolina
- Oregon Health Sciences University
- Scripps Mercy Hospital
- Stanford University
- University of California, San Diego
- University of California, San Francisco
- University of Florida College of Medicine, Jacksonville
- University of Florida, Gainesville
- University of Maryland
- University of Texas, Houston
- University of Utah

While most studies have examined early initiation of VTE prophylaxis within either 48 or 72 hours of admission in specific patient groups, 2 recent studies examined the benefit of initiating pharmacologic VTE prophylaxis within 24 hours of admission. Both studies examined all patients with trauma rather than specific patient groups. The first study was a retrospective review of a prospectively collected database that examined a quality metric they called door-to-prophylaxis time and demonstrated that patients with earlier door-to-prophylaxis time (25 vs 35 hours) had fewer VTE [58]. Additionally, they found that each hour of delay after admission was associated with a 1.5% increase in the risk of VTE. The second study was from the CLOTT study group [59]. It also examined initiation of prophylaxis within 24 hours of admission for all patients. Similar to the first study, the initiation of pharmacologic VTE prophylaxis within 24 hours of admission was safe and effective. It was associated with a 42% lower rate of VTE. Bleeding complications, including progression of ICH, following initiation of prophylaxis, were rare in both groups. Interestingly, patients in the group with prophylaxis initiated greater than 24 hours after admission had a higher incidence of ICH progression than those with initiation in less than 24 hours (0.5% vs 0.2%). Together, these 2 studies provide strong evidence that initiating pharmacologic VTE prophylaxis in all major trauma patients is safe and effective, and that a door-to-prophylaxis time of less than 24 hours is a good quality metric for trauma programs to follow.

SUMMARY

VTE has been recognized as a feared complication following major trauma for nearly 100 years. Prophylaxis has been studied extensively to prevent unnecessary morbidity and mortality. Clinicians must weigh the risks of bleeding from injuries after initiating prophylaxis against the benefits of prophylaxis to identify the appropriate initiation time.

The definition of early initiation of prophylaxis has varied depending on specific patient injuries. Multiple authors have demonstrated that initiation of pharmacologic VTE prophylaxis within 48 hours of admission for patients is safe and effective for patients with solid organ injuries, spinal cord injuries, and traumatic brain injuries. However, more recent data [58,59] suggest that initiation of prophylaxis within 24 hours of admission is safe and effective and should be implemented as a quality metric for trauma programs.

CLINICS CARE POINTS

- Patients who suffer major trauma are at risk of developing VTE, which can have significant morbidity and mortality.
- The risk of morbidity and mortality increases without the use of pharmacologic VTE prophylaxis.
- Clinicians concerned with the progression of bleeding from injuries may delay the initiation of prophylaxis for as long as 72 hours following admission.
- The risk of progression of bleeding from injuries, including blunt solid organ injuries, traumatic brain injuries, and spinal cord injuries, after initiation of pharmacologic VTE prophylaxis is low.
- Initiating pharmacologic VTE prophylaxis within 24 hours of admission is safe and effective.
- Using a door-to-prophylaxis time of less than 24 hours is a reasonable quality metric for trauma programs to implement and track.

Acknowledgments

The CLOTT Study Group investigators and their current affiliations are Scott Brakenridge, University of Washington, Seattle, WA. Brandon Bruns, UT Southwestern Medical School, Dallas, TX. Mark D. Cipolle, Lehigh Valley Health Network, Allentown, PA. Todd W. Constantini, University of California, San Francisco, San Francisco, CA. Bruce Crookes, Medical University of South Carolina, Charleston, SC. Andrew J. Kerwin, University of Tennessee Health Science Center. Laszlo N. Kiraly Oregon Health & Science University, Portland, OR. Lisa Marie Knowlton, Stanford University, Stanford, CA. Margaret M. Knudson, University of California, San Francisco. Matthew J. Martin,

LAC + USC, Los Angeles, CA. Michelle K. McNutt, University of Texas Health Science Center at Houston, Houston, TX. David J. Milia, Medical College of Wisconsin, Milwaukee, WI. Alicia Mohr, University of Florida College of Medicine, Gainesville, FL. Ernest E. Moore, University of Colorado, Denver, CO. Frederick Rogers, Lancaster General Hospital, Lancaster, PA. Thomas Scalea, University of Maryland School of Medicine, Baltimore, MD. Sherry Sixta, St Anthony Hospital & Medical Campus, Lakewood, CO. David Spain, Stanford University, Stanford, CA. George C. Velmahos, Massachusetts General Hospital, Boston, MA.

Disclosure

The authors have nothing to disclose.

References

[1] McCartney JS. Pulmonary embolism following trauma. Surg Gynecol Obstet 1935;61:369–79.
[2] Barnes AR. Pulmonary embolism. JAMA 1937;109(17):1347–53.
[3] Fitts WT Jr, Lehr HB, Bitner RL, et al. An analysis of 950 fatal injuries. Surgery 1964;56:663–8.
[4] Freeark RJ, Boswick J, Fardin R. Posttraumatic venous thrombosis. Arch Surg 1967;95(4):567–75.
[5] Sevitt S, Gallagher N. Venous thrombosis and pulmonary embolism. A clinico-pathological study in injured and burned patients. Br J Surg 1961;48:475–89.
[6] Kudsk KA, Fabian TC, Baum S, et al. Silent deep vein thrombosis in immobilized multiple trauma patients. Am J Surg 1989;158(6):515–9.
[7] Geerts WH, Code KI, Jay RM, et al. A prospective study of venous thromboembolism after major trauma. N Engl J Med 1994;331(24):1601–6.
[8] Hamada SR, Espina C, Guedj T, et al. High level of venous thromboembolism in critically ill trauma patients despite early and well-driven thromboprophylaxis protocol. Ann Intensive Care 2017;7(1):97.
[9] Centers for Disease Control. Venous thromboembolism (blood clots). Available at: https://www.cdc.gov/blood-clots/data-research/facts-stats/index.html2024. Accessed July 5, 2024.
[10] Glazier CR, Baciewicz FA Jr. Epidemiology, etiology, and pathophysiology of pulmonary embolism. Int J Angiol 2024;33(2):76–81.
[11] Heit JA, Spencer FA, White RH. The epidemiology of venous thromboembolism. J Thromb Thrombolysis 2016;41(1):3–14.
[12] Huang W, Goldberg RJ, Anderson FA, et al. Secular trends in occurrence of acute venous thromboembolism: the Worcester VTE study (1985-2009). Am J Med 2014;127(9):829–39.e5.
[13] Dasta JF, Pilon D, Mody SH, et al. Daily hospitalization costs in patients with deep vein thrombosis or pulmonary embolism treated with anticoagulant therapy. Thromb Res 2015;135(2):303–10.
[14] Schultz DJ, Brasel KJ, Washington L, et al. Incidence of asymptomatic pulmonary embolism in moderately to severely injured trauma patients. J Trauma 2004;56(4):727–31 [discussion: 31–3].
[15] Menaker J, Stein DM, Scalea TM. Incidence of early pulmonary embolism after injury. J Trauma 2007;63(3):620–4.
[16] Lundy JB, Oh JS, Chung KK, et al. Frequency and relevance of acute peritraumatic pulmonary thrombus diagnosed by computed tomographic imaging in combat casualties. J Trauma Acute Care Surg 2013;75(2 Suppl 2):S215–20.

[17] Knudson MM, Moore EE, Kornblith LZ, et al. Challenging traditional paradigms in posttraumatic pulmonary thromboembolism. JAMA Surg 2022;157(2):e216356.
[18] Guyatt GH, Akl EA, Crowther M, et al. Executive summary: Antithrombotic therapy and prevention of thrombosis, 9th ed: American college of chest physicians evidence-based clinical practice guidelines. Chest 2012;141(2 Suppl):7S–47S.
[19] Rogers FB, Cipolle MD, Velmahos G, et al. Practice management guidelines for the prevention of venous thromboembolism in trauma patients: the EAST practice management guidelines work group. J Trauma 2002;53(1):142–64.
[20] Haut ER, Schneider EB, Patel A, et al. Duplex ultrasound screening for deep vein thrombosis in asymptomatic trauma patients: a survey of individual trauma surgeon opinions and current trauma center practices. J Trauma 2011;70(1):27–33 [discussion: 4].
[21] Haut ER, Chang DC, Pierce CA, et al. Predictors of posttraumatic deep vein thrombosis (DVT): hospital practice versus patient factors-an analysis of the national trauma data bank (NTDB). J Trauma 2009;66(4):994–9 [discussion: 9–1001].
[22] Bandle J, Shackford SR, Kahl JE, et al. The value of lower-extremity duplex surveillance to detect deep vein thrombosis in trauma patients. J Trauma Acute Care Surg 2013;74(2): 575–80.
[23] Roberts L, Rozen T, Murphy D, et al. A preliminary study of intensivist-performed DVT ultrasound screening in trauma ICU patients (APSIT study). Ann Intensive Care 2020;10(1):122.
[24] Knudson MM, Gomez D, Haas B, et al. Three thousand seven hundred thirty-eight posttraumatic pulmonary emboli: a new look at an old disease. Ann Surg 2011;254(4):625–32.
[25] Knudson MM, Ikossi DG, Khaw L, et al. Thromboembolism after trauma: an analysis of 1602 episodes from the American College of Surgeons National Trauma Data Bank. Ann Surg 2004;240(3):490–6 [discussion: 6–8].
[26] Nichols C, Schellenberg M, Lewis MR, et al. Venous thromboembolism chemoprophylaxis compliance in the surgical intensive care unit. Am Surg 2023;89(10):4050–4.
[27] Louis SG, Sato M, Geraci T, et al. Correlation of missed doses of enoxaparin with increased incidence of deep vein thrombosis in trauma and general surgery patients. JAMA Surg 2014;149(4):365–70.
[28] Schellenberg M, Costantini T, Joseph B, et al. Timing of venous thromboembolism prophylaxis initiation after injury: findings from the consensus conference to implement optimal VTE prophylaxis in trauma. J Trauma Acute Care Surg 2023;94(3):484–9.
[29] Sumislawski JJ, Kornblith LZ, Conroy AS, et al. Dynamic coagulability after injury: is delaying venous thromboembolism chemoprophylaxis worth the wait? J Trauma Acute Care Surg 2018;85(5):907–14.
[30] Coleman JR, Kay AB, Moore EE, et al. It's sooner than you think: blunt solid organ injury patients are already hypercoagulable upon hospital admission - results of a bi-institutional, prospective study. Am J Surg 2019;218(6):1065–73.
[31] Joseph B, Pandit V, Harrison C, et al. Early thromboembolic prophylaxis in patients with blunt solid abdominal organ injuries undergoing nonoperative management: is it safe? Am J Surg 2015;209(1):194–8.
[32] Skarupa D, Hanna K, Zeeshan M, et al. Is early chemical thromboprophylaxis in patients with solid organ injury a solid decision? J Trauma Acute Care Surg 2019;87(5):1104–12.
[33] Schellenberg M, Inaba K, Biswas S, et al. When is it safe to start VTE prophylaxis after blunt solid organ injury? A prospective study from a level I trauma center. World J Surg 2019;43 (11):2797–803.
[34] Schellenberg M, Owattanapanich N, Emigh B, et al, AAST VTE Prophylaxis Study Group. When is it safe to start venous thromboembolism prophylaxis after blunt solid organ injury? A prospective American Association for the Surgery of Trauma multi-institutional trial. J Trauma Acute Care Surg 2024;96(2):209–15.
[35] Rafieezadeh A, Prabhakaran K, Jose A, et al. Early versus late venous thromboembolism prophylaxis in patients with severe blunt solid organ injury. Injury 2025;56 (9):112524.

[36] Yorkgitis BK, Berndtson AE, Cross A, et al. American Association for the Surgery of Trauma/American College of Surgeons-Committee on Trauma Clinical Protocol for inpatient venous thromboembolism prophylaxis after trauma. J Trauma Acute Care Surg 2022;92(3):597–604.
[37] Ley EJ, Brown CVR, Moore EE, et al. Updated guidelines to reduce venous thromboembolism in trauma patients: a Western trauma association critical decisions algorithm. J Trauma Acute Care Surg 2020;89(5):971–81.
[38] Benjamin E, Aiolfi A, Recinos G, et al. Timing of venous thromboprophylaxis in isolated severe pelvic fracture: effect on mortality and outcomes. Injury 2019;50(3):697–702.
[39] Salottolo K, Carrick M, Nwafo N, et al. Timing of venous thromboembolism chemoprophylaxis with major surgery of lower-extremity long bone fractures. J Trauma Acute Care Surg 2023;94(1):169–76.
[40] Kobzeva-Herzog AJ, Smith SM, Counihan DR, et al. Timing of venous thromboembolism prophylaxis initiation and complications in polytrauma patients with high-risk bleeding orthopedic interventions: a nationwide analysis. J Trauma Acute Care Surg 2024;97(1):96–104.
[41] Gould MK, Garcia DA, Wren SM, et al. Prevention of VTE in nonorthopedic surgical patients: Antithrombotic Therapy and Prevention of Thrombosis, 9th ed: American College of Chest Physicians Evidence-Based Clinical Practice Guidelines. Chest 2012;141(2 Suppl):e227S–77S.
[42] Burczak KW, Van Gent JM, Bavishi D, et al. Risk factors for progression of intracranial hemorrhage after initiation of VTE chemoprophylaxis: an evaluation of 1390 TBI patients. Trauma Surg Acute Care Open 2025;10(3):e001606.
[43] Norwood SH, Berne JD, Rowe SA, et al. Early venous thromboembolism prophylaxis with enoxaparin in patients with blunt traumatic brain injury. J Trauma 2008;65(5):1021–6 [discussion: 6–7].
[44] Norwood SH, McAuley CE, Berne JD, et al. A potentially expanded role for enoxaparin in preventing venous thromboembolism in high risk blunt trauma patients. J Am Coll Surg 2001;192(2):161–7.
[45] Norwood SH, McAuley CE, Berne JD, et al. Prospective evaluation of the safety of enoxaparin prophylaxis for venous thromboembolism in patients with intracranial hemorrhagic injuries. Arch Surg 2002;137(6):696–701 [discussion: 2].
[46] Pastorek RA, Cripps MW, Bernstein IH, et al. The Parkland Protocol's modified Berne-Norwood criteria predict two tiers of risk for traumatic brain injury progression. J Neurotrauma 2014;31(20):1737–43.
[47] Joseph B, Aziz H, Pandit V, et al. Prospective validation of the brain injury guidelines: managing traumatic brain injury without neurosurgical consultation. J Trauma Acute Care Surg 2014;77(6):984–8.
[48] American College of Surgeons, American Congress of Rehabilitation Medicine. *American College of Surgeons Trauma Quality Improvement Program Best Practices Guidelines: The Management Of Traumatic Brain Injury,* 2024. Accessed December 20, 2025.
[49] Dengler BA, Haight T, Fu A, et al. Safety of early chemoprophylaxis for venous thromboembolism after traumatic brain injury: a systematic review and meta-analysis. A military traumatic brain injury initiative study. J Neurosurg 2025;142(4):1046–57.
[50] Karmur BS, Mann JA, Leung AA, et al. Early versus late initiation of chemical venous thromboembolism prophylaxis in adult patients with severe traumatic brain injury: a systematic review and meta-analysis. Neurocrit Care 2026;44(2):427–44.
[51] Bryson DJ, Uzoigwe CE, Braybrooke J. Thromboprophylaxis in spinal surgery: a survey. J Orthop Surg Res 2012;7:14.
[52] Glotzbecker MP, Bono CM, Harris MB, et al. Surgeon practices regarding postoperative thromboembolic prophylaxis after high-risk spinal surgery. Spine (Phila Pa 1976) 2008;33(26):2915–21.

[53] Sharpe JP, Gobbell WC, Carter AM, et al. Impact of venous thromboembolism chemoprophylaxis on postoperative hemorrhage following operative stabilization of spine fractures. J Trauma Acute Care Surg 2017;83(6):1108–13.
[54] Dornbush C, Maly C, Bartschat N, et al. Chemoprophylaxis timing is not associated with postoperative bleeding after spinal trauma surgery. Clin Neurol Neurosurg 2023;225:107590.
[55] Mohanty S, von Riegen H, Akodu M, et al. Timing of chemical anticoagulant administration in spine trauma and its impact on VTE, bleeding, and mortality: a systematic review and meta-analysis. Glob Spine J 2025;16(1):21925682251353138.
[56] Godat LN, Haut ER, Moore EE, et al. Venous thromboembolism risk after spinal cord injury: a secondary analysis of the CLOTT study. J Trauma Acute Care Surg 2023;94(1):23–9.
[57] Wu YT, Chien CY, Matsushima K, et al, CLOTT Study Group. Early venous thromboembolism prophylaxis in patients with trauma intracranial hemorrhage: analysis of the prospective multicenter consortium of leaders in traumatic thromboembolism study. J Trauma Acute Care Surg 2023;95(5):649–56.
[58] Van Gent JM, Clements TW, Lubkin DE, et al. Door-to-prophylaxis' as a novel quality improvement metric in prevention of venous thromboembolism following traumatic injury. Trauma Surg Acute Care Open 2024;9(1):e001297.
[59] Kerwin AJ, Byerly S, Filiberto DM, et al, CLOTT Study Group. Timing is everything: early initiation of VTE prophylaxis following major trauma is effective and safe. Ann Surg 2025;282(3):382–8.

Advances in Surgery 60 (2026) 183–196

ADVANCES IN SURGERY

Is Pyloroplasty Necessary During Esophagectomy? Review of Literature and Technical Considerations

Ian G. Christie, MD[a], Evan T. Alicuben, MD[b], Arjun Pennathur, MD[b], Samuel Luketich[c], James D. Luketich, MD[a,*]

[a]Division of Thoracic and Foregut Surgery, Department of Cardiothoracic Surgery, University of Pittsburgh, Pittsburgh, PA, USA; [b]Division of Thoracic and Foregut Surgery, University of Pittsburgh Medical Center, Pittsburgh, PA, USA; [c]Department of Biology, University of Pittsburgh, Pittsburgh, PA, USA

Keywords

• Esophagectomy • Pyloroplasty • Pyloric drainage • Delayed gastric emptying • Minimally invasive surgery • Esophageal cancer

Key points

- Optimal outcomes after esophagectomy include both oncologic resection and optimized gastric conduit emptying to reduce aspiration and pulmonary complications.
- Pyloroplasty, particularly the Heineke–Mikulicz technique, has the strongest evidence for reducing delayed gastric emptying and gastric outlet obstruction.
- Modern minimally invasive esophagectomy with a narrow, straight conduit, the routine need for pyloric drainage remains debated, though recent randomized data favor pyloroplasty.
- Meticulous conduit construction, routine postoperative assessment, and consideration for pyloric intervention are essential for durable functional outcomes.

*Corresponding author. University of Pittsburgh Medical Center: Shadyside Campus, 5200 Center Avenue, 7th Floor POB, Pittsburgh, PA 15232. *E-mail address:* luketichjd@upmc.edu

https://doi.org/10.1016/j.yasu.2026.03.015

Abbreviations

botox	botulinum toxin
G-POEM	gastric peroral endoscopic myotomy of the pylorus
MIE	Mckeown and Ivor Lewis esophagectomy

INTRODUCTION

Esophagectomy is the gold standard local therapy for localized and resectable locally advanced esophageal cancer. The principal goal of esophagectomy is complete tumor excision and adequate lymphadenectomy. However, functional outcomes after esophagectomy are also important. The goal is to create a conduit that empties well and minimizes reflux symptoms. Creation of a thin conduit with a straight trajectory and a high intrathoracic or cervical anastomosis has been used to promote emptying and avoid reflux. However, unlike the native esophagus, a gastric tube lacks peristaltic contractile function. Pyloric drainage is often performed as an adjunct to esophagectomy. However, many surgeons have proposed a selective use of pyloric drainage during esophagectomy. We will review options for pyloric drainage procedures including pyloroplasty, surgical pyloromyotomy, gastric peroral endoscopic myotomy of the pylorus (G-POEM), pyloric botulinum toxin (botox) injection, and endoscopic balloon dilation. We will review the data evaluating the impact of routine pyloric drainage during esophagectomy.

HEINEKE–MIKULICZ PYLOROPLASTY

The preferred technique for pyloroplasty during esophagectomy is the Heineke–Mikulicz pyloroplasty. Dr Heineke first described this approach in 1886 for treatment of gastric outlet obstruction and peptic ulcer disease [1]. This technique involves longitudinal full-thickness incision over the pylorus extending from the antrum extending onto duodenum, with a transverse closure (Fig. 1). This effectively widens the pyloric channel and is associated with low risk of stricture or other wound healing complications. In a laparoscopic approach, stay sutures are first placed on the superior and inferior aspect of the pylorus, aiding in exposure of the pylorus, place it on stretch and orient it at a right angle to the surgeon's working arm. The pylorus is opened using ultrasonic shears. Closure is performed in interrupted fashion transversely, taking care to incorporate mucosal and muscular layers on all suture bites (Fig. 2). An omental pedicle flap may also be used to buttress the closure, which is tacked over the pylorus anteriorly (Fig. 3).

JABOULAY GASTRODUODENOTOMY

Dr Jaboulay described his approach to pyloric drainage augmentation in 1892, with an enterotomy along the distal greater curvature of the stomach and a duodenotomy along the D1, D2 segment with a side to side anastomosis [1]. This approach is of historical interest and may be considered in cases of peptic ulcer

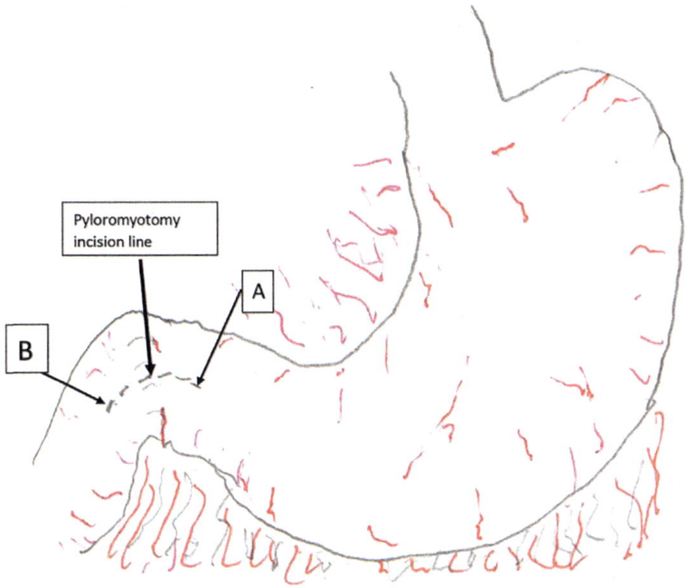

Fig. 1. Heineke–Mikulicz pyloroplasty: the dashed line denotes full-thickness incision across pylorus from antrum (*A*) to duodenum (*B*). (*Figure courtesy* Sam Luketich.)

disease or gastric outlet obstruction where there is a severe inflammatory process in the pylorus that contraindicates pyloric incision. This is not a preferred approach for use during esophagectomy given the need for an enterotomy along the greater curvature of the stomach in the area of the right gastroepiploic arcade, the key blood supply to the gastric conduit.

FINNEY PYLOROPLASTY

Dr Finney proposed his approach for pyloroplasty in 1902, using a longitudinal *U* shaped along the greater curvature of the stomach across the pylorus and onto the medial duodenum with a side to side closure of the antral side of the incision to the duodenal side, creating an enlarged gastroduodenal channel [1]. This approach may be advantageous in cases that demand a larger gastroduodenal incision, such as for management of bleeding peptic ulcer disease or in the severely scarred pylorus that is not amenable to a Heineke–Mikulicz pyloroplasty. Again, this is not the preferred approach for use during pyloroplasty given the need for extended incision onto the greater curvature of the stomach.

PYLOROPLASTY DURING ESOPHAGECTOMY: HISTORICAL PERSPECTIVE

While the importance of conduit emptying and function is universally recognized, there are many factors that contribute. The necessity of routine inclusion

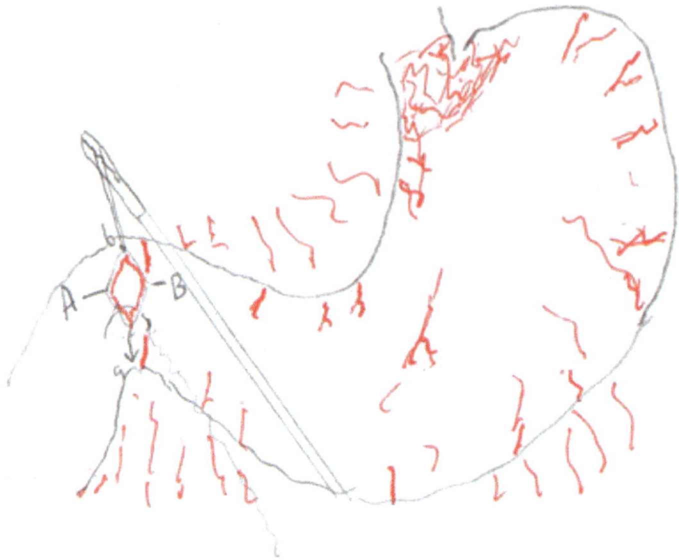

Fig. 2. Heineke–Mikulicz Pyloroplasty: Interrupted Transverse Closure of Pyloroplasty. "A" and "B" denote borders of longitudinal incision, lower case "a" and "b" denote stay sutures to provide traction and countertraction to facilitate transverse closure. (*Figure courtesy* Sam Luketich.)

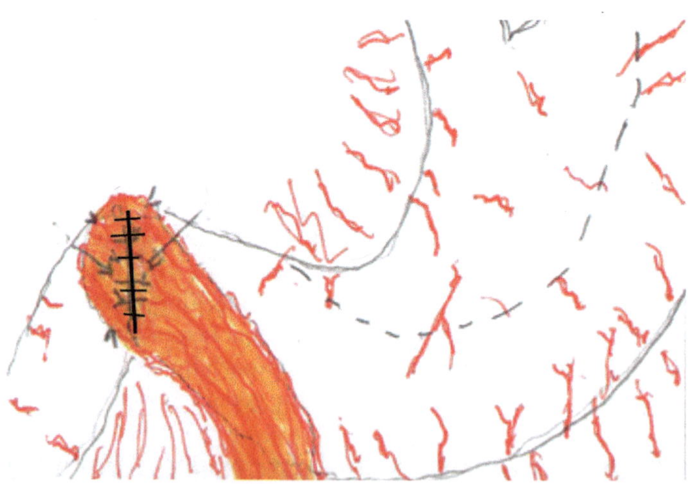

Fig. 3. Heineke–Mikulicz pyloroplasty: interrupted transverse closure of pyloroplasty with pedicled omental flap buttressing repair. (*Figure courtesy* Sam Luketich.)

of a pyloroplasty during esophagectomy is not universally recognized. There have been several trials over various periods examining this topic with mixed results.

In 1987, Cheung and colleagues reported a randomized clinical trial of 72 patients undergoing transthoracic esophagectomy with use of the whole stomach as a conduit in the right chest. Patient was randomized to inclusion or omission of pyloroplasty [2]. There were no pyloroplasty-related complications. They found that postoperative gastric emptying was significantly delayed in the no pyloroplasty group. Ultimately, the authors recommended routine inclusion of pyloroplasty given that it was performed safely and could improve gastric emptying.

In 1989, Gupta and colleagues prospectively studied gastric emptying 24 patients who were status postesophagectomy and gastric reconstruction with and without pyloroplasty [3]. They observed delay in gastric emptying compared to preoperative baseline in both groups. The pyloroplasty group had improved gastric emptying as compared to the control group.

In 1990, Mannell and colleagues performed a randomized trial of 40 patients undergoing esophagectomy with substernal gastric reconstruction randomized with or without pyloroplasty [4]. They observed increased pulmonary complications and symptoms of gastric stasis in the early postoperative period among the control arm. The authors recommended use of pyloroplasty.

In 1991, Chattopadhyay and colleagues performed a trial of 24 patients undergoing esophagectomy with cervical anastomosis randomized to with or without pyloroplasty [5]. The authors noted increase delay in gastric emptying in the no pyloroplasty group but no difference in clinical outcomes. The authors also observed no difference in bile content of gastric juices after surgery between groups [6]. Thus, they concluded that there was no benefit to pyloroplasty.

In 1991, Fok and colleagues published a larger trial of 200 patients undergoing esophagectomy with whole stomach reconstruction randomized 1:1 to with or without pyloroplasty [7]. The authors noted improved diet tolerance in the pyloroplasty group and reduced symptoms of delayed gastric emptying. They also observed a higher rate of pulmonary complications and need for parenteral nutrition in the no pyloroplasty group. The authors recommended inclusion of pyloroplasty during esophagectomy.

In 1994, Kao and colleagues reported a trial of 38 patients undergoing esophagectomy with or without pyloroplasty [8]. The authors found that use of pyloroplasty was associated with improvement in gastric emptying, and recommended its use during esophagectomy.

In 1995, Zieren and colleagues studied 52 patients undergoing esophagectomy with cervical anastomosis randomized with and without pyloroplasty [9]. In this study, there was no observed benefit in gastric emptying nor patient symptoms associated with pyloroplasty. On the other hand, one patient had a fatal pyloroplasty leak, and 2 patients had severe pyloroplasty stricture. The authors did not recommend use of pyloroplasty.

In 1996, Kobayashi and colleagues reported a trial of 67 patients undergoing esophagectomy randomized with or without pyloroplasty [10]. The pyloroplasty group had reduction in early symptoms of regurgitation, reduction in delayed gastric emptying, but no differences in objective nutrition parameters. The authors concluded that pyloroplasty effectively improves quality of life and gastric emptying.

In light of the multiple small trials reported above with varying results, Urschel and colleagues performed a systematic review and meta-analysis of 9 randomized trials including 533 patients comparing pyloroplasty to no pyloroplasty at time of esophagectomy [11]. Outcomes including mortality, anastomotic leak, pulmonary complications, and gastric outlet obstruction. The study found a significant reduction in gastric outlet obstruction in favor of the pyloroplasty cohort, but no significant differences in any other endpoints. The authors concluded that pyloric drainage reduces the occurrence of gastric obstruction postesophagectomy.

PYLOROPLASTY DURING ESOPHAGECTOMY IN THE MODERN ERA

Development and clinical implementation of the totally minimally invasive McKeown and Ivor Lewis esophagectomy (MIE) was pioneered by Dr Luketich and colleagues. In 2002, the first large experience of MIE in 222 patients, reporting only 1.4% operative mortality and 11% rate of anastomotic leak. Notably, pyloroplasty or pyloromyotomy was performed in 74% of these cases. In 2010, Dr Luketich published a report of over 1000 minimally invasive esophagectomies, reporting 1.7% mortality and leak requiring surgery in 5% of cases. Over 85% of these patients underwent pyloric drainage procedure. These reports were followed by a prospective multicenter trial including 17 sites and 104 patients who underwent MIE with 2.9% mortality and 8.6% anastomotic leak. Pyloroplasty was undertaken in 64% of these patients [12].

In 2010, Nguyen and colleagues published a retrospective review of 109 minimally invasive esophagectomy cases comparing outcomes with or without pyloroplasty [13]. The authors observed no differences in clinical outcomes and shorter operative times in the no pyloroplasty cases. They concluded that omission of pyloroplasty was safe.

In 2014, Antonoff and colleagues published a retrospective study examining outcomes after esophagectomy in 293 patients undergoing various pyloric drainage strategies including no intervention, pyloroplasty, pyloromyotomy, pyloric dilation, and pyloric botox [14]. They observed greater pulmonary complications in the group who did not undergo pyloric drainage. Major complications related to pyloric drainage were very rare (0.6%) cases. They authors concluded that pyloric drainage was useful in avoiding pulmonary complications after esophagectomy, and that short-term outcomes were similar among the various drainage procedures.

In 2024, Doran and colleagues published a large retrospective analysis of 207 consecutive patients undergoing esophagectomy with or without pyloroplasty

[15]. They found no difference in overall clinical outcomes between the groups but noted a higher incidence of need for pyloric dilation in the no pyloroplasty group. Among the subgroup of patients who required postoperative dilation, there were increased odds of respiratory complication and greater weight loss. Thus, the authors concluded that pyloroplasty is a useful adjunct to avoid the need for pyloric dilation postoperatively, which is a negative prognostic predictor.

Arya and colleagues reported a meta-analysis comprising 25 studies and over 3000 patients all published since 2000 comparing pyloric drainage strategies at time of esophagectomy including: no intervention, botox injection, finger fracture, pyloroplasty, and pyloromyotomy [16]. Although there were trends toward lower pulmonary complications, anastomotic leak, and improved gastric emptying for the pyloric drainage arm, none of these trends were statistically significant. The authors concluded that the ideal technique remains undefined and that rigorous prospective evaluation is needed to determine the role of pyloric drainage in the modern era of esophagectomy. Major studies are summarized in Table 1.

UNIVERSITY OF PITTSBURGH RANDOMIZED CLINICAL TRIAL

While a number of randomized trials reviewed above had demonstrated the benefit of pyloroplasty in the 1980s to 1990s, the benefit remained questionable in the modern era. In many of these older trials, the entire stomach was used as a conduit. In the modern era of minimally invasive Ivor Lewis and Mckeown esophagectomy, surgeons create a narrow conduit with a high intrathoracic or cervical anastomosis, paying special attention to avoid redundancy and tortuosity of the conduit. Thus, many surgeons feel that their conduit empties well without pyloric drainage augmentation. Previous data in the modern era of esophagectomy were limited to retrospective comparisons.

Luketich, Pennathur, and colleagues sought out to perform a large, single institutional randomized trial to compare use and omission of pyloroplasty during minimally invasive Ivor Lewis or Mckeown esophagectomy. This was a phase III randomized control trial with evaluation of 134 patients, who underwent MIE and were randomized using a Bayesian model resulting in 90 patients with pyloroplasty and 44 patients without. All cases were performed minimally invasively with a consistent technique for creation of the gastric tube starting within 5 cm of the pylorus and with a consistent tube diameter 3 cm. Pyloroplasty was done using Heineke–Mikulicz technique.

The primary endpoint was a composite outcome of pulmonary complication and/or anastomotic leak requiring surgery. This was significantly greater in the no pyloroplasty arm, occurring in 27% of patients, as compared to 18% in the no pyloroplasty group. Incidence of delayed gastric emptying seen on postoperative esophagram was also increased in the no pyloroplasty arm. There were no significant differences in mortality, quality of life, duration of nasogastric tube drainage, nor length of stay. Over 2 year follow-up, 7 patients (16%) in

Table 1
Major studies evaluating the impact of pyloroplasty during esophagectomy

Study	Study type	Patients, studies	Pyloric intervention	Major outcomes	Conclusion
Fok et al [7] 1991	Single-center RCT	200 patients	Pyloroplasty vs no pyloric drainage	Pyloroplasty reduced delayed gastric emptying, pulmonary complications, need for tpn	Favors pyloroplasty
Urschel et al [11] 2002	Meta-analysis of RCTs	9 trials, 533 patients	Pyloroplasty vs no pyloric drainage	Reduction in gastric outlet obstruction for pyloroplasty	Favors pyloroplasty
Nguyen et al [13] 2010	Retrospective single center	109 patients, all MIE	Pyloroplasty vs no pyloric drainage	No difference in mortality, leak, gastric emptying	No benefit to pyloroplasty
Antonoff et al [14] 2014	Retrospective single center	293 patients, transhiatal and transthoracic	Pyloric drainage vs no pyloric drainage	Reduction in pulmonary complications after pyloric drainage	Favors pyloroplasty
Doran et al [15] 2025	Retrospective single center	207 patients, Ivor Lewis Esophagectomy	Pyloroplasty vs no pyloric drainage	Significant need for postoperative pyloric intervention	Favors pyloroplasty
Arya et al [16] 2015	Meta-analysis of retrospective studies	25 studies, 3172 patients	Pyloric drainage vs no pyloric drainage	No difference pulmonary complications, leak, gastric emptying	No benefit to pyloroplasty
Luketich et al [17] 2026	Single-center RCT	134 patients, all MIE	Pyloroplasty vs no pyloric drainage	Pyloroplasty decreased composite outcome: leak and/or pulmonary complication	Favors pyloroplasty

Abbreviation: RCT, randomized controlled trial; TPN, total parenteral nutrition.

the no pyloroplasty cohort required pyloric intervention including dilation (n = 6), and surgical conduit revision with pyloroplasty (n = 1).

This study provided level I evidence in favor of pyloroplasty during esophagectomy in a center with significant experience in MIE. The study primarily focused on short term outcomes. Further studies to assess longer term outcome are warranted. Multicenter prospective evaluation is also indicated to validate these results. The Japanese Trial PYNI-GAREREO Phase III Randomized Controlled Trial (Pyloroplasty vs No Intervention in GAstric REmnant REconstruction after Oesophagectomy) is enrolling patients toward this aim, with a proposed study group of 140 patients.

COMPLICATIONS OF PYLOROPLASTY

Pyloroplasty leak is exceedingly rare (<1% patients) given the robust blood supply of the antrum and pylorus. Furthermore, placement of a pedicled omental flap to buttress pyloroplasty closure may help to prevent clinically significant leak [18]. Pyloroplasty may contribute to *dumping* syndrome. In this phenomenon, rapid transit of hyperosmolar chyme into the small bowel causes osmotic fluid shifts into the small bowel contributing to cramping, nausea, tachycardia, and diarrhea [19]. Intake of smaller protein rich meals and avoidance of excess simple carbohydrates can combat this effect. Finally, pyloroplasty may be implicated in bilious reflux. These cases are rare and generally are managed successfully using dietary modification, ursodiol, and bile acid sequestrant therapy. Again, creation of a narrow conduit with a high intrathoracic anastomosis may limit symptoms of acid and bile reflux.

In 2007, Palmes and colleagues retrospectively analyzed 198 patients undergoing esophagectomy, comparing patients undergoing pyloroplasty, pyloromyotomy, and no pyloric drainage [20]. They observed no differences in anastomotic leakage, gastrointestinal leakage, or length of stay. On the other hand, patients with pyloric drainage had higher incidence of reflux seen on endoscopy. They cautioned that routine pyloric drainage should be omitted due to lack of benefit and risk of bilious reflux.

OTHER PYLORIC DRAINAGE PROCEDURES

Pyloromyotomy

Development of the pyloromyotomy is attributed to Dr Harold Stiles in 1910, although was widely attributed to Dr Ramstedt, who described the procedure in 1911 [21]. This procedure involves a 2.0 cm length of myotomy across the pyloric muscularis, leaving the mucosal layer intact. It is classically indicated in infantile hypertrophic pyloric stenosis. In the native pylorus during a laparoscopic approach, full-thickness pyloromyotomy without risk of mucosal injury can be challenging. Full-thickness pyloroplasty guarantees a complete myotomy and does not risk a delayed leak secondary to unrecognized mucosal injury.

In 1997, Law and colleagues report a trial of 92 patients undergoing esophagectomy randomized to undergo either pyloroplasty or pyloromyotomy [22].

The authors noted increased time for gastric emptying in the pyloromyotomy groups, but no differences in complications, mortality, or other clinical outcomes. They concluded that both procedures were effective.

In 2007, Lanuti and colleagues reported a retrospective review of 242 patients who underwent esophagectomy, comparing cohorts with and without pyloromyotomy [23]. They noted no difference in incidence gastric outlet obstruction comparing the groups. Patients in both groups who did develop gastric outlet obstruction were successfully managed with conservative measures and endoscopic pyloric dilation in the majority of cases.

Pyloric digital fracture

During open esophagectomy, digital fracture of the pylorus has been described as a procedure in which the surgeon identifies the pylorus muscle, then firmly pinches the anterior pyloric wall and lateral wall for 10 to 20 seconds each until they feel the pylorus relax.

In 2010, Deng and colleagues reported a study of 78 patients undergoing esophagectomy who were prospectively enrolled and underwent either no pyloric drainage procedure or digital pyloric fracture [24]. They noted improved gastric emptying in the group who underwent pyloric fracture.

Gastric peroral endoscopic myotomy of the pylorus

G-POEM was first reported by Dr Khasab and colleagues in 2013, proposing a totally endoscopic means of pyloromyotomy [25]. This technique involves creation of a mucosotomy 5 cm proximal to the pylorus, then a tunneled creation of a submucosal tunnel extending across the pylorus. Myotomy is performed either at full-thickness or of the inner circular muscle fibers alone, extending 2 to 3 cm onto the antrum and across the entire length of pylorus onto the proximal duodenum. Following myotomy, the mucosotomy site is closed using endoscopic clips.

Nammour and colleagues recently published a series of 11 patients with delayed gastric emptying after Ivor Lewis esophagectomy treated with G-POEM [26]. They observed improvement in gastric emptying in 88% of patients and no treatment related adverse events.

Endoscopic pyloric botulinum toxin injection

Pyloric botox injection is an endoscopic adjunct for pyloric drainage augmentation. This procedure involves direct visualization of the pylorus under endoscopic view, 4 quadrant injection of the pylorus in the muscularis layer with botox. Typically, 25 units of botox are injected into each quadrant for a 100-unit total dosage. The duration of benefit expected from this procedure is typically on the order of months. Benefit from botox can be a valuable diagnostic tool in workup for more invasive and definitive pyloric drainage procedure.

In 2009, Cerfolio and colleagues reported a retrospective review of 221 patients undergoing esophagectomy were retrospectively evaluated, including cohorts that underwent pyloroplasty, pyloromyotomy, pyloric botox, and no drainage adjunct [27]. They found that patients who underwent botox injection had improved gastric emptying as compared to all other subgroups, and also had shorter operative time and reduced length of postoperative hospital stay.

Endoscopic pyloric dilation

Pyloric dilation provides yet another endoscopic adjunct to augment pyloric drainage [28]. An endoscopically deployed balloon is positioned across the pylorus and inflated with liquid to perform a pneumatic dilation. Use of contrast enhanced saline for balloon filling facilitates fluoroscopic imaging to ensure appropriate balloon position during dilation. Given the lack of feedback regarding resistance to dilation when using the pressure-filled balloon, serial dilation starting with a conservative balloon diameter such as 1.5 cm with inspection between dilations is recommended. Most patients can be dilated to a 2 cm size. In cases of severe stricture staged progressive dilations may be indicated. Duration of benefit after dilation may be limited, but can serve as a prognostic tool in selection for definitive pyloric drainage procedure.

In 1996, Manjari and colleagues reported a trial of 30 patients undergoing esophagectomy randomized to pyloroplasty, pyloromyotomy, or pyloric dilation [29]. There were no significant differences in gastric emptying or quality of life observed in 3-month follow-up. The authors concluded that early outcomes are equivalent among the various pyloric drainage procedures evaluated.

Technical pearls to optimize conduit function

Conduit emptying is dependent on multiple factors beyond just inclusion of a pyloric drainage procedure. Creation of a straight and narrow conduit is key to optimize conduit emptying and functional outcome. In our center, the gastric conduit is created within 5 cm of the pylorus, so as to minimize the size of antral reservoir, which may dilate or be a lead point for herniation and conduit redundancy, particularly after Ivor Lewis esophagectomy [18]. We also create a narrow gastric conduit with a 3 cm diameter, which is less subject to food stasis and dilation over time. Another key principle is to avoid axial rotation or excessive length of the conduit while it is brought into the chest. During a Mckeown esophagectomy, excess conduit can be reduced back into the abdomen and a crural closure can be performed. However, during an Ivor Lewis esophagectomy, it is difficult to reduce excess conduit once it is pulled into the chest, and so it is paramount to avoid this. In an Ivor Lewis case, use a tacking suture of the conduit to the diaphragm may help to prevent conduit herniation.

Postoperative assessment of conduit emptying

Postoperative assessment of conduit emptying should be done routinely and used to guide patient management. High-volume nasogastric drainage, presence of a dilated conduit on chest radiograph, and poor passage of contrast through the pylorus on postoperative esophagram all herald poor conduit emptying. Adjustment of postoperative pathway including prolonged nasogastric drainage and delayed progression of per oral diet are indicated. For patients who did not undergo pyloric drainage during index procedure, these signs may warrant postoperative pyloric intervention. Failure to diagnose and intervene on a poorly emptying conduit may predispose patients to aspiration and postoperative pulmonary complications. Furthermore, a dilated conduit may be subject to impaired perfusion or radial pressure on the anastomosis, with increased potential for postoperative anastomotic leak.

Delayed presentation of poor conduit emptying

Delayed gastric emptying may manifest not only in the acute postoperative period but also in the long term. This may manifest with dysphagia, weight loss, regurgitation, aspiration, and recurrent pneumonia. In addition to the pylorus, pathology of the conduit such as dilation, torsion, redundancy, or para conduit hernia should be considered. Workup includes esophagram, CT imaging, and endoscopy with consideration for endoscopic dilation for palliation of dysphagia. When workup suggests pyloric obstruction, pyloric interventions are indicated. Management of the dilated or tortuous conduit is more challenging. Our center has described an emerging technique for surgical revision of herniated and redundant conduits for patients with severe anatomic abnormality and symptoms refractory to endoscopic palliation and dietary modification [30].

SUMMARY

The debate over pyloroplasty versus no emptying procedure is far from over. In our randomized trial (Luketich, et al.), we found that a composite outcome of pulmonary complication and/or anastomotic leak requiring surgery was significantly greater in the no pyloroplasty arm, occurring in 27% of patients, as compared to 18% in the no pyloroplasty group. In addition, the incidence of delayed gastric emptying seen on postoperative esophagram was also increased in the no pyloroplasty arm. This article summarizes the data, and recent level I evidence that favors pyloroplasty. Meta-analysis and older randomized studies also favor pyloroplasty; however, there have been retrospective trials supporting use of no drainage procedure. We are in the planning phases of a follow-up randomized trial after MIE, designed to determine if other methods of pyloric emptying, such as myotomy and botox injection might be equally effective in the era of a narrow conduit reconstruction. Whether or not surgeons use pyloric drainage routinely, they are encouraged to refine a consistent technique during esophagectomy and to perform careful follow-up, both short term and long term. If clinical evidence of poor gastric emptying occurs, intervention should be considered. At the index operation of MIE, creation of a straight and narrow conduit with pyloroplasty or G-POEM, with a high intrathoracic anastomosis is our preferred technique. Careful assessment of short-term outcome as well as long term quality of life are indicated in the follow-up of esophagectomy patients as other causes of poor gastric emptying and problems with alimentation can occur, such as conduit shelving, strictures and other factors. As esophageal cancer care improves, new challenges emerge in the long-term survivors of esophagectomy who may face numerous issues, most recently more attention has been given to the actual lie of the conduit and its follow-up trajectory and diameter, all of which can contribute to dysphagia and poorly emptying conduit. Thoracic surgeons are rising to these challenges with new interventions such as endoscopic (G-POEM) and surgical pyloric drainage and conduit revision procedures [30].

CLINICS CARE POINTS

- Our randomized trial of pyloroplasty versus no pyloroplasty after MIE provides level I evidence that including a pyloroplasty lowers the risk of serious anastomotic leaks and pulmonary complications.
- Our review of other trials and meta-analyses on this topic favors performing a pyloric drainage procedure in conjunction with MIE.
- Other methods of pyloric emptying such as G-POEMS and botulinum toxin injection were not evaluated in our study but there is some evidence these interventions may provide some degree of improved gastric emptying after esophagectomy.
- For future reference, we look forward to the results of another randomized trial of pyloroplasty versus no intervention after esophagectomy (PYNI-GAREREO Trial.

Disclosure

The authors have nothing to disclose.

References

[1] Lovasik BP, Dodson TF, Srinivasan JK. Heineke, mikulicz, jaboulay, and finney: innovators of surgical pyloroplasty. Am Surg 2021;87(5):737–40.
[2] Cheung HC, Siu KF, Wong J. Is pyloroplasty necessary in esophageal replacement by stomach? A prospective, randomized controlled trial. Surgery 1987;102(1):19–24.
[3] Gupta S, Chattopadhyay TK, Gopinath PG, et al. Emptying of the intrathoracic stomach with and without pyloroplasty. Am J Gastroenterol 1989;84(8):921–3.
[4] Mannell A, McKnight A, Esser JD. Role of pyloroplasty in the retrosternal stomach: results of a prospective, randomized, controlled trial. Br J Surg 1990;77(1):57–9.
[5] Chattopadhyay TK, Gupta S, Padhy AK, et al. Is pyloroplasty necessary following intrathoracic transposition of stomach? Results of a prospective clinical study. Aust N Z J Surg 1991;61(5):366–9.
[6] Chattopadhyay TK, Shad SK, Kumar A. Intragastric bile acid and symptoms in patients with an intrathoracic stomach after oesophagectomy. Br J Surg 1993;80(3):371–3.
[7] Fok M, Cheng SW, Wong J. Pyloroplasty versus no drainage in gastric replacement of the esophagus. Am J Surg 1991;162(5):447–52.
[8] Kao CH, Chen CY, Chen CL, et al. Gastric emptying of the intrathoracic stomach as oesophageal replacement for oesophageal carcinomas. Nucl Med Commun 1994;15(3):152–5.
[9] Zieren HU, Müller JM, Jacobi CA, et al. [should a pyloroplasty be carried out in stomach transposition after subtotal esophagectomy with esophago-gastric anastomosis at the neck? A prospective randomized study]. Chirurg 1995;66(4):319–25.
[10] Kobayashi A, Ide H, Eguchi R, et al. [The efficacy of pyloroplasty affecting to oral-intake quality of life using reconstruction with gastric tube post esophagectomy]. Nihon Kyobu Geka Gakkai Zasshi 1996;44(6):770–8.
[11] Urschel JD, Blewett CJ, Young JEM, et al. Pyloric drainage (Pyloroplasty) or no drainage in gastric reconstruction after esophagectomy: a meta-analysis of randomized controlled trials. Dig Surg 2002;19(3):160–4.

[12] Luketich JD, Pennathur A, Franchetti Y, et al. Minimally invasive esophagectomy: results of a prospective phase II multicenter trial-the eastern cooperative oncology group (E2202) study. Ann Surg 2015;261(4):702–7.
[13] Nguyen NT, Dholakia C, Nguyen XMT, et al. Outcomes of minimally invasive esophagectomy without pyloroplasty: analysis of 109 cases. Am Surg 2010;76(10):1135–8.
[14] Antonoff MB, Puri V, Meyers BF, et al. Comparison of pyloric intervention strategies at the time of esophagectomy: is more better? Ann Thorac Surg 2014;97(6):1950–8.
[15] Doran SLF, Digby MG, Green SV, et al. Effect of pyloroplasty on clinical outcomes following esophagectomy. Surg Endosc 2025;39(1):432–9.
[16] Arya S, Markar SR, Karthikesalingam A, Hanna GB. The impact of pyloric drainage on clinical outcome following esophagectomy: a systematic review. Dis Esophagus 2015;28(4): 326–35.
[17] Luketich JD, Sarkaria ID, Levy RM, et al. A phase III randomized controlled trial of pyloroplasty versus no pyloroplasty in patients undergoing minimally invasive esophagectomy or robot-assisted minimally invasive esophagectomy. Ann Surg 2026;283(4):569–80.
[18] Pennathur A, Awais O, Luketich JD. Technique of minimally invasive Ivor Lewis esophagectomy. Ann Thorac Surg 2010;89(6):S2159–62.
[19] Hui C, Bauza GJ. Dumping syndrome. In: StatPearls. StatPearls Publishing; 2025. Available at: http://www.ncbi.nlm.nih.gov/books/NBK470542/. Accessed December 1, 2025.
[20] Palmes D, Weilinghoff M, Colombo-Benkmann M, et al. Effect of pyloric drainage procedures on gastric passage and bile reflux after esophagectomy with gastric conduit reconstruction. Langenbecks Arch Surg 2007;392(2):135–41.
[21] Mazurak M, Patkowski D. A history of the surgical correction of pyloric stenosis. J Pediatr Surg 2021;56(10):1904–7.
[22] Law S, Cheung MC, Fok M, et al. Pyloroplasty and pyloromyotomy in gastric replacement of the esophagus after esophagectomy: a randomized controlled trial. J Am Coll Surg 1997;184(6):630–6.
[23] Lanuti M, de Delva PE, Wright CD, et al. Post-esophagectomy gastric outlet obstruction: role of pyloromyotomy and management with endoscopic pyloric dilatation. Eur J Cardio Thorac Surg 2007;31(2):149–53.
[24] Deng B, Tan QY, Jiang YG, et al. Prevention of early delayed gastric emptying after high-level esophagogastrostomy by "pyloric digital fracture.". World J Surg 2010;34(12): 2837–43.
[25] Khashab MA, Ngamruengphong S, Carr-Locke D, et al. Gastric per-oral endoscopic myotomy for refractory gastroparesis: results from the first multicenter study on endoscopic pyloromyotomy (with video). Gastrointest Endosc 2017;85(1):123–8.
[26] Nammour T, Nishimura M, Zbib N, et al. Gastric peroral endoscopic pyloromyotomy as an effective treatment for symptomatic delayed gastric emptying following ivor Lewis esophagectomy. iGIE 2025; https://doi.org/10.1016/j.igie.2025.09.005.
[27] Cerfolio RJ, Bryant AS, Canon CL, et al. Is botulinum toxin injection of the pylorus during Ivor Lewis [corrected] esophagogastrectomy the optimal drainage strategy? J Thorac Cardiovasc Surg 2009;137(3):565–72.
[28] Kochhar R, Kochhar S. Endoscopic balloon dilation for benign gastric outlet obstruction in adults. World J Gastrointest Endosc 2010;2(1):29–35.
[29] Manjari R, Padhy AK, Chattopadhyay TK. Emptying of the intrathoracic stomach using three different pylorus drainage procedures–results of a comparative study. Surg Today 1996;26 (8):581–5.
[30] Kim S, Luketich JD, Gutierrez E, et al. Robotic transhiatal revision of gastric conduit after esophagectomy: experience in 15 patients. Ann Thor Surg Short Reports 2025; https://doi.org/10.1016/j.atssr.2025.11.004.

Advances in Surgery 60 (2026) 197–232
ADVANCES IN SURGERY

Minimally Invasive Approaches to Complex Abdominal Wall Reconstruction

Kaela E. Blake, MD[a,*], Benjamin K. Poulose, MD, MPH[b], Courtney E. Collins, MD[b]

[a]The University of Tennessee Health Sciences College of Medicine, Knoxville, TN, USA; [b]Center for Abdominal Core Health, The Ohio State University College of Medicine, Columbus, OH, USA

Keywords

• Robotic • Abdominal wall reconstruction • Hernia • Repair • Minimally invasive • Ventral • Incisional

Key points

- Robotic platforms have enabled the replication of open abdominal wall reconstruction (AWR) principles with minimally invasive surgery (MIS) benefits, driving rapid adoption over the last decade.
- The optimal repair (not the platform) must remain the priority—which includes patient factors, defect complexity, the need for soft tissue contouring, and available surgical expertise.
- MIS AWR offers fewer wound complications, shorter length of stay, and smaller scars at the expense of longer operative times, higher costs, steep learning curve, and uncertain long-term superiority.
- AWR techniques should be reserved for large, complex hernias in carefully selected cases and only performed by surgeons with appropriate expertise or those within a structured training program.
- Robotic AWR shows similar recurrence with improved short-term recovery, but needs high-quality, long-term data and continued refinement in training and cost-efficiency.

Video content accompanies this article at http://www.advancessurgery.com.

*Corresponding author. *E-mail address:* kblake@utmck.edu

https://doi.org/10.1016/j.yasu.2026.05.002

Abbreviations

AWR	abdominal wall reconstruction
eTEP	extended totally extraperitoneal
EHS	European Hernia Society
IPOM	intraperitoneal onlay mesh
MIS	minimally invasive surgery
rTAR	robotic transversus abdominis release
TAPP	transabdominal preperitoneal

BACKGROUND

Definition of abdominal wall reconstruction

Hernia repair is one of the most performed elective general surgical procedures in the country. Every surgical trainee graduates with at least a rudimentary knowledge of how to address abdominal wall defects. However, hernia disease is a very broad spectrum, and it can be difficult to ascertain what is a "repair" versus a "reconstruction" and when each is clinically indicated. The most widely accepted definition of abdominal wall reconstruction (AWR) stems from the Quality Collaborative coding consensus [1] published in *Hernia*, which closely aligns with the Centers for Medicare & Medicaid Services quality measures and reporting standards. In this framework, AWR refers to "the operative restoration of abdominal wall continuity and function using component separation (myofascial release), mesh reinforcement, or equivalent reconstructive techniques for complex or large hernias." This excludes simple primary closures or simple sublay mesh placements that do not involve myofascial release or retromuscular reconstruction. This is an important distinction because advanced hernia repair techniques such as component separation confer a much higher risk of complications and long-term sequelae and so should only be undertaken by surgeons who feel comfortable with these techniques. Additionally, the decision-making required to manage complex AWR patients is very intricate, and should only be undertaken by those with experience not only with repair approaches but also with the complications of the various techniques.

Evolution and trends toward robotic abdominal wall reconstruction

Hernia repair and AWR have undergone profound paradigm shifts as surgical technology has advanced. In the 1990s, the proliferation of the laparoscopic platform demonstrated fewer wound complications and shorter rates of hospital length of stay. However, it became apparent that despite some benefits, traditional laparoscopic intraperitoneal onlay mesh (IPOM) techniques had significant limitations, such as the confinement of mesh placement to the intraperitoneal position, limited ability to close the fascia, and challenging adhesiolysis using "straight sticks," which proved to be extremely difficult and time consuming. The role of laparoscopy for hernia repair operations was generally restricted to smaller defects amenable to either a bridging IPOM or transfascial sutures placed under direct visualization, while more complex defects required an open approach.

The advent of robotic platforms offered a dramatic paradigm shift. The enhanced dexterity, three-dimensional visualization, and improved ergonomics made it possible to replicate open retromuscular principles such as Rives-Stoppa and posterior component separations through small incisions in a way that was not possible on the laparoscopic platform. Early reports of robotic transabdominal Rives-Stoppa and robotic transversus abdominis release (rTAR) appeared in the mid-2010s, followed soon by extended totally extraperitoneal (eTEP) adaptations. The improvement of ergonomics on the robotic platforms also made the classic IPOM repair easier to perform, particularly for adhesiolysis and fascial closure. As a result, there has been a significant increase in the usage of robotic platforms for abdominal wall operations, mirroring trends seen in other surgical disciplines such as colorectal, urology, and gynecology. Between 2011 and 2018 the proportion of patients undergoing robotic ventral hernia repair increased from 0.5% to 13.8% (a 28 fold increase) [2]. This has largely come at the expense of laparoscopic repairs, which decreased from 25.8% to 15.9% in the same time period [2]. Open approaches to hernia repair have also decreased, but to a lesser extent (73.7% to 70.2%) [2]. If these trends continue, it is possible that laparoscopy will largely be replaced by robotic platforms in the coming years.

Benefits and drawbacks of minimally invasive abdominal wall reconstruction

As with all emerging technologies it is important to understand both the benefits and potential pitfalls of minimally invasive hernia repair, especially when it comes to complex procedures. Minimally invasive (now largely robotic) AWR has many potential benefits, including:

- *Decreased wound complications:* Hernia repair operations using MIS techniques demonstrate lower rates of wound complications and skin dehiscence compared with open approaches. These benefits are especially worth considering in high-risk patient populations such as those with obesity, diabetes mellitus, tobacco use, immunosuppression, and nutritional deficiencies.
- *Shorter hospital stays:* Patients undergoing minimally invasive AWR demonstrate shorter hospital lengths of stay, ranging between 1.5 and 3 days compared with those undergoing open AWR, which ranges between 5.3 and 9.6 days [3,4]. Reasons for this are multifactorial, but likely include reduced pain at discharge, earlier return of appetite and bowel function, less wound care needs, and overall improved function in the immediate post-operative period.
- *Improved surgeon ergonomics:* The robotic platform allows for improved ergonomics for surgeons, which is especially important for longer, complex reconstructions. Over the course of a surgical career, the strain placed on the surgeon by long, open operations is an important consideration, especially as more surgeons start to specialize specifically in complex hernia repairs.

- *Improved esthetic results:* One of the most (visually) obvious advantages to any MIS approach is the lack of a large incision. Besides the decreased risk of wound complications, many patients also find small, MIS incisions preferable to a large laparotomy incision, especially if their hernia stems from a prior laparotomy that resulted in a wound complication.

However, like all things, the benefits of minimally invasive AWR come with important drawbacks that warrant careful considerations. The disadvantages include:

- *Learning curve:* Learning safe and effective robotic AWR requires time, patience, appropriate supervision, and ongoing proctoring with mentorship. To become proficient at simple robotic hernia repair operations (excluding AWR), surgeons need to perform approximately 20 cases [5]. For more complex operations, including robotic AWR with transversus abdominis release (TAR), true proficiency requires 70 cases or more [6,7]. Furthermore, learning complex reconstruction techniques requires a "step up" approach with intentional patient selection to achieve expertise in an efficient and safe manner.
- *Increased operative time and cost:* Even after overcoming the learning curve and establishing proficiency, robotic hernia repairs continue to have longer operative times compared with open approaches, especially as the complexity of procedures increases [3,4,8]. This reduces operative efficiency for surgeons and lengthens the time that patients spend under general anesthesia. Furthermore, the increased operative time combined with the cost of using robotic platforms significantly increases the total intra-operative cost for robotic cases compared with open cases [3]. Although this is somewhat offset by the potential savings conferred by the decreased length of hospital stay, it continues to represent a significant upfront financial burden for hospital systems.
- *Limited ability to address soft tissue:* While one benefit of MIS approaches is the lack of a large incision, this also means that surgeons are unable to address soft tissue problems like unattractive scars, redundant skin, large areas of subcutaneous dead space after hernia reduction, and other soft tissue contouring complaints. Combining skin and soft tissue contouring procedures to improve the aesthetic outcome of ventral hernia repairs have been shown to improve patient quality of life [9].
- *Unclear long-term benefits:* Despite promising results in the immediate postoperative period, long-term results for MIS, particularly robotic approaches to hernia repair, are less clear. An analysis of the 10 year outcomes for over 161,000 patients using Medicare claims data demonstrated that robotic hernia repairs have a small but statistically significantly increased rate of hernia recurrence (13.43%) compared with both laparoscopic (12.33%) and open approaches (12.74%) [2]. Albeit, long-term quality of life results appear to be similar between robotic and open approaches [10–12].
- *Difficult access and enterolysis:* MIS techniques for intra-abdominal access can be challenging, especially in patients with a history of multiple prior hernia repairs and indwelling mesh. Furthermore, MIS enterolysis can be tedious and technically difficult. The risk of bowel injuries, particularly unrecognized bowel injuries, has been reported to be higher in MIS operations compared with open operations.

Safely learning minimally invasive abdominal wall reconstruction

The rapid adoption of MIS techniques, specifically robotic approaches, has made video-based learning for abdominal wall reconstruction more feasible and accessible. There has been a rapid influx of surgical videos available on the internet, which allows surgeons worldwide to view and potentially replicate complex robotic AWR techniques.

As previously mentioned, the case volume necessary to achieve comfort and proficiency with complex minimally invasive AWR is high. It is possible that video-based learning may help "flatten" the learning curve by providing examples of key steps and troubleshooting techniques explained by experts in the field, particularly for surgeons who do not practice at high volume centers. However, it is important to keep in mind several key points when using videos on the internet to learn surgical techniques. First, there is no standardization or peer-review process that ensures the quality and educational content of a video uploaded independent of a recognized surgical society. Second, there is an inherent risk of selection bias for these videos in terms of not only patient selection, but also editing choices with omissions that may obscure the technical challenges, troubleshooting maneuvers and detailed nuances of a procedure. This can lead to the portrayal of a very difficult operation appearing to be simpler and easily replicable, which can fail to accurately represent the true complexity of the operation. Lastly, videos alone do not capture the multifaceted decision making required in the pre-operative, intra-operative, and post-operative periods that are required to achieve safe, durable, and positive outcomes for patients.

Thoughtful case selection with the appropriate degree of complexity, and a "step up" approach to learn each surgical technique should be 2 foundational pillars for surgeons interested in learning advanced MIS AWR. Table 1 provides detailed pre-operative considerations that require a thorough understanding to achieve proficiency in AWR.

MINIMALLY INVASIVE APPROACHES TO VENTRAL HERNIA REPAIR

Abdominal access: transabdominal versus extended totally extraperitoneal

There are advantages and disadvantages to consider when choosing access for MIS AWR. Although technically challenging, eTEP access with extraperitoneal dissection allows for retromuscular mesh placement with minimal to no violation of the posterior sheath, allowing surgeons to largely avoid both adhesiolysis and posterior sheath closure. However, patient selection for eTEP is key, which requires:

1. Wide rectus abdominis musculature to facilitate access and space for dissection
2. Hernias with contents that can be reduced from the relatively small retrorectus space
3. A safe zone for the "crossover" from one retrorectus space to the other

Table 1
Important considerations when selecting the optimal approach for AWR patients

Indications for patient and approach selection	
Choosing Between MIS, open, and hybrid approaches • The type of repair—including type of mesh, mesh placement, and approach to fascial closure with or without component separation must be decided before (or simultaneously) with the decision about which platform to use—laparoscopic, robotic, open, hybrid. • The top priority should always be which type of repair (primary, onlay, retromuscular, intraperitoneal, etc.) will provide the best outcome for the patient. • The platform is secondary, and should be adjusted to ensure that the optimal repair is provided. • When deciding the best approach, several patient factors and technical steps must be considered (listed below)	
Patient considerations	**Technical considerations**
Wound risk: Patients at risk for wound complications or those with a history of wound healing issues may especially benefit from a minimally invasive approach. Social factors like the type of work patients perform and their ability to complete wound care at home must be considered.	*Foreign bodies:* Patients with a significant amount of foreign material (old mesh, tacks causing pain, suture abscesses, etc.) may be more appropriate for an open approach as these can be tedious to remove with an MIS approach and difficult to identify without the tactile feedback of palpation.
Cosmesis: While MIS may seem like it always confers a cosmetic benefit to patients, this is not always the case. Patients should be asked how they feel about any existing scars and how they would feel about having redundant skin after an MIS operation. Sometimes patients prefer a larger scar in order to excise more soft tissue to optimize the abdominal wall contour.	*Soft tissue:* After considering the patients' cosmetic wishes, surgeons should develop a plan for the soft tissue component of the operation after hernia reduction to address issues like redundant skin, thin skin prone to ischemia, and large areas of subcutaneous "dead space." While some of these issues can be mitigated with MIS approaches, others may warrant an open approach (potentially with plastic surgery) to achieve the best results.
Surgical risk: Complex AWR on the robotic platform, particularly early in the learning curve, can significantly add anesthesia time and potentially surgical risk to the patient. Patients at higher risk, particularly those with cardiopulmonary disease who cannot tolerate a long operation, may be more appropriate for an open approach.	*Anterior release vs posterior release:* The superiority of anterior vs posterior component separation has long been debated and is beyond the scope of this article. However, it is important to note that anterior component separation does confer many benefits such as more medialization of the rectus complex and less need for enterolysis. Additionally, for patients with large hernia sacs who already have significant subcutaneous dissection from the hernia itself, and for whom an open approach has been deemed preferable, an anterior component separation should be considered.

(*continued on next page*)

Table 1
(*continued*)

Patient considerations	Technical considerations
	Posterior sheath: For patients undergoing posterior component separation [transversus abdominis release with retromuscular mesh], achieving posterior sheath approximation is paramount to exclude the viscera from the uncoated mesh. However, when defects are not large enough to require a TAR (ie, those under 8–10 cm) but with too much tension to approximate the posterior sheaths after the retrorectus dissection, surgeons must anticipate this challenge and choose the approach that will still allow them to achieve posterior closure. This may require bridging the posterior sheaths with the hernia sac, omentum. or absorbable mesh. This is often more difficult with MIS approaches, given the pneumoperitoneum, which increases tension on the posterior sheath, and may require more robotic sewing, thus prolonging the operation.

Although eTEP access may help avoid adhesiolysis in patients with hostile abdomens, this approach should be used judiciously in these patients as they are at high risk for unrecognized bowel injuries during what essentially amounts to a blind dissection. When difficult adhesions are anticipated, the transabdominal approach is recommended since it allows for better visualization of the abdominal contents. This may reduce the risk of a bowel injury, facilitate the reduction of herniated contents, and save operative time, particularly for those early in the learning curve. However, the transabdominal approach requires closure of the posterior sheaths, which adds operative time to the case.

Transabdominal approach

Technical considerations

Technique. The patient should be positioned supine with arms tucked at the side. The peritoneal cavity is accessed in a minimally invasive fashion, typically at Palmer's point in the left upper quadrant. Three trocars are placed along the lateral abdominal wall, similar to conventional laparoscopic or robotic IPOM configuration (Fig. 1). After adhesiolysis, the medial border of the contralateral rectus abdominis muscle is identified, and the posterior rectus sheath is incised approximately 1 cm lateral to the linea alba. The posterior sheath is then mobilized laterally away from the rectus abdominis muscle, taking care to preserve

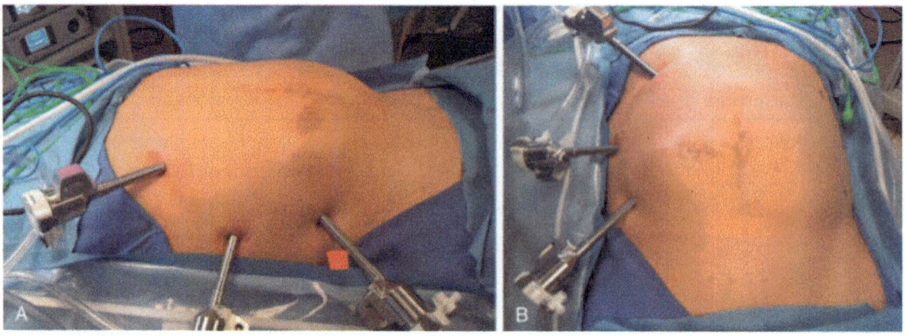

Fig. 1. Port positioning for rTAR with transabdominal access. rTAR, robotic transversus abdominis release. (Vahagn C. Nikolian, Yuri W. Novitsky, Dina Podolsky, 14 - Robotic transversus abdominis release (r-TAR) procedure, in Yuri W. Novitsky, Atlas of Robotic General Surgery, 2022, Elsevier.)

all neurovascular bundles along the linea semilunaris. Dissection is continued to obtain a mesh overlap of approximately 8 to 10 cm in all directions around the hernia defect, often extending down to the space of Retzius and superiorly to the xiphoid process.

Approach to transversus abdominis release. Top-Down Approach: The posterior lamella of the internal oblique and the transversus abdominus muscle are incised 1 cm medial to the linea semilunaris, ensuring to protect all neurovascular bundles (Fig. 2). The transversus abdominis muscle is elevated away from the transversalis fascia laterally. To avoid creating holes in the peritoneum, we recommend to dissect between the transversalis fascia and bare muscle fibers of the

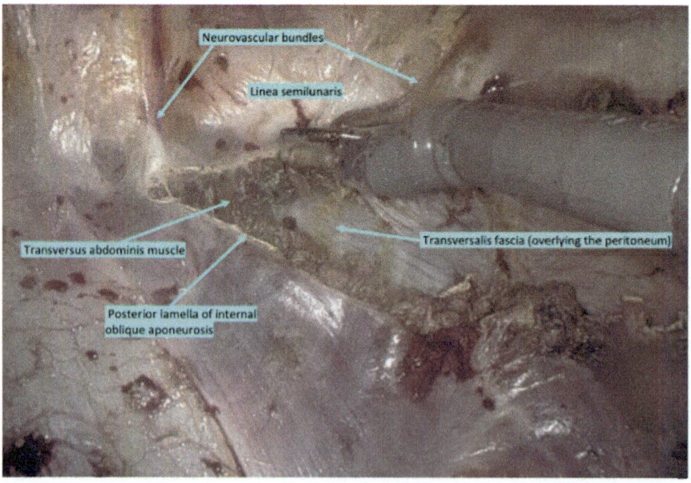

Fig. 2. Starting the TAR medial to the neurovascular bundles in the upper abdomen. TAR, transversus abdominis release.

transversus abdominis muscle, which will keep the transversalis fascia attached to the peritoneum for a thicker posterior layer. It is also acceptable to dissect between the peritoneum and transversalis fascia. However, the peritoneum becomes very thin and holes in the peritoneum are more likely with this approach. This dissection is carried caudally for the length of the posterior sheath mobilization (Fig. 3) and laterally out to the retroperitoneal fat. If mesh needs to wrap under the costal margin, is important to note that the neurovascular bundles are located along the costal margin, and must be protected. The incision for the TAR must similarly start 1 cm medial to the costal margin in the subcostal region to avoid injuring the superior epigastric vessels and neurovascular bundles overlying the rib (Fig. 4). The diaphragm inserts deep to the transversus abdominis muscle along the upper midline (Fig. 5), and it must be divided along its distal insertion to the posterior sheath (Fig. 6). This will allow the dissection to continue under the costal margin, below the muscle fibers and central tendon of the diaphragm. Failure to recognize this step can lead to dissection above the diaphragm muscle fibers, causing inadvertent entry into the pleural cavity and mediastinum.

Bottom up Approach: For patients with upper abdominal wall scarring or other contraindications to a top down approach, the TAR can be initiated inferiorly. Caudal to the arcuate line, the deep inferior epigastric vessels are first mobilized with the rectus abdominis muscle within the retrorectus space, until reaching the linea semilunaris (approximately 1 cm lateral to the deep inferior epigastric vessels). At this location, the transversalis fascia must be divided along its insertion to the linea semilunaris, which grants access to the lateral preperitoneal space of Bogros (Fig. 7). Dissection is then continued cranially until reaching the arcuate line. The transversalis fascia is mobilized away

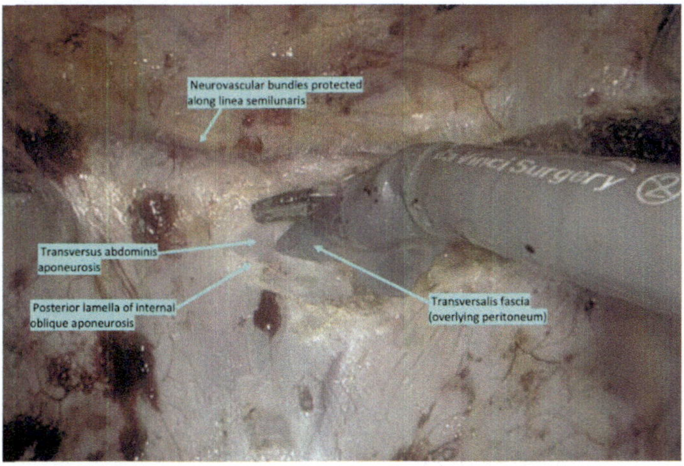

Fig. 3. Continuing the TAR caudally along the middle portion of the abdominal wall. TAR, transversus abdominis release.

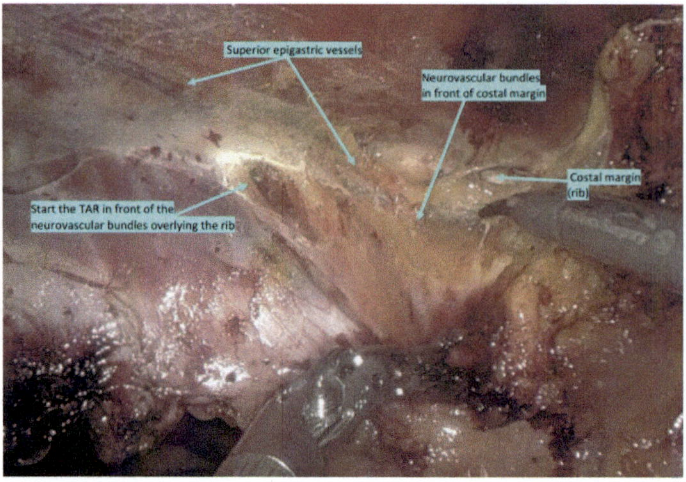

Fig. 4. Start the TAR medial to the costal margin in the subcostal region to avoid injuring the neurovascular bundles. TAR, transversus abdominis release.

from the undersurface of the posterior rectus sheath at the arcuate line. This allows the surgeon to incise the posterior rectus sheath medial to the linea semilunaris without making a hole in the peritoneum. The TAR can then be extended cranially until the desired amount of space is created for wide mesh overlap. Once the dissection is completed, 3 additional trocars are placed

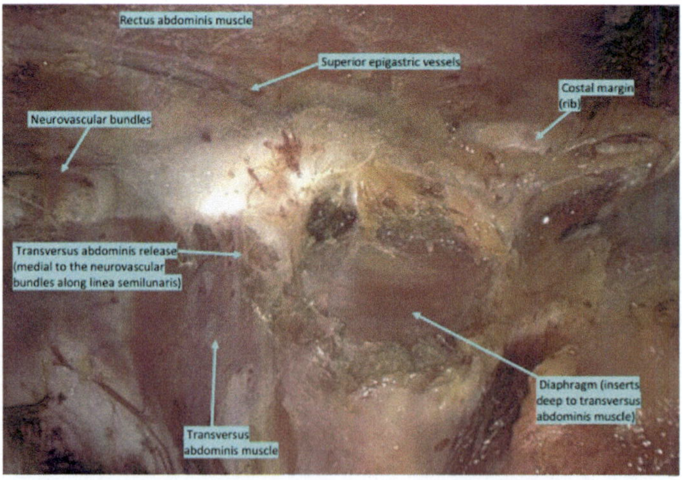

Fig. 5. The diaphragm inserts deep to the transversus abdominis muscle along the upper midline.

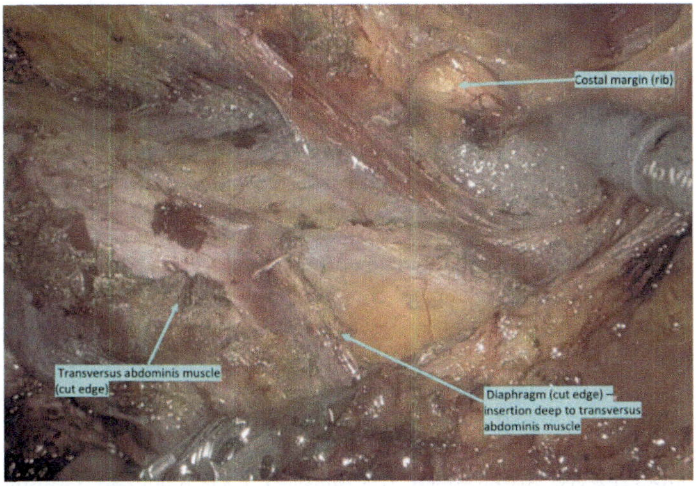

Fig. 6. The diaphragm must be divided along its distal insertion to the posterior sheath to continue under the costal margin.

along the contralateral abdominal wall and the robotic is undocked, rotated and redocked to perform the same dissection on the second side.

Posterior sheath closure. Once the dissection has been completed on both sides, the posterior sheath is closed with a running, absorbable, barbed suture. All significant holes in the peritoneum should be closed. If the posterior sheaths do not

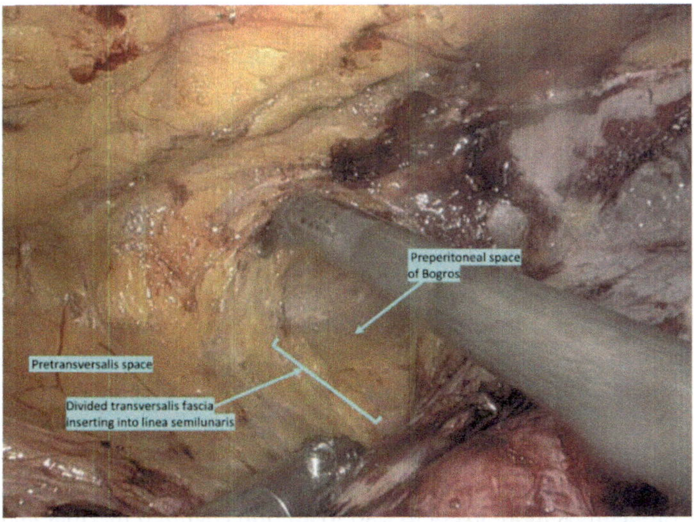

Fig. 7. Caudal to the arcuate line, divide the attachments of the transversalis fascia to the linea semilunaris to access the lateral preperitoneal space of Bogros.

approximate easily without tension, a wider dissection should be performed, or the posterior rectus sheaths can be bridged with an absorbable mesh, omentum, falciform ligament, or the hernia sac as needed.

Anterior sheath closure. The anterior sheath is closed with a large (0 or number 1) running barbed suture. To facilitate closure, reduce the pneumoperitoneum to as low as 6 to 8 mm Hg, and start a running suture both at the top and the bottom of the hernia defect, running toward each other.

Mesh placement. An uncoated, macroporous mesh is recommended when placing it in the retromuscular space. Coated meshes or microporous meshes have a higher risk of developing seromas in this location. Mesh can be placed at multiple timepoints during the operation, including after the dissection has been completed on the first retromuscular side (prior to redocking on the contralateral side), after the posterior rectus sheath closure, or after the anterior rectus sheath closure. Measure the length and width of the retromuscular space to determine the size of the mesh. If a bilateral TAR has been completed, measure from the midline to the lateral edge of one side of the dissection and double it to obtain the total width. Roll the mesh and insert it into the abdomen, which often requires upsizing the trocar to a 12 mm port.

If the mesh is placed before re-docking to the contralateral side, place the mesh as far lateral in the retromuscular dissection. To avoid mesh slippage, secure the mesh to the lateral abdominal wall musculature in 1 to 2 places using an absorbable suture (taking care not to injure enteric structures). Then re-dock the robotic platform on the contralateral side. Complete the dissection on the contralateral side, and then unroll the mesh into the newly formed retromuscular pocket.

If the mesh is placed after both retrorectus dissections are performed, the mesh is introduced in the same way, however it may be difficult to fully deploy the mesh underneath the working robotic trocars. Laparoscopic instruments through the contralateral side may help facilitate this step, or if needed, the robot can be redocked a third time. For patients undergoing a unilateral TAR, it is recommended that the TAR be completed after re-docking to allow for better visualization of the pocket for mesh placement. Refer to "Video 1 Robotic TAR" to view the full operation.

Tips and troubleshooting

When placing trocars, be mindful of collision with the patient's lower extremities. The lower trocar may need to be placed higher and more medial than expected, and the bed should be slightly flexed to help with clearance and to elongate the abdomen. If there continues to be a concern for clearance, a bariatric trocar is recommended, and the patient's legs can be dropped.

Adhesiolysis must be carried out laterally to safely clear the extent of the intended retromuscular dissection. Performing a TAR with bowel adherent to the underside of the peritoneum is more likely to lead to an unrecognized thermal injury to the viscera. However, if a TAR is not planned, there is no need to divide adhesions along the lateral abdominal wall and risk a bowel injury during adhesiolysis.

The decision about which side to start the case on should be considered with care. For example, if it has been pre-determined that only a unilateral TAR is to be performed, it is best to complete that dissection last to allow for better visualization during mesh placement.

Minimally invasive transabdominal TAR

- Retrorectus dissection: Incise posterior sheath just lateral to linea alba and dissect to the neurovascular bundles.
- Top down TAR: Incise the posterior lamella of internal oblique and transversus abdominis muscle 1 cm medial to the neurovascular bundles along the linea semilunaris and costal margin.
- Preserve posterior layer: Keep transversalis fascia attached to peritoneum to prevent holes
- Medial subcostal dissection: divide the distal diaphragm muscle fibers inserting into the posterior sheath to ensure dissection continues below the diaphragm.
- Bottom up TAR: Incise the transversalis fascia along the linea semilunaris to enter the lateral preperitoneal space. Mobilize the peritoneum cranially away from the underside of the posterior rectus sheath until the posterior rectus sheath can be divided medial to the neurovascular bundles.
- Tension-free posterior closure: Use wide dissection or bridge—using the hernia sac, falciform, omentum, or absorbable mesh
- Adequate overlap: Achieve 8–10 cm retromuscular dissection circumferentially.
- Mesh choice: Use uncoated macroporous mesh in the retromuscular plane.

Extended totally extraperitoneal approach

Technical considerations

Technique. Patient positioning is similar to the transabdominal approach with the same consideration for trocar clearance. Although we will describe this procedure using a lateral dock, trocars can be placed in various configurations depending on the location of the defect.

The most common access site for an eTEP is in the subcostal position of the upper abdominal wall. A 5 mm incision is made just below the costal margin and an Optiview trocar is used to dissect down to the retrorectus space. Once the rectus abdominis muscle fibers are identified, start the insufflation and carefully advance the trocar into the retrorectus space. Care should be taken not to rupture the posterior sheath as insufflation of the peritoneal cavity can limit working space. Once the retrorectus space is entered, the camera is used to dissect a pocket large enough to place the first robotic trocar. This should be placed at the lateral border of the rectus abdominis muscle as superiorly as possible and just medial to the linea semilunaris. To facilitate accuracy of port placement, we recommend using a long spinal needle to test the location an angle of entry prior to port placement. The retrorectus space is developed using a combination of blunt dissection and electrocautery until 2 additional trocars are placed, again at the lateral border of the rectus abdominis, just medial to the linea semilunaris. Once 3 robotic trocars are placed, the robotic platform can then be docked. There are multiple options for port configuration during eTEP approaches based on the location of the hernia defect (Fig. 8).

Once docked, the ipsilateral retrorectus dissection is completed with care taken to clearly identify the linea alba. The crossover location is then selected.

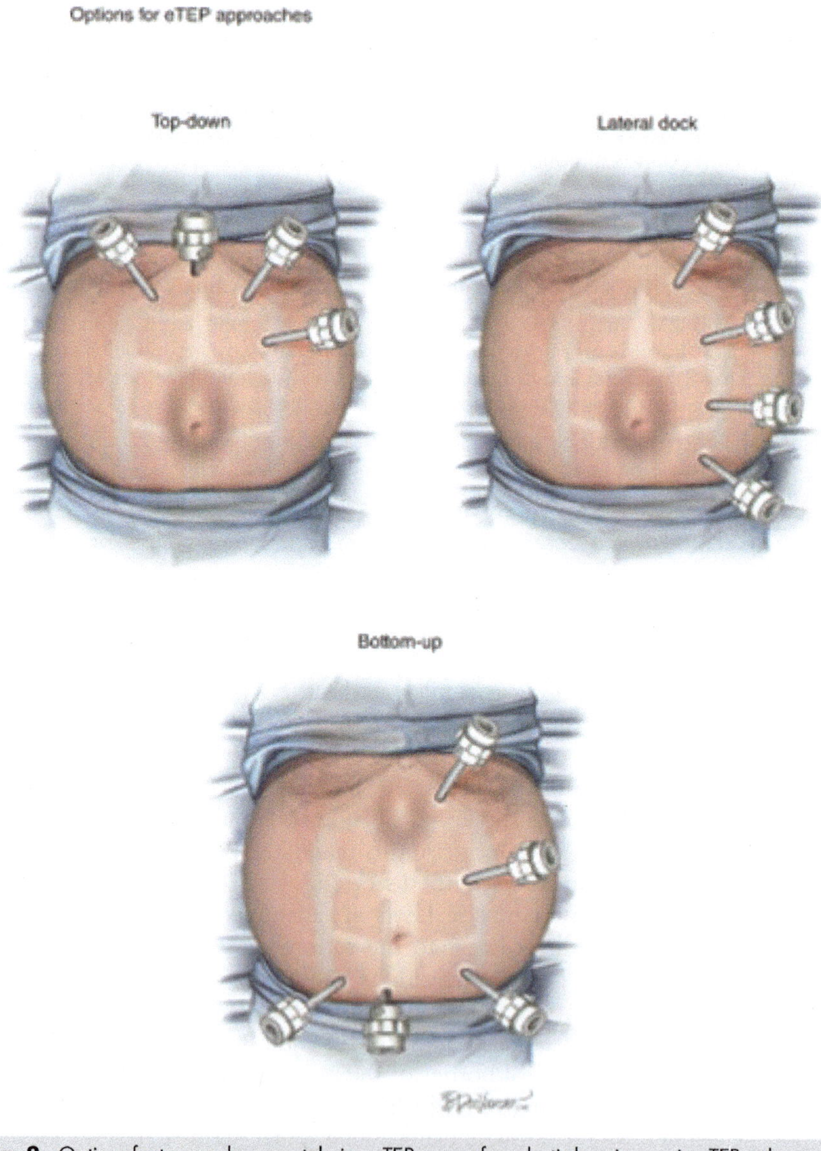

Fig. 8. Options for trocar placement during eTEP access for robotic hernia repair. eTEP, enhanced totally extraperitoneal. (Michael J. Rosen, Chapter 7 - Robotic Extended-View Totally Extraperitoneal Ventral Hernia Repair, in Atlas of Abdominal Wall Reconstruction, 3rd Edition, 2025, Elsevier.)

The most common location to crossover is superiorly at the level of the falciform ligament. However, inferiorly (caudal to the arcuate line along the median umbilical ligament), or in the mid-abdomen (along the hernia itself) are also options. When crossing over superiorly, the posterior rectus sheath is incised just lateral to the linea alba, and the preperitoneal fat of the falciform ligament is identified. Care should be taken dissect the preperitoneal fat away from the linea alba without injuring the linea alba. The contralateral posterior rectus sheath is incised, and the contralateral retrorectus space is developed. When crossing over inferiorly, below the arcuate line, the transversalis fascia is incised along its attachments to the linea alba. The preperitoneal fat surrounding the median umbilical fold is kept intact, and dissected away from the linea alba until reaching the contralateral transversalis fascia. The contralateral transversalis fascia is incised, and the retrorectus space is similarly developed. When crossing over directly over the hernia defect, the hernia sac is sharply incised without electrocautery to avoid thermal injury to the herniated viscera. The hernia contents are reduced, and the hernia sac in circumferentially mobilized out of the hernia defect until reaching the contralateral side. The contralateral posterior rectus sheath is incised to enter and dissect the retrorectus space.

Once bilateral retrorectus spaces are mobilized, the anterior fascia is closed in a similar manner as described in the transabdominal approach. The posterior sheath is then reapproximated and uncoated mesh is placed in the retrorectus position (Fig. 9). Refer to "Video 2 Robotic eTEP" for the complete operation. When a TAR is not performed and the dissection is confined to the retrorectus spaces, sometimes the posterior rectus sheaths have too much tension to reapproximate primarily. If re-approximation of the posterior rectus sheaths is attempted in the setting of excessive tension, there is a high risk for posterior sheath disruption and an interparietal hernia with bowel exposed to uncoated mesh. To avoid risking this complication, the surgeon may leave the posterior rectus sheaths in a bridged configuration with the intact falciform ligament and median umbilical ligament bridging the posterior rectus sheaths along the midline. This will safely exclude the viscera from the uncoated mesh. When a TAR is performed after eTEP access with retrorectus dissection, there is enough laxity to reapproximate the posterior rectus sheaths once the dissection is complete.

Mesh fixation and drain placement are considered in the same manner. The authors typically place one drain in the retrorectus space, which is removed prior to the patients' discharge home.

Tips and troubleshooting

Access for the eTEP approach is key, as puncturing the posterior sheath will create significant difficulty during the case with limited working space. If a hole in the posterior sheath is incidentally created, there are several maneuvers that may help. Small holes may be repaired with either a suture or a clip. Alternatively, a Veress needle or a 5 mm trocar can be introduced into the peritoneal cavity and used to ventilate.

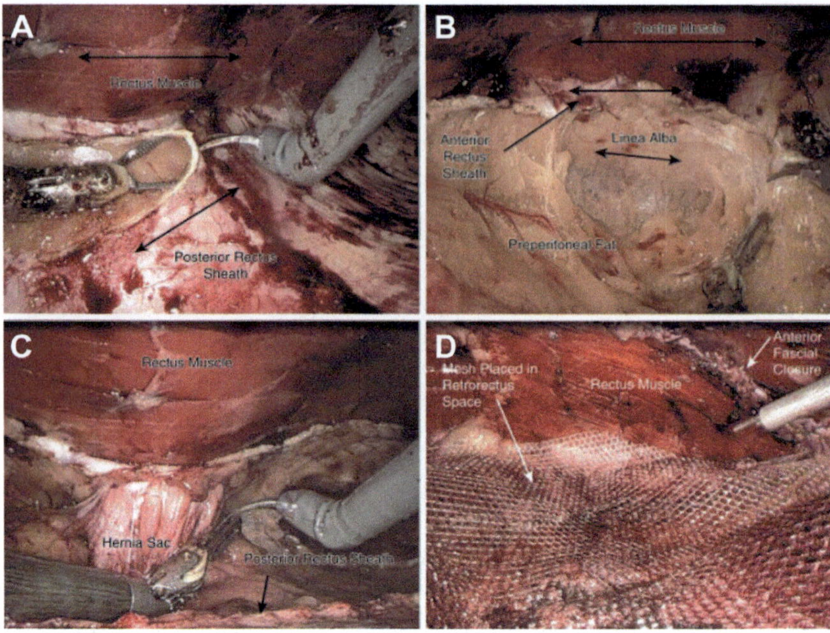

Fig. 9. eTEP technique. (*A*) After "crossing over" the linea alba, the rectus sheath is incised and preperitoneal fat is dissected. (*B*) Here the plane has been dissected showing the critical structures. (*C*) The hernia sac is revealed and will be reduced. (*D*) The anterior fascia has been closed (seen in upper right-hand corner) and mesh has been placed. eTEP, enhanced totally extraperitoneal. (Syed A. Ahmad, Aurora D. Pryor, Shackelford's Surgery of the Alimentary Tract, 2 Volume Set, 9th Edition, 2025, Elsevier.)

A minimally invasive TAR can be performed with an eTEP approach, although if a bilateral TAR is to be performed a double dock is still required with eTEP access. If a unilateral TAR is planned, access should be obtained on the side opposite of the planned TAR.

It is important to note that the eTEP approach is essentially a blind procedure, as visualization of the abdominal cavity is limited. Therefore, use of electrocautery on the posterior sheath, especially during the crossover step, should be limited as it is not known if bowel is lying directly beneath it. If there is any concern for injury, the posterior sheath should be opened to allow for adequate inspection. Some surgeons routinely perform an intraperitoneal diagnostic laparoscopy at the conclusion of the case that can also be considered.

eTEP access for minimally invasive AWR

- Precise retrorectus access is key: Avoid posterior sheath injury to preserve working space, and place ports as lateral as possible within the retrorectus space.

- Controlled crossover: Transitioning between the retrorectus spaces (superiorly, inferiorly, or via the defect) with careful tissue handling, avoiding electrocautery is important to prevent bowel injury.
- Bridged posterior closure: When the dissection is limited to the retrorectus spaces, bridge the posterior rectus sheaths using the intact falciform and median umbilical ligaments to avoid excessive tension on the closure.
- Exclude the viscera from the mesh: Close any holes in the hernia defect or peritoneum.
- Mesh choice: Use uncoated macroporous mesh in the retromuscular plane.

MINIMALLY INVASIVE SURGERY APPROACHES TO HERNIAS IN CHALLENGING LOCATIONS

Subxiphoid hernias

Subxiphoid hernias are classified as "M1" defects, located within 3 cm of the xiphoid process according to the European Hernia Society (EHS) classification [13] (Fig. 10). These hernias commonly result from prior cardiac operations requiring a median sternotomy or isolated upper abdominal wall operations. This can be a difficult location to reapproximate the fascial defect due to the insertion of the rectus abdominis complex onto the costal margin, which limits mobility of the linea alba. Since there is often tension on the fascial closure, wide mesh overlap is essential for the durability of this repair. Botox injections to bilateral rectus abdominis muscles along the costal margin can be considered preoperatively to facilitate primary fascial closure. When deciding between MIS and open approaches, an open approach is favored when redundant

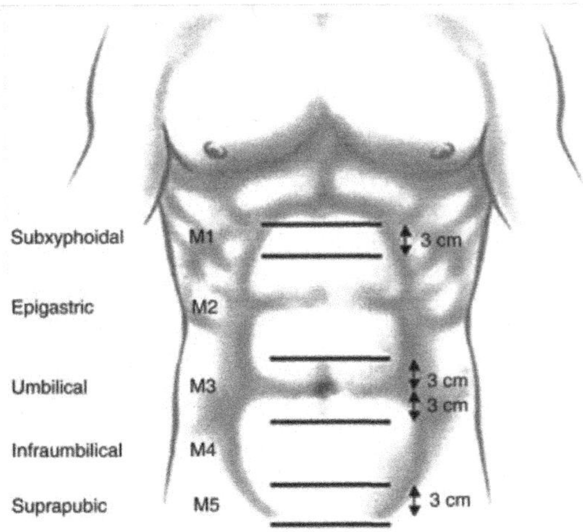

Fig. 10. European Hernia Society classification of primary and incisional abdominal wall hernias. (Syed A. Ahmad, Aurora D. Pryor, Shackelford's Surgery of the Alimentary Tract, 2 Volume Set, 9th Edition, 2025, Elsevier.)

skin and/or soft tissue excision is anticipated. Due to the technical difficulty of suturing the fascia laparoscopically, a robotic approach is the favored minimally invasive approach.

Patients are positioned supine, arms tucked and with their hips at the break of the operating table. The break of the table is flexed to elongate the patients' abdomen. A transabdominal preperitoneal (TAPP) approach, transabdominal retrorectus approach with upper TAR, or eTEP technique can all be used with good outcomes. For the transabdominal approaches, 3 robotic trocars are placed transversely across the lower abdomen just caudal to the umbilicus to allow space to start the flap (Fig. 11). For a TAPP approach, the peritoneum is divided in a transverse fashion in the supraumbilical position at least 10 cm away from the inferior edge of the hernia defect (Video 3 Subxiphoid TAPP). A preperitoneal flap is created and the dissection is carried cranially, being careful to avoid making holes in the peritoneum. Once the hernia contents are reduced, the superior edge of the fascial defect is identified. At this point, the subxiphoid fat and transversalis fascia are divided and the dissection must drop into the true preperitoneal plane. Transitioning into the true preperitoneal plane at the xiphoid process is important to avoid injuring the diaphragmatic attachments to the posterior rectus sheath (pars abdominalis) and erroneously dissecting above the diaphragm that will lead into the thoracic cavity. The peritoneum is then mobilized away from the undersurface of the diaphragmatic muscle fibers bilaterally and the central tendon of the diaphragm along the midline (Fig. 12). The peritoneal dissection must stop prior to reaching the esophageal hiatus and vena cava. Once a large preperitoneal pocket has been

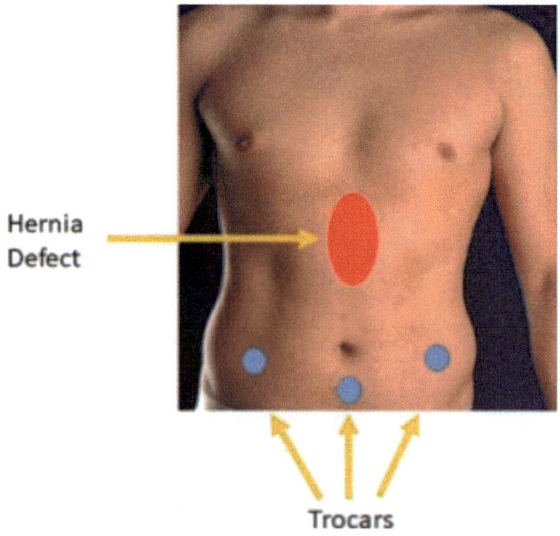

Fig. 11. Port placement for robotic subxiphoid hernia repair. (Hamid Reza Zahiri, Igor Belyansky, Adrian Park, Abdominal Wall Hernia, Current Problems in Surgery, 55 (8), 2018, 286-317, https://doi.org/10.1067/j.cpsurg.2018.08.005.)

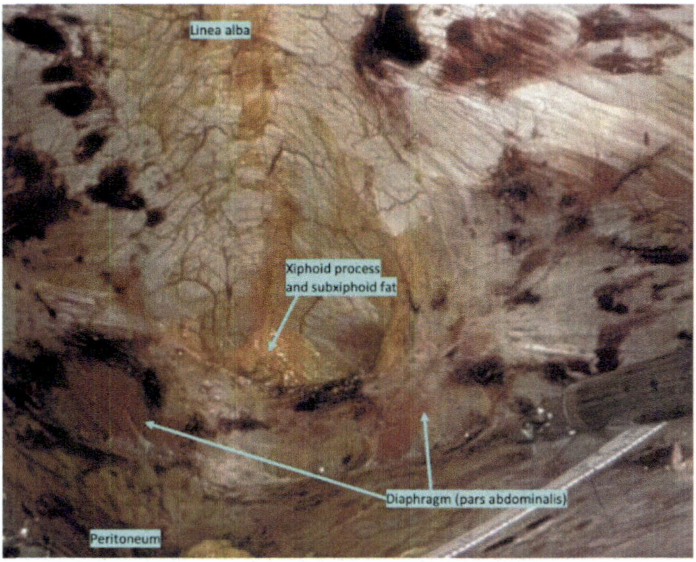

Fig. 12. View of subxiphoid region of abdominal wall. Pars abdominalis is the insertion of the diaphragm to the posterior rectus sheath. (*Photo courtesy of* Dr David Lourié.)

created, close the hernia defect with a running barbed suture and place mesh to widely cover the defect by approximately 8 to 10 cm in all directions (Fig. 13). Lastly, close the peritoneal flap with a running absorbable barbed suture.

A transabdominal retrorectus approach with an upper TAR can be used when the peritoneal flap is too thin to develop (Video 4 Subxiphoid TAR). This is achieved by incising the posterior rectus sheath in a transverse fashion

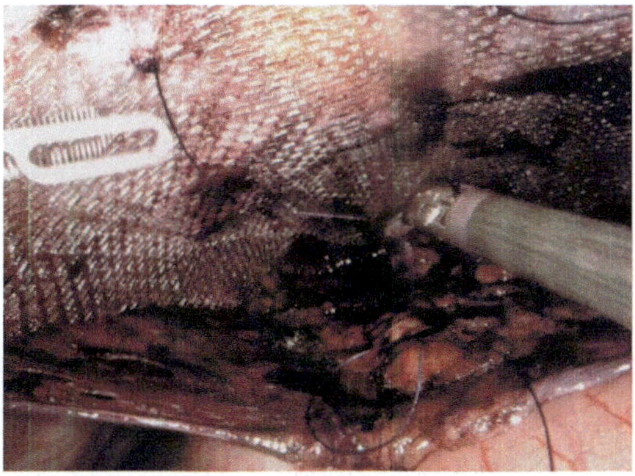

Fig. 13. A large sheet of uncoated mesh is placed in the preperitoneal plane to widely cover the defect. (*Photo courtesy of* Dr Sabrina Drexel.)

and entering the retrorectus plane (Fig. 14). Bilateral retrorectus spaces are developed in a cranial direction. The preperitoneal fat along the falciform ligament is preserved and kept attached to the posterior rectus sheath. Continue the dissection laterally on each side by performing a TAR in the subcostal region (Fig. 15). It is important to first identify the superior epigastric vessels and costal margin. All neurovascular bundles overlying the costal margin and semilunar line must be preserved. The posterior rectus sheath (posterior lamella internal oblique aponeurosis and transversus abdominis muscle) is incised medial to the neurovascular bundles until reaching the pre-transversalis plane. It is important to note that after the transversus abdominis muscle has been divided, the diaphragm inserts deep to the transversus abdominis muscle along the midline. In order to fully expose the medial insertion of the diaphragm along the posterior sheath, the hernia contents must be reduced and the xiphoid process visualized. At this point, the dissection must transition into the true preperitoneal plane (below the preperitoneal fat) along the midline by dividing the subxiphoid fat pad. This allows for visualization of the medial diaphragm fibers (pars abdominalis) (Fig. 16). The distal insertion of the diaphragm is divided, and the preperitoneal dissection continues cranially under the diaphragm muscle fibers until reaching the central tendon of the diaphragm (Fig. 17). Again, ensure that the peripheral insertion of the diaphragm at this location has been identified and the dissection continues in the true preperitoneal plane under the diaphragm muscle fibers. Otherwise, erroneous dissection into the pleural cavity and mediastinum could occur if the dissection continues above the diaphragm. The remaining steps are similar to those described for a TAPP approach with defect closure (Fig. 18) and mesh placement.

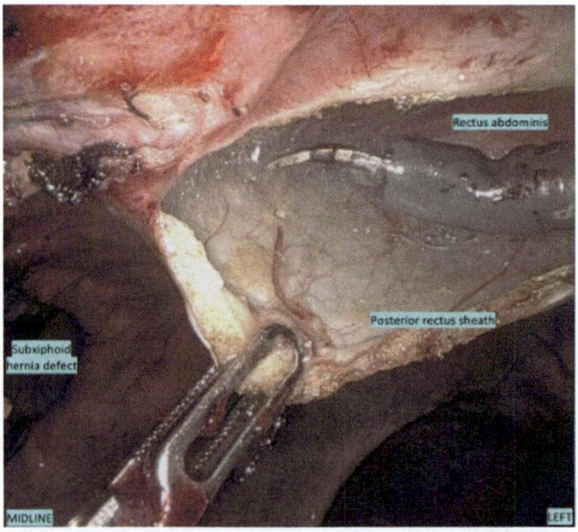

Fig. 14. Make a transverse incision along posterior rectus sheath to enter retrorectus plane to repair a subxiphoid hernia using a TAR approach. TAR, transversus abdominis release. (*Photo courtesy of* Dr Charlotte Horne.)

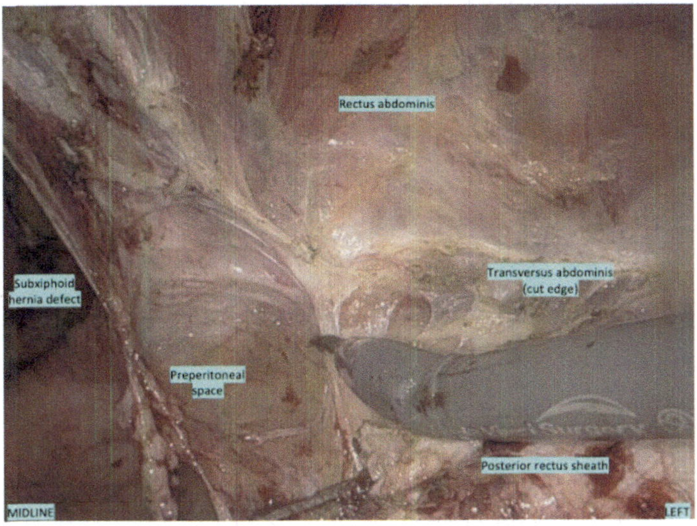

Fig. 15. Perform a TAR to enter the preperitoneal plane in the subxiphoid region. TAR, transversus abdominis release. (*Photo courtesy of* Dr Charlotte Horne.)

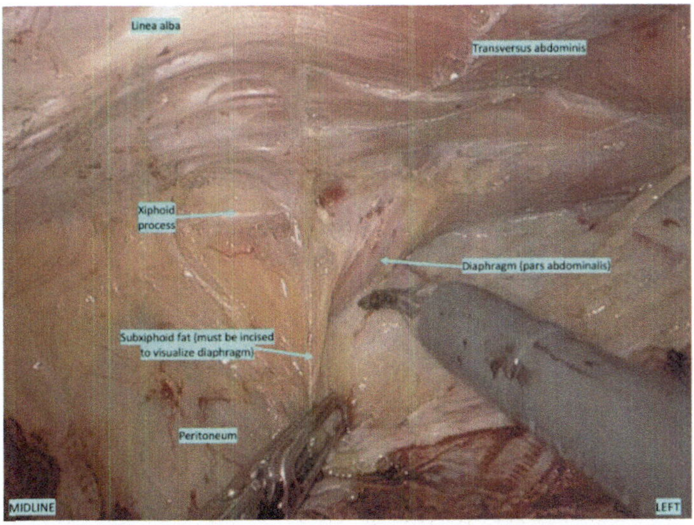

Fig. 16. The subxiphoid preperitoneal fat must be incised to visualize the diaphragm fibers (pars abdominalis) inserting deep to the subxiphoid preperitoneal fat along the midline. (*Photo courtesy of* Dr Charlotte Horne.)

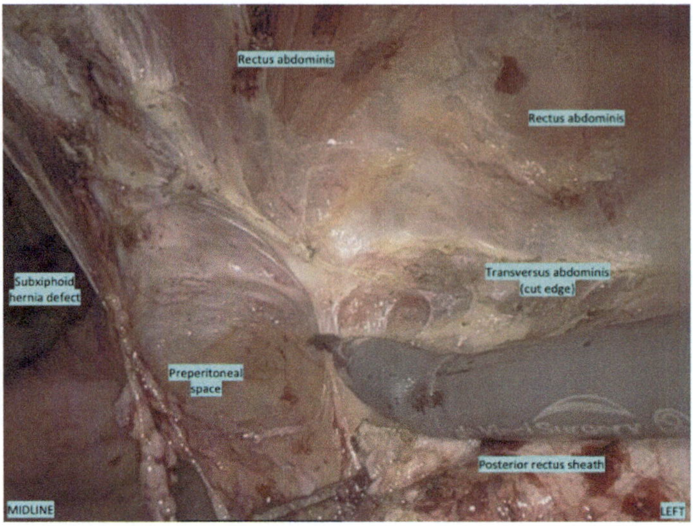

Fig. 17. Completed subxiphoid preperitoneal dissection, exposing a large portion of the central tendon of the diaphragm to allow for wide mesh overlap. (*Photo courtesy of* Dr Charlotte Horne.)

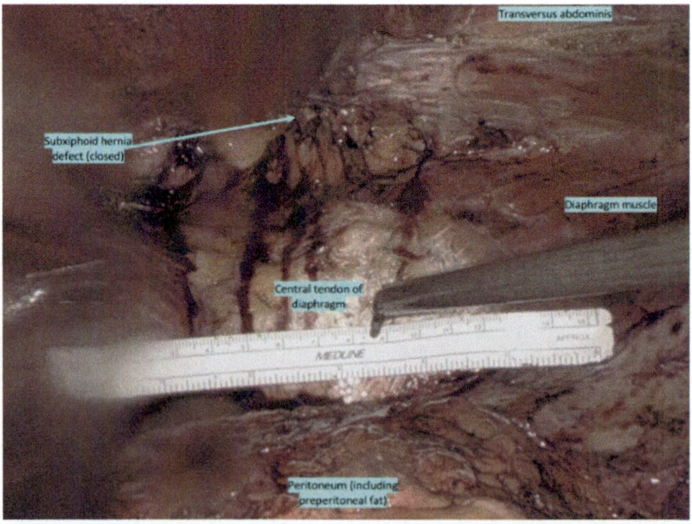

Fig. 18. Subxiphoid defect closure with a large preperitoneal flap ready for wide mesh placement. (*Photo courtesy of* Dr Charlotte Horne.)

When performing eTEP access, the surgeon should first gain access to the retrorectus space in the left or right upper quadrant, medial to the linea semilunaris and caudal to the hernia defect. Once the retrorectus space is accessed, blunt dissection using the camera and pneumoperitoneum are used to dissect the posterior sheath away from the rectus abdominis musculature and create working room for two additional caudal ports in the retrorectus space. The robot is docked, and the crossover is performed by incising the medial insertion of the posterior rectus sheath. The contralateral posterior rectus sheath is incised while preserving the preperitoneal fat along the linea alba. The contralateral retrorectus space is developed until there is enough working room to place 2 additional robotic ports transversely across the abdomen, which results in a total of 3 robotic ports placed transversely along the infraumbilical abdominal wall (Fig. 19). The robot is undocked and redocked into the 3 lower transverse ports for a "bottom up" approach. The remainder of the operation continues as described in the transabdominal retrorectus with TAR description with the exception of closing the peritoneal flap at the end.

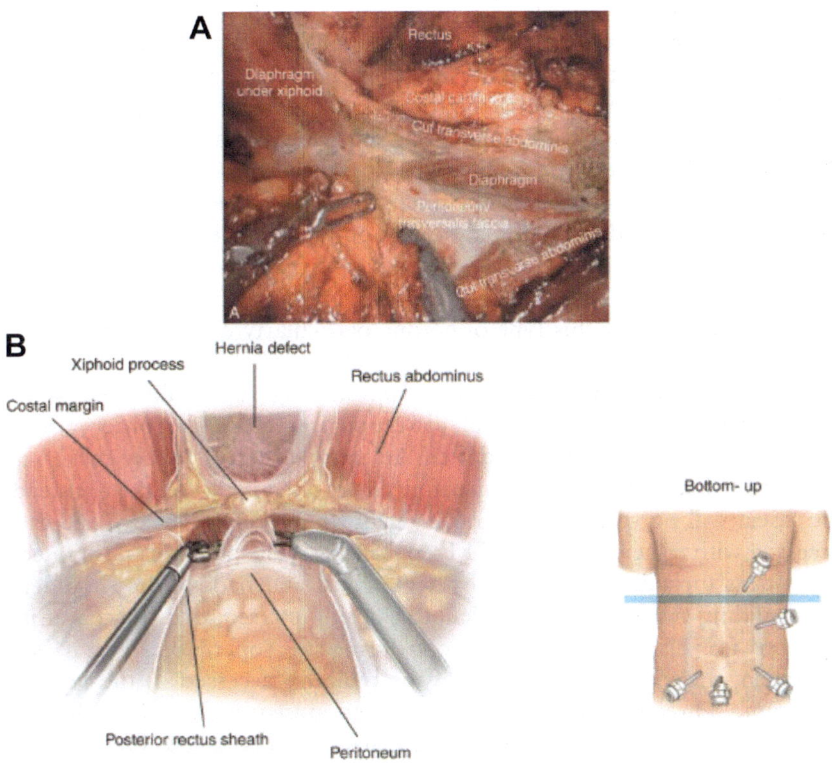

Fig. 19. Port placement for robotic subxiphoid hernia repair with eTEP access. eTEP, enhanced totally extraperitoneal. (Michael J. Rosen, Chapter 7 - Robotic Extended-View Totally Extraperitoneal Ventral Hernia Repair, in Atlas of Abdominal Wall Reconstruction, 3rd Edition, 2025, Elsevier.)

Robotic subxiphoid hernia repair

- TAPP, transabdominal retrorectus with upper TAR, and eTEP approaches are all good options for repair.
- At the xiphoid process, transition the dissection from the pre-transversalis plane (above the preperitoneal fat) to below/under the preperitoneal fat to the true preperitoneal plane in order to stay below the diaphragm and avoid entering the thoracic cavity
- When performing a retromuscular approach with TAR, divide the transversus abdominis muscle medial to the linea semilunaris and costal margin to avoid injuring the neurovascular bundles.
- Mobilize the peritoneum below the xiphoid process, along the central tendon of diaphragm for approximately 8–10 cm past the defect.
- Wide mesh overlap using an uncoated, macroporous mesh is recommended at this location.

Suprapubic hernias

Suprapubic hernias are located in the "M5" location, within 3 cm of the pubic bone, according to the EHS Classification [13] (see Fig. 10). These hernias can result after incisions along the lower midline, such as caesarean sections or extraction locations for colorectal operations. When considering open or minimally invasive approaches, similar to other types of hernias, open approaches are preferred when concomitant soft tissue excision or panniculectomy is planned. Additionally, an open approach is preferred for large, loss of domain defects in which wide mesh coverage from the medial aspect of each psoas muscle is needed. Otherwise, minimally invasive approaches are a great option for this type of hernia, particularly a robotic preperitoneal approach.

It is important to note that when approaching suprapubic defects minimally invasively, a preperitoneal dissection is required in order visualize, close and reinforce the fascial defect. An intraperitoneal sublay mesh repair with mesh fixation to the intraperitoneal portion of the bladder instead of the fascia will not provide a durable repair. The preperitoneal plane can be accessed with either TAPP or eTEP approaches. The patient is positioned supine, arms tucked, with a strap over the chest and pads at the shoulders to avoid sliding since steep Trendelenburg position is required. Place a urinary catheter for bladder decompression during the operation. For a TAPP approach, the intra-abdominal cavity is typically accessed in the left upper quadrant. Three robotic trocars are placed transversely across the upper abdomen (Fig. 20) and the patient is transitioned to steep Trendelenburg. A preperitoneal flap just caudally the umbilicus is created and carried down to the pubic bone. When starting the preperitoneal flap, we recommend to access and mobilize the pre-transversalis fascial plane (superficial to the preperitoneal fat) instead of the preperitoneal plane in order to keep

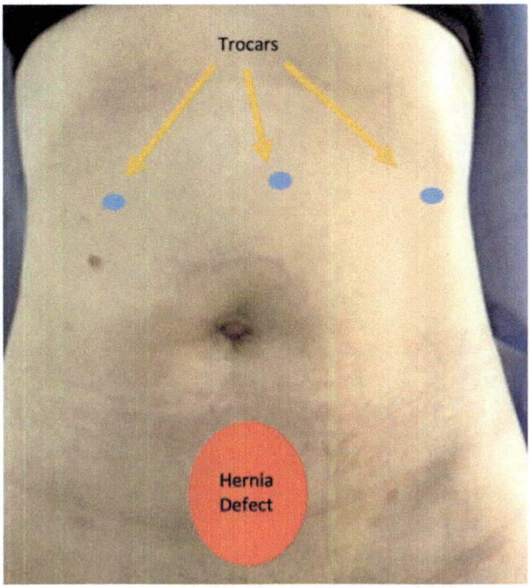

Fig. 20. Port placement along the upper abdomen, directed toward the pelvis for a suprapubic hernia repair.

the flap thicker. This will decrease the likelihood of creating holes in the peritoneum. If the peritoneal flap becomes very thin and holes develop despite using the pre-transversalis fascial plane, we recommend to transition into the retrorectus plane by incising the posterior rectus sheath (Fig. 21). This is especially important if the bladder is fused to the anterior abdominal wall. To avoid injuring the bladder, mobilize the retrorectus planes bilaterally to the pubis, which facilitates mobilization of an adherent bladder anteriorly along the midline. The flap is then carried down to the pubic bone and the hernia contents are reduced, which usually contain the bladder and incarcerated preperitoneal fat. Once the hernia contents are reduced, the dissection is continued inferiorly approximately 1 to 2 cm below the pubic bone. This is the maximum extent of the inferior dissection to avoid injuring the prostate or urethra. The dissection is then carried laterally toward bilateral Spaces of Bogros until a wide pocket for mesh overlap can be achieved of approximately 5 to 8 cm in both directions. Be careful to avoid injuring the external iliac vein and venous branches along Cooper's ligament during this dissection. We recommend to avoid disrupting or excising the fatty lymphatic tissue within the femoral canal to avoid a lymphocele. When performing the lateral dissection, if the mesh needs to extend to the psoas muscle, the transversalis fascia must be divided along its attachment to the linea semilunaris in order to enter the lateral preperitoneal plane (Fig. 22). The hernia defect is then repaired by reapproximating the linea alba using a large, barbed self-

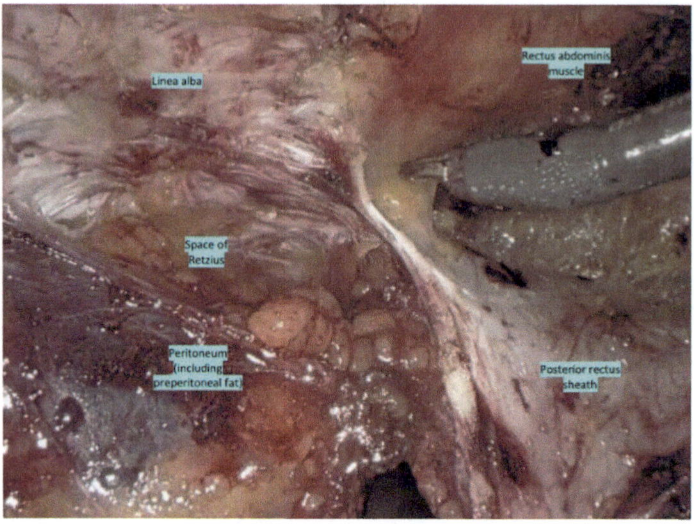

Fig. 21. Creating a flap using the preperitoneal space along the linea alba and retrorectus space laterally. (*Photo courtesy of* Dr Sabrina Drexel.)

locking suture (Fig. 23). A macroporous, uncoated mesh is placed in the preperitoneal/retromuscular plane (Fig. 24). We recommend fixation of the mesh in multiple places along bilateral Cooper's ligaments and the pubic tubercle with a slowly absorbable suture. A drain is not normally left in this location

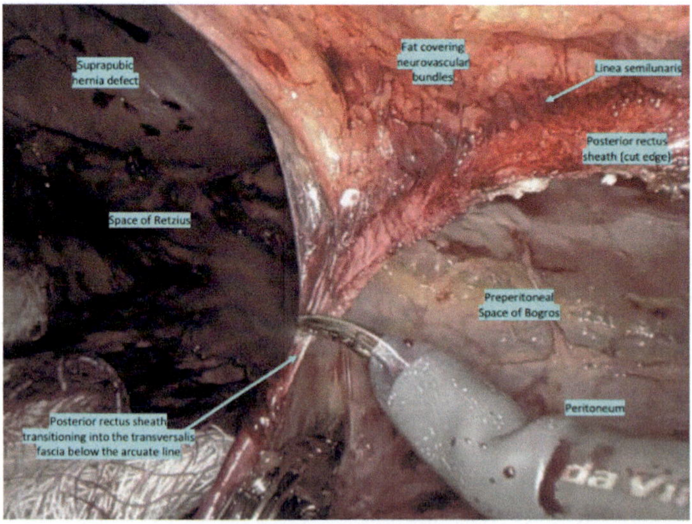

Fig. 22. Transversus abdominis release along the lower abdomen. (*Photo courtesy of* Dr Sabrina Drexel.)

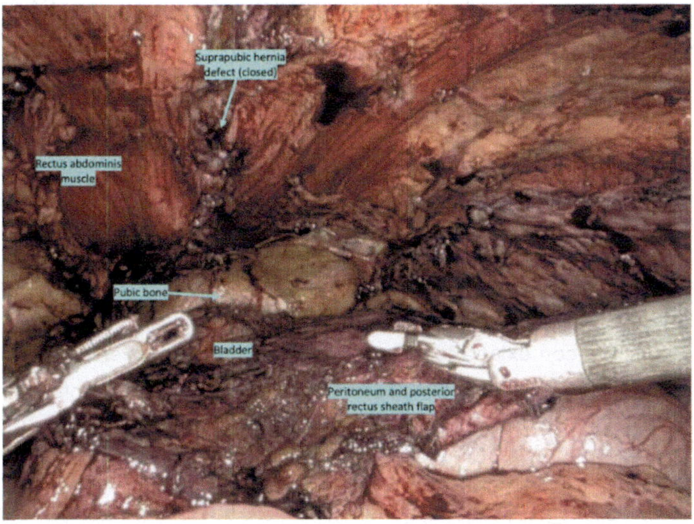

Fig. 23. Completed suprapubic preperitoneal dissection and closure of fascial defect. (*Photo courtesy of* Dr Sabrina Drexel.)

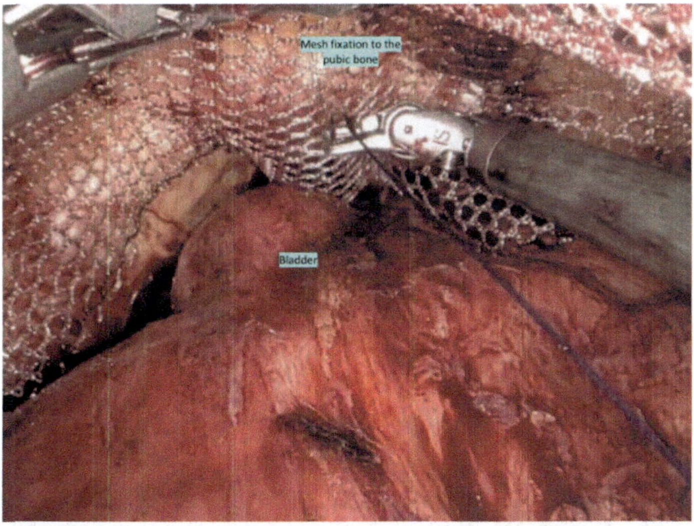

Fig. 24. Mesh placement for a suprapubic hernia repair in the preperitoneal space with fixation sutures to the pubic bone and Cooper's ligaments. (*Photo courtesy of* Dr Sabrina Drexel.)

and the preperitoneal flap is closed. See "Video 5 Suprapubic TAR" for the full operation.

Robotic suprapubic hernia repair

- Position patient in steep Trendelenburg with a urinary catheter in place.
- A preperitoneal approach is required to visualize and repair the fascia in the suprapubic location. This requires bladder mobilization.
- Caudal to the arcuate line, the transversalis fascia must be divided along its insertion into the linea semilunaris to gain access to the lateral preperitoneal space of Bogros.
- The dissection can extend to the psoas muscle for wide overlap.
- Obtain a wide preperitoneal dissection, extending 1 to 2 cm inferior to pubic bone and bilaterally at least approximately 5 to 8 cm to achieve wide mesh overlap around the anterior pelvis.
- A uncoated, macroporous mesh with fixation to the pubic bone and bilateral Cooper's ligaments is recommended.

Flank hernias

A flank hernia is classified as L1 to 3 according to the EHS classification system [13] (Fig. 25). This can be a difficult location due to the boney structures of the costal margin and pelvis, as well as limited posterior/lateral space for wide mesh

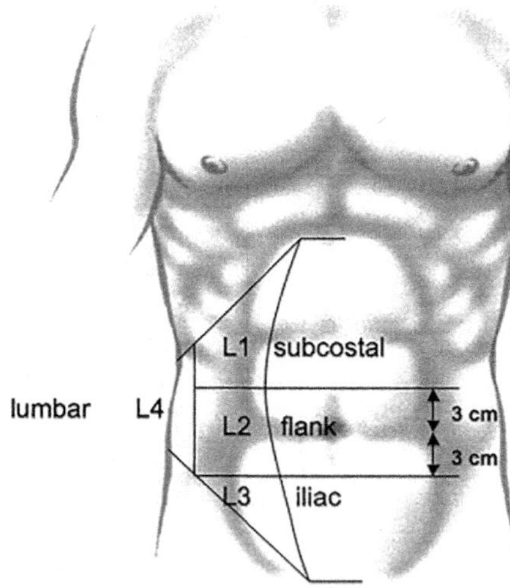

Fig. 25. European Hernia Society classification of lumbar (L1-3) and flank (L4) hernias. (Muysoms, F.E., Miserez, M., Berrevoet, F. et al. Classification of primary and incisional abdominal wall hernias. Hernia 13, 407–414 (2009). https://doi.org/10.1007/s10029-009-0518-x.)

overlap. Often times, primary fascial closure is not technically feasible when the hernia defect is in close proximity to the boney structures. Therefore, the strength of the repair depends on wide mesh overlap with a heavyweight, macroporous, permanent synthetic mesh. A preperitoneal repair is the recommended approach for a flank hernia defect, in order to visualize and reduce the hernia contents, reapproximate the fascia and achieve wide mesh overlap (Video 6 Flank TAPP). MIS approach is a good option when the hernia defect is located more posterior, and the mesh will not need to extend across the linea alba to the contralateral side. A more posterior defect will allow more working space for trocar placement when the patient is in lateral decubitus positioning. If a lateral flank defect and a concomitant midline defect exists, we recommend an open approach with midline access in order to widely wrap mesh in both directions.

Position the patient in lateral decubitus position and widely prep to expose all landmarks: spine, costal margin, anterior superior iliac spine, inguinal ligament and umbilicus. Place 3 ports longitudinally along the abdomen, as medial as possibly, away from the hernia defect, to allow working room within the abdominal cavity to start the flap (Fig. 26). Start the operation by reducing the hernia contents from the hernia defect. However, if the colon or another retroperitoneal structure is incarcerated within the hernia defect, we recommend to first start the preperitoneal flap and wait to reduce the retroperitoneal viscera after the flap has been matured and the defect has been exposed. If the peritoneum is durable, a trans-abdominal preperitoneal repair is recommended. This is accomplished by carefully peeling the peritoneum away from the abdominal wall (Fig. 27), starting far enough away from the defect to gain 8 to 10 cm of mesh overlap. However, often times the peritoneum underlying the posterior rectus sheath is very thin, and it is difficult to start a preperitoneal plane without creating holes. In this case, start a retrorectus flap and perform a

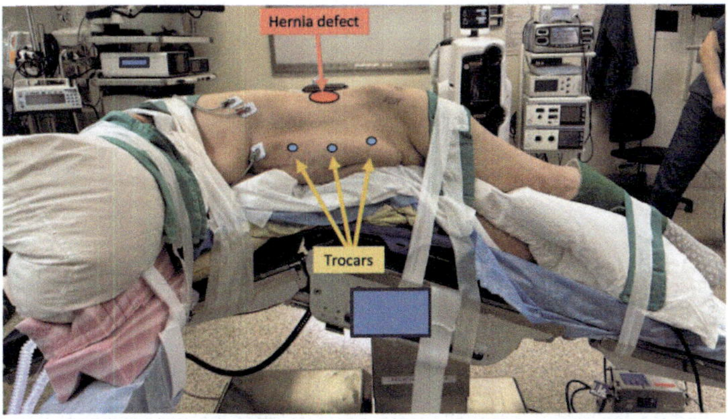

Fig. 26. Patient positioning and port placement for a robotic flank hernia repair. (*Photo courtesy of* Dr Lucas Beffa.)

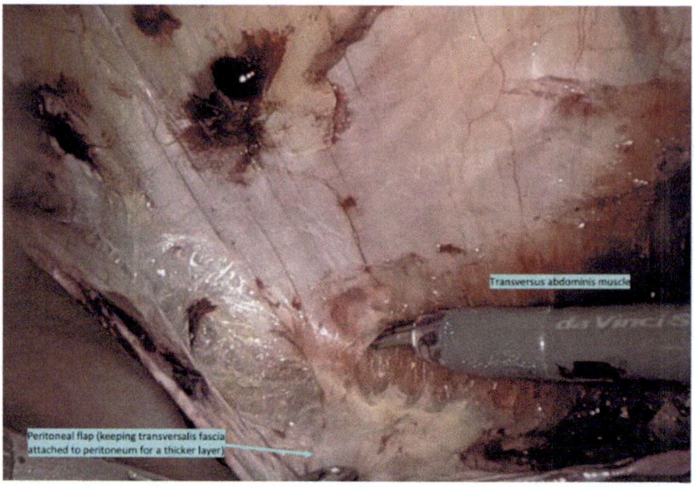

Fig. 27. Start with a preperitoneal flap to allow wide mesh overlap medial to the flank defect. (*Photo courtesy of* Dr Lucas Beffa.)

unilateral transversus abdominis release to access the retroperitoneum. Once the retroperitoneum has been accessed, reduce the contents of the hernia sac (Fig. 28). Expose the medial aspect of the psoas muscle along the length of the hernia defect, being careful to not injure the lateral sidewall nerves, ureter and external iliac vessels (Fig. 29). The key to this step is staying close to the

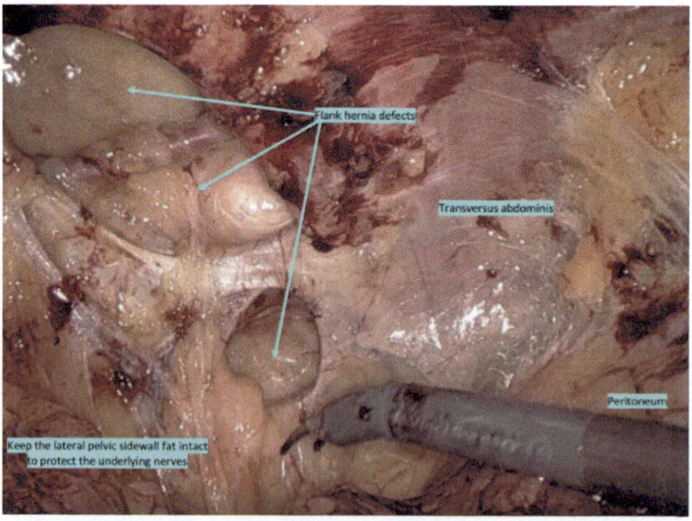

Fig. 28. Reduce the retroperitoneal hernia contents after the preperitoneal flap has been created. Continue the dissection to the psoas muscle while keeping the lateral pelvic sidewall fat intact to protect the underlying nerves. (*Photo courtesy of* Dr Lucas Beffa.)

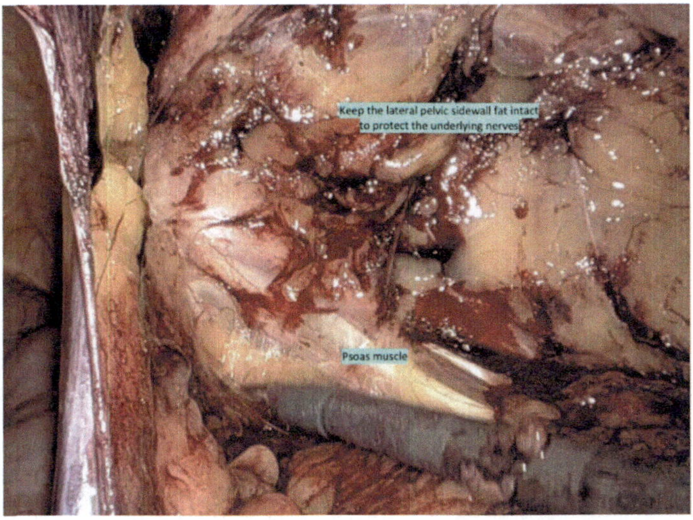

Fig. 29. Posterior/lateral dissection should continue until reaching the medial aspect of the psoas muscle. (*Photo courtesy of* Dr Lucas Beffa.)

peritoneum during the dissection and leaving retroperitoneal fat in place along the pelvic sidewall (triangle of pain). Use minimal electrocautery in this location to reduce the risk of a thermal injury to the colon. Continue the preperitoneal flap until the medial aspect of the psoas muscle is exposed, which is furthest extent of the posterior/lateral dissection. The dissection should continue cranially below the costal margin and diaphragm and inferiorly into the Space of Bogros for 8 to 10 cm of wide mesh overlap in all directions. Close the fascial defect primarily with a large, barbed, self-locking suture (Fig. 30) and then place mesh (Fig. 31). Typically, fixation is not necessary once wide mesh

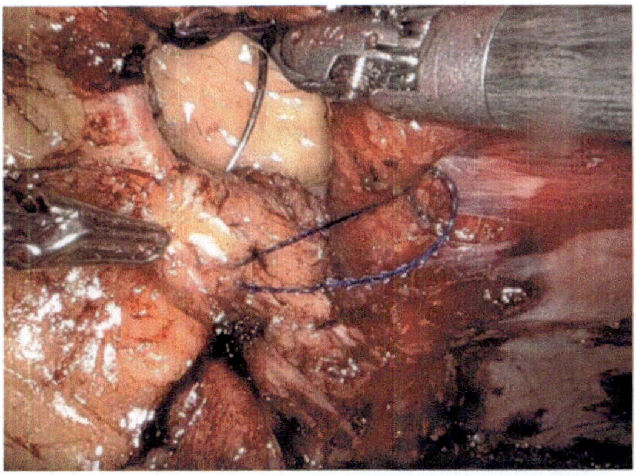

Fig. 30. Close the flank hernia defect primarily with large barbed sutures. (*Photo courtesy of* Dr Lucas Beffa.)

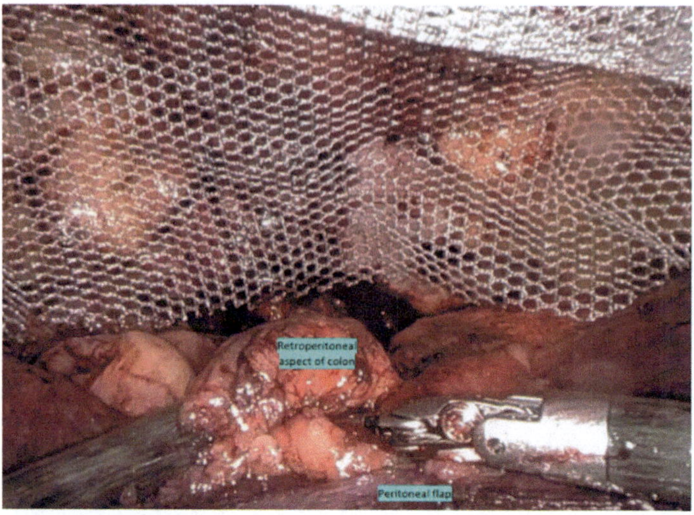

Fig. 31. Ensure the mesh reaches to the medial aspect of the psoas muscle, posterior to the colon in order to accomplish wide overlap. (*Photo courtesy of* Dr Lucas Beffa.)

overlap has been achieved. However, if fixation is deemed necessary, the mesh can be fixated to the costal margin, anterior superior iliac spine, Cooper's ligament, and transfascial locations, ensuring to protect the lateral sidewall nerves.

Robotic flank hernia repair

- Position patient in lateral decubitus position with a urinary catheter in place and prep all landmarks: spine, umbilicus, costal margin, ASIS, inguinal ligament.
- Develop a large preperitoneal plane for mesh placement, reducing the retroperitoneal viscera after the flap has been created.
- If the edge of the peritoneal flap is thin, consider starting the flap using the retrorectus plane and performing a unilateral transversus abdominis release to access the retroperitoneum.
- Keep the lateral pelvic sidewall fat intact to protect the underlying nerves.
- The most posterior extent of the dissection is the medial aspect of the psoas, and 8 to 10 cm in all directions to ensure wide mesh overlap. Fixation is not needed if wide mesh overlap has been achieved.
- A heavyweight, macroporous permanent synthetic mesh is recommended.

DISCUSSION

Robotic surgery has recently changed the landscape of hernia surgery, allowing complex abdominal wall reconstruction techniques to be approached in a minimally invasive fashion. With appropriate expertise and resources, minimally invasive abdominal wall reconstruction can be an excellent option in carefully selected patients. Patients who benefit the most from MIS AWR are those who do not need soft tissue resection, extensive gastrointestinal surgery, or dense adhesiolysis, along with those who are at a higher risk for wound complications with open techniques. MIS AWR has been shown to be safe and effective for both midline and atypical hernias. However, hernia pathology should be considered a long-term disease process with significant rates of recurrence. Therefore, as stewards of the abdominal wall, complex reconstruction techniques should not be applied to simple, straightforward hernias.

Post-operative considerations after minimally invasive AWR are similar to those undergoing open AWR. Patients are admitted to the hospital after surgery for observation. Pain control is the mainstay of post-operative care, which typically includes a multi-modal pain regimen. Appropriate pain control will improve early ambulation, quality of life, and can reduce the length of hospital stay. Patients are discharged once pain is controlled with oral medications and they are tolerating diet. Abdominal binders can provide comfort and support during the initial post-operative period. While no specific activity restrictions have been shown to impact outcomes, patients are typically counseled to limit heavy lifting for 4 to 6 weeks after major hernia operations.

After the initial post-operative period, patients should be followed at 6 months and annually after surgery to in order to track and improve both short-term and long-term outcomes. Robotic abdominal wall reconstruction generally shows a consistent pattern across the most-cited systematic reviews and meta-analyses: procedures take longer in the operating room but are associated with shorter hospital stays and fewer wound-related complications than open repairs [14,15]. There is only one published randomized controlled trial comparing the outcomes of robotic versus open retromuscular ventral hernia repair, and it similarly shows a longer operative time (median 206 vs 156 min; $P < .001$) but shorter length of hospital stay for the robotic cohort (1 vs 2 days; $P < .001$) [16]. The trial found no difference in the primary composite outcome including SSI, SSOPI, readmission, and hernia recurrence at 1 year and 2 year follow-up, and there was no difference in quality of life between the two groups [16]. The benefits of the robotic approach must be balanced against higher in-hospital charges and increased procedural costs driven by robotic capital and disposables. Economic analyses have found that the net cost-effectiveness depends heavily on local costs, reimbursement, and whether shorter stays or fewer wound complications offset operating room expense [17]. Importantly, available data show similar hernia-recurrence rates with short-to-medium follow-up between robotic and open repairs, but long-term, high-quality randomized evidence remains limited. Much of the current literature is observational or from single centers with variable surgeon experience. Therefore, the choice between robotic and open AWR is best individualized to patient risk for wound complications, defect complexity, and local surgical expertise and resources [14].

Future research should focus on generating high-quality, long-term data through multicenter, randomized controlled trials to define the true clinical and cost-effectiveness of robotic compared with open abdominal wall reconstruction. Additionally, research should evaluate strategies to shorten the learning curve, improve operative efficiency, and reduce costs through optimization of robotic workflows and training programs. As robotic platforms and imaging technologies advance, future studies may also explore integration of augmented reality, intraoperative navigation, and artificial intelligence to enhance precision and standardize outcomes in complex abdominal wall reconstruction.

SUMMARY

Robotic abdominal wall reconstruction offers short-term advantages over open repair, including shorter hospital stay and fewer wound complications, albeit with longer operative times and higher procedural costs. Current evidence suggests comparable hernia recurrence rates between approaches, but long-term, high-quality data remain limited. The future of robotic AWR lies in prospective research to clarify its cost-effectiveness, optimal patient selection, and its ability to leverage emerging technologies such as advanced imaging and artificial intelligence to enhance surgical precision and outcomes.

CLINICS CARE POINTS

- Minimally invasive AWR can be achieved using a transabdominal or eTEP approach.
- The eTEP technique decreases the time required for adhesiolysis and posterior sheath closure at the cost of less visualization and the potential for an unrecognized bowel injury due to thermal energy.
- The TAR may start at the cranial or caudal aspect of the retrorectus space, but must start medial to the neurovascular bundles along the linea semilunaris and costal margin.
- Pneumoperitoneum during MIS AWR increases tension on the posterior closure, therefore a wide dissection or bridged approach should be used to close the posterior layer in a tension-free manner.
- Adequate mesh overlap requires 8 to 10 cm of retromuscular dissection in all directions to decrease the risk of hernia recurrence.
- Uncoated macroporous mesh is recommended in the retromuscular plane.
- Minimally invasive AWR techniques can be used for hernias in challenging locations, such as subxiphoid, flank and suprapubic defects.

Acknowledgments

The authors thank Drs. Dina Podolsky, Sabrina Drexel, David Lourié, Charlotte Horne, and Lucas Beffa for providing video and/or photographic content to support this article. We greatly appreciate their contributions and support.

Disclosure

K.E. Blake receives honorarium from Gore and BD for consulting and speaking engagements. B.K. Poulose has received research funding from BD Interventional and Advanced Medical Solutions; has received consulting fees from Abbvie/Allergan; receives salary support from the Abdominal Core Health Quality Collaborative and is Chief Medical Officer of EndoEvolve. C.E. Collins has nothing to disclose.

SUPPLEMENTARY DATA

Supplementary data to this article can be found online at https://doi.org/10.1016/j.yasu.2026.05.002.

References

[1] Abdominal Core Health Quality Collaborative. A pragmatic, evidence-based approach to coding for abdominal wall reconstruction. Hernia 2022;26(2):589–97; https://doi.org/10.1007/s10029-021-02458-w.
[2] Fry BT, Howard RA, Thumma JR, et al. Surgical approach and long-term recurrence after ventral hernia repair. JAMA Surg 2024;159(9):1019–28.
[3] Belyansky I, Weltz AS, Sibia US, et al. The trend toward minimally invasive complex abdominal wall reconstruction: is it worth it? Surg Endosc 2018;32(4):1701–7.
[4] Nguyen B, David B, Shiozaki T, et al. Comparisons of abdominal wall reconstruction for ventral hernia repairs, open versus robotic. Sci Rep 2021;11(1):8086.
[5] Loh WS, Howard RA, Fry BT, et al. Learning curves for robotic-assisted ventral hernia repair. JAMA Netw Open 2024;7(12):e2448521; https://doi.org/10.1001/jamanetworkopen.2024.48521.
[6] Irfan A, Cochrun S, He K, et al. Towards identifying a learning curve for robotic abdominal wall reconstruction: a cumulative sum analysis. Hernia 2023;27(3):671–6.
[7] Kudsi OY, Gokcal F, Bou-Ayash N, et al. Learning curve of robotic transversus abdominis release in ventral hernia repair: a cumulative sum (CUSUM) analysis. Surg Endosc 2022;36(5):3480–8.
[8] González De Godos A, Sánchez González J, López Rodríguez B, et al. Comparative approach for abdominal wall reconstruction after ventral hernia: open versus minimally invasive surgery. Hernia 2025;29(1):69.
[9] Amro C, Ryan IA, Elhage SA, et al. Comparative analysis of ventral hernia repair and transverse abdominis release with and without panniculectomy: a 4-Year match-pair analysis. Ann Plast Surg 2024;92(4S Suppl 2):S80–6.
[10] Guzman-Pruneda FA, Huang LC, Collins C, et al. Abdominal core quality of life after ventral hernia repair: a comparison of open versus robotic-assisted retromuscular techniques. Surg Endosc 2021;35(1):241–8.
[11] Asencio F, Carbó J, Ferri R, et al. Laparoscopic versus open incisional hernia repair: long-term Follow-up results of a randomized clinical trial. World J Surg 2021;45(9):2734–41.
[12] Rogmark P, Petersson U, Bringman S, et al. Quality of life and surgical outcome 1 year after open and laparoscopic incisional hernia repair: PROLOVE: a randomized controlled trial. Ann Surg 2016;263(2):244–50.
[13] Muysoms FE, Miserez M, Berrevoet F, et al. Classification of primary and incisional abdominal wall hernias. Hernia 2009;13(4):407–14.
[14] Lima DL, da Silveira CAB, de Oliveira CNB, et al. Open versus robotic transversus abdominis release for ventral hernia repair: an updated systematic review, meta-analysis, and meta-regression. Surg Endosc 2024;38(12):7083–92.
[15] Henriksen NA, Helgstrand F, Jensen KK. Short-term outcomes after open versus robot-assisted repair of ventral hernias: a nationwide database study. Hernia 2024;28:233–40.

[16] Warren JA, Blackhurst D, Ewing JA, et al. Open versus robotic retromuscular ventral hernia repair: outcomes of the ORREO prospective randomized controlled trial. Surg Endosc 2024;38(12):7466–74.
[17] Kudsi OY, Kaoukabani G, Bou-Ayash N, et al. A comparison of clinical outcomes and costs between robotic and open ventral hernia repair. Am J Surg 2023;226(1):87–92.

Advances in Surgery 60 (2026) 233–250

ADVANCES IN SURGERY

Do Surgical Patients Feel They Are Adequately Informed of Decision-making Prior to Surgery?

Daniel I. Hoffman, MD[a], Elizabeth J. Lilley, MD, MPH[b,c,d], Matthew Bartek, MD, MPH[e,f,*]

[a]Department of Surgery, Center for Surgery and Public Health, Brigham and Women's Hospital, Boston, MA, USA; [b]Harvard Medical School, Boston; [c]Department of Supportive Oncology, Center for Surgery and Public Health, Dana Farber Cancer Institute, Boston, USA; [d]Division of Surgical Oncology, Department of Surgery, Brigham and Women's Hospital, Boston, MA, USA; [e]Division of Palliative Care and Geriatrics, Department of Surgery, Massachusetts General Hospital, Harvard Medical School, Boston, MA, USA; [f]Division of Trauma, Emergency Surgery, and Surgical Critical Care, Department of Surgery, Massachusetts General Hospital, Harvard Medical School, Boston, MA, USA

Keywords

• Shared decision-making • Informed consent • Communication • Goals of care • Patient-reported outcome measures • Palliative care

Key points

- Even when formal informed consent requirements are satisfied, many surgical patients do not *feel* fully informed, especially about nonoperative options, long-term functional outcomes, and what life might look like if serious complications occur.
- Informed consent, informed decision-making, and shared decision-making (SDM) are distinct concepts: current practice emphasizes disclosure and documentation over deliberation and value-concordant decision-making.
- Heterogeneous metrics exist to measure both subjective and objective adequacy of decision-making, including experiential satisfaction (ie, patient surveys and decisional regret), factual elements (ie, knowledge recall), and SDM behaviors (ie, observer or patient-reported scales).

Continued

*Corresponding author. Division of Palliative Care and Geriatrics, Department of Surgery, Massachusetts General Hospital, Harvard Medical School, Boston, MA. *E-mail address:* mbartek@mgb.org

https://doi.org/10.1016/j.yasu.2026.05.001

Continued

- Structured tools can improve preoperative decision-making, including patient decision aids, risk calculators with visual displays, and conversation frameworks such as Best Case/Worst Case and the Better Conversations model.
- Best Case/Worst Case and Better Conversations can reframe the informed consent process from a technical lecture and complication list to a goals-focused, scenario-based, deliberative discussion that integrates professional judgment with patient values.
- Major knowledge gaps remain in special populations such as emergency surgery or cognitively impaired patients, and most systems do not yet routinely measure SDM or decision quality—leaving substantial room for implementation, evaluation, and improvement.

Abbreviations

AI	artificial intelligence
BC/WC	Best Case/Worst Case
ICU	intensive care unit
PROMs	patient-reported outcome measures
QPLs	question prompt lists
SDM	shared decision-making

INTRODUCTION

In most surgical settings, obtaining informed consent is woven into daily workflow: a standardized form, a rehearsed conversation, a signature. Yet when patients are interviewed after surgery, many report that they did not fully understand key elements of the decision–particularly long-term functional outcomes, nonoperative alternatives, and what life might look like if complications occur [1,2]. These deficits are not merely academic. They can contribute to decisional regret, dissatisfaction, allegations of inadequate consent, and most importantly treatments that are misaligned with patients' values and goals. Several trends magnify the importance of this topic for practicing surgeons:

- *Demographic shifts:* Populations are aging, with rising numbers of frail, multimorbid older adults undergoing major surgery. High-stakes operations near the end of life are increasingly common [3].
- *Complex options:* For many conditions, there is no single "right" operation; instead, surgeons and patients must navigate multiple approaches, varying risk profiles, and nonoperative options.
- *Accountability and measurement:* regulatory agencies, payers, and health systems increasingly scrutinize informed consent processes, shared decision-making (SDM), and patient-reported experiences.

Within this context, asking "Do surgical patients feel they are adequately informed?" means much more than "Did they sign the consent form?" Furthermore, determining whether patients *feel* informed of decision-making requires examination of their subjective experiences, which should be differentiated from whether they *are* informed (ie, objective recall of elements of the decision-making process).

Key concepts

Several related but distinct concepts on preoperative decision-making are essential for this article (Table 1).

- *Informed consent:* Rooted in legal and ethical doctrine informed consent requires disclosure of the nature and purpose of the intervention; risks and benefits; reasonable alternatives, including no intervention; and assessment of comprehension and voluntariness [4]. In many hospitals, this has become a form-driven, risk-enumeration exercise, that is, "disease, operation, risks, benefits, alternatives, signature."
- *Informed decision-making:* This concept broadens focus from disclosure to deliberation: the patient not only receives information but also has sufficient understanding and support to weigh options, clarify goals, and formulate preferences. [5].
- *SDM:* A collaborative process in which clinicians and patients exchange information, discuss options and outcomes, and agree on a plan that is concordant with the patient's values and goals [6]. A key feature is that there are genuinely reasonable options; if one option is clearly superior on medical grounds, the emphasis shifts from "sharing" to "explaining and advising."
- *Patient-reported outcome measures (PROMs):* PROMs capture patients' health status (ie, pain, function, and quality of life) from their perspective. The emergence and use of PROMs has broadened the assessment of outcomes of surgical decisions beyond simply the impact on "morbidity and mortality" to include patient experiences in a rigorous, data-driven manner. The expansion of surgical research to include PROMs may support SDM by incorporating patient perspectives into clinical decision processes [7].

Scope of this article

This article focuses on elective and urgent adult surgical patients. We will

1. Summarize what is known about patients' and families' perceptions of preoperative information and decision-making.
2. Describe determinants of patients' and families' perceived adequacy of informed decision-making, including patient-level, clinician-level, and system-level factors.
3. Review instruments and approaches used to measure whether patients feel informed or involved.
4. Highlight communication tools and interventions—particularly decision aids, risk visualization, and structured conversation frameworks such as Best Case/Worst Case (BC/WC) and the Better Conversations model.
5. Identify gaps and propose evidence-informed strategies for practicing surgeons.

DISCUSSION

Do surgical patients feel adequately informed?

Across multiple settings and specialties, a considerable proportion of surgical patients are or feel incompletely informed at the time of consent or in the early

Table 1
Key concepts in surgical decision-making

Concept	Core definition	Primary focus	Typical measures or indicators	Implications
Informed consent	Legal–ethical requirement to disclose nature, purpose, risks, benefits, and alternatives of treatment	Disclosure, comprehension, and voluntariness	Signed consent form; patient recall of risks/benefits	Ensuring minimum legal standards; protecting patient autonomy and liability
Informed decision-making	Process in which the patient receives adequate information, understands options, and forms a preference consistent with their goals	Understanding and deliberation	Knowledge scores; decision quality scales; decisional conflict	Bridging the gap between "told" and "truly understands"
SDM	Collaborative process where clinician and patient exchange information and jointly agree on a plan consistent with patient values and best evidence	Collaboration and value concordance	SDM-Q-9, collaboRATE, OPTION scales	Emphasizes discussion of options, values, and patient role preferences

postoperative period. One study noted that self-reported decisional regret was present in about 1 in 7 surgical patients; another commented that in major abdominal/thoracic surgery reported, regret was expressed in 37%, with substantial regret in about 1 in 12 [1,2,5,7–10]. Common findings include

- *Variable recall of risks and alternatives:* Shortly after consent—and even more so postoperatively—patients demonstrate variable recall of major risks that were documented or nonoperative options [2,11,12].
- *Blindsided to negative experiences of surgery:* While surgeons do enumerate risks during informed consent, patients may be left blindsided to negative experiences of surgery that do not rise to the level of reportable complications (ie, urinary retention and incisional scars) [13]. Some of these physiologic and functional outcomes are expected changes related to the operation. However, patients may view these as complications rather than the expected surgical course.
- *Overly optimistic expectations:* Patients may assume that surgery will "fix the problem" and restore them to baseline or better, even when surgeons might view stable function or modest improvement as success; this may lead to decisional regret in as much as 20% of patients [1,14]. Moreover, surgeons regularly use language, which suggests that surgery will "fix" their patients' medical problems, even when they themselves admit to the limitations of surgery to do so [15].
- *Variable satisfaction with involvement:* Patients experience variable degrees of involvement with care, which may be associated with differences in overall satisfaction [3,16].

These patterns appear across informed consent settings ranging from ambulatory hernia repair and elective orthopedic procedures to major oncologic and vascular surgery. Differences in literacy, education, and language proficiency [17] may also influence perceived adequacy of consent, even in highly educated patients. Observational, interview-based, and mixed-methods studies with patients, family members, and surgeons--in conjunction with expert viewpoints--have added nuance to our understanding of barriers to perceived adequacy of informed decision-making. Common themes include

- *The "mini-medical school" lecture:* During surgical consultations, surgeons reliably provide extensive explanations of diagnosis, anatomy, imaging, and technical details. While patients may sometimes appreciate this, information on patient values, nonoperative options, or what life will be like after the operation is frequently omitted [3,18–21].
- *Silences around goals and downsides:* Explicit goals of surgery and long-term consequences (ie, loss of independence, chronic symptoms, or the possibility that the operation will not achieve their goals) are not clearly discussed in as many as 80% of surgical consent discussions [18–20,22].
- *Trust, deference, and paternalism:* Patients may express profound trust in their surgeons and a tendency to defer, especially in high-risk settings or when they feel acutely ill. Consent may be viewed as an opportunity to "go along" with what the surgeon thinks is best rather than as a moment of choice [3,23,24]. When clinicians themselves are uncertain about the best course, SDM

behaviors may be more common; however, if they strongly favor surgery, the conversation may shift toward persuasion rather than deliberation [3,21,25].
- *Form versus conversation:* Patients distinguish signing the consent form from the "real conversation." If the conversation feels rushed or fragmented, the signed form may do little to mitigate their sense of being underinformed. The focus of the form is often "can we operate safely?" rather than "should we operate at all, given this person's goals and trajectory?" [19,20,23,26,27].

Taken together, these data suggest that *many patients do not experience preoperative conversations as genuinely informative or shared, particularly for preference-sensitive, high-stakes decisions.* From the surgeon's side, a box may be checked; from the patient's side, important questions may remain unanswered.

Determinants of perceived adequacy

Patient-level factors

Several patient characteristics influence whether individuals feel informed:

- *Health literacy:* Patients with limited health literacy may struggle with written forms and statistical risk communication. They may benefit disproportionately from plain language, teach-back, and visual aids [2,11,12].
- *Language and culture:* Non–English speaking patients and those from cultures that emphasize deference to medical authority may be less likely to ask clarifying questions or express disagreement [2,11,28].
- *Decision-making preference:* Some patients prefer to delegate decisions to the surgeon, while others want explicit SDM. Importantly, many may want a combination of guidance and involvement—not one or the other [3,16,29].
- *Emotional state:* Anxiety, pain, and acute illness may diminish capacity to process information, especially when conversations occur on the day of surgery or during an emergency admission [2,11].

Clinician-level factors

On the clinician side, key determinants include

- *Who obtains consent:* In many institutions, junior residents or advanced practice providers obtain consent for common operations. Informed consent processes may be user-dependent and influence variability in measures of quality [5,21,30].
- *Comfort with prognostic uncertainty and bad news:* Surgeons may vary in how explicitly they address key components of informed decision-making, including discussion of poor outcomes, long-term functional decline, or the possibility that surgery will not help [27,31].
- *Attitudes toward SDM:* Surgeons who see SDM as central to professionalism may be more likely to invite questions, elicit values, and present nonoperative options; others may not value SDM or feel that it is too time consuming [3,16,25].

System-level factors

More broadly, systemic factors within the hospital or health system landscape can shape these conversations [12,26,27]:

- *Time pressure:* Tight clinic schedules, overlapping OR responsibilities, and add-on cases constrain preoperative conversations.
- *Fragmentation:* Patients may see one surgeon in clinic, a different one on the ward, and yet another on the day of surgery, which may lead to diffused responsibility.
- *Form-driven processes:* Organizational focus on signed consent forms and preoperative checklists can inadvertently signal that documentation, not deliberation, is the priority.

What are the core elements of high-quality preoperative discussions?

Synthesizing survey, interview, and observational data, several consistent preferences emerge:

- *Honesty about prognosis and uncertainty:* Patients prefer realistic descriptions of potential outcomes over vague reassurance. While providers aim to support and promote hope among their patients, this can be manifested by neglecting to convey medical truths, transparently [32–34].
- *Functional and quality-of-life framing:* Patients want to know whether they will be able to live independently, walk, think clearly, or continue valued activities—not just survival or technical success.
- *Explicit consideration of nonoperative options:* Many patients, especially older adults with serious illness, may want to hear that "doing less" or focusing on comfort is a legitimate choice.
- *Guided participation:* Most do not want to make decisions in isolation; they want surgeons to share their recommendation and reasoning, then invite discussion and modification.
- *Time, continuity, and support:* Adequate time to process information, involvement of family or trusted others, and consistency in messaging across the team are all highly valued.

When these elements are present, patients may be more likely to describe themselves as informed, even if they ultimately choose burdensome treatments.

How do we measure whether patients feel adequately informed?

Because "feeling informed" is subjective and experiential, measurement is challenging. Several complementary approaches exist.

Consent-focused questionnaires

Numerous studies use adapted questionnaires [2,11,12] that ask patients:

- Whether the surgeon explained the procedure, benefits, risks, and alternatives.
- Whether they had enough time to ask questions.
- Whether they understood the information.
- Whether they felt involved in the decision.

These instruments vary in quality and often emphasize recall of facts rather than deeper understanding of implications or alignment with values. Systematic reviews of such tools note variable psychometric rigor and limited use outside research settings [12].

Shared decision-making measures

Several validated instruments capture aspects of SDM:

- *SDM-Q-9* (patient) and *SDM-Q-Doc* (clinician): Nine items each, covering information exchange, deliberation, and joint decision. Widely used in outpatient settings, including some surgical clinics [35,36].
- *collaboRATE:* A 3 item, ultrabrief patient measure of involvement; feasible for routine clinic use [37].
- *OPTION scale:* Observer-rated measure of clinician behaviors that support SDM (eg, presenting options and eliciting preferences) [38].

Of note, these instruments are not surgery-specific but have been applied in perioperative studies and can serve as pragmatic tools for surgeons to track and improve their communication.

Patient-reported outcome measures

Although PROMs are primarily intended to track outcomes (eg, pain, disability, and quality of life), they can also serve as an adjunct to help support and frame decision-making:

- Baseline PROMs and expected trajectories help set realistic expectations about recovery.
- Postoperative PROMs can feed back into conversations with future patients, providing concrete data about typical course and variability.

At present, however, there is no widely adopted, surgery-specific PROM that directly measures the adequacy of preoperative decision-making, and few institutions systematically collect SDM-specific measures in surgical practice.

Interventions and tools to improve preoperative decision-making

Patient decision aids for surgical choices

Patient decision aids are structured tools (ie, booklets, videos, and web-based modules) designed to help patients make specific decisions (Table 2). Across many conditions, a Cochrane review [39] showed that decision aids

- Improve knowledge and risk understanding
- Reduce decisional conflict
- Increase alignment between chosen option and patient values
- Sometimes lead to more conservative treatment choices when appropriate

Specific decision aids have been developed for a variety of surgical decisions [39], such as

- Repair versus surveillance of abdominal aortic aneurysm
- Lumpectomy versus mastectomy for early breast cancer
- Joint replacement versus nonoperative management for advanced arthritis

Although uptake remains uneven, the evidence suggests that well-designed decision aids can meaningfully improve patients' understanding and satisfaction, particularly when integrated into clinic workflows rather than offered as stand-alone handouts [39].

Table 2
Selected tools and interventions to improve preoperative decision-making

Tool or intervention	Primary purpose	Target population or setting	Evidence summary	Practical tips for implementation
Generic patient decision aids	Improve knowledge, risk understanding, and alignment with values for specific treatment choices	Preference-sensitive surgical decisions (eg, AAA repair, breast surgery, and joint replacement)	Cochrane review shows improved knowledge, more accurate risk perception, reduced decisional conflict; some shift toward more conservative options [39]	Integrate into clinic workflow (sent before visit or used in visit); pair with focused Q&A rather than handing out alone
ACS NSQIP risk calculator	Provide individualized estimates of morbidity/mortality and selected outcomes	Broad elective or nonelective surgery, often inpatient	Validated across large surgical cohorts; improves calibration of predicted risk vs observed outcomes [40]	Use as a starting point for discussion; avoid "numbers dump," ie, translate into plain language and functional implications
Visual consent tools and risk charts	Make risks more understandable via icon arrays or charts; support preference-sensitive risk discussion	Patients with limited numeracy; complex risk profiles	Early pilot work suggests improved satisfaction without increased visit length [41]	Coview visual display with patient; explicitly ask which outcomes matter most to them
BC/WC	Structure high-stakes decisions around best, worst, and most likely trajectories for each option	High-risk surgery in frail or seriously ill older adults	Pre–post intervention study showed improvements in observed SDM behaviors and richer discussion of tradeoffs [20,31]	Draw trajectories in real time; emphasize function, location of care, and burdensome treatments, not only survival

(*continued on next page*)

Table 2
(*continued*)

Tool or intervention	Primary purpose	Target population or setting	Evidence summary	Practical tips for implementation
Better Conversations framework	Reorient consent from technical explanation to goal-focused deliberation about whether surgery is worth the downsides	High-risk and preference-sensitive surgical decisions	Built on qualitative analysis of >500 recorded conversations; offers a conceptual core for improved consent [19]	Five broad steps: Show your cards → state goals → describe all downsides → deliberate → agree on a plan
QPLs	Empower patients to ask focused questions and engage in deliberation	Older adults considering major surgery; general surgery clinics	Randomized trial showed feasibility but did not increase patient well-being, although may be confounded by ceiling effects. QPL was associated with higher OPTION5 scores [42].	Give QPL prior to visit; explicitly invite patients to use it ("Let's go through your list")
SDM measurement tools (SDM-Q-9, collaboRATE, OPTION)	Monitor and improve decision-making quality over time	Any outpatient surgical practice or perioperative clinic	Validated measures correlate with patient involvement and satisfaction; limited routine use in surgery [35–38]	Start with brief tools (eg, collaboRATE) for periodic clinic audits; use results in feedback and teaching

Risk calculators and visual consent tools

Modern surgical practice increasingly relies on risk calculators (ie, ACS NSQIP [40]) to estimate individualized probabilities of morbidity and mortality. These can help surgeons calibrate their own estimates and provide more personalized risk information. However, listing percentages alone does little to help patients imagine how those complications will feel or what they would mean for their lives. Visual risk communication tools can help bridge this gap by

- Displaying personalized risk estimates using icon arrays, bar graphs, or other intuitive graphics
- Allowing patients to choose which outcomes (ie, loss of independence and need for dialysis) they care about most
- Structuring the subsequent conversation around these priorities

Early pilot studies of visual consent interfaces suggest improved satisfaction without substantial increases in visit length [41]. They can help shift the dialog from "here is the risk" to "which risks matter most to you?"

Structured conversation frameworks: Best Case/Worst Case and Better Conversations

BC/WC is a scenario-based framework developed and prospectively studied by Schwarze and colleagues specifically for high-stakes surgical decisions in older, frail patients [20]. Key features of BC/WC include

- Presenting at least 2 authentic options (ie, surgery vs nonoperative management).
- Using a hand-drawn graphic with separate trajectories for each option (best case outcome, worst case outcome, and most likely outcome).
- Describing outcomes narratively in terms of functional status, place of care (home, hospital, and nursing facility), burdensome interventions (intensive care unit [ICU], dialysis, and tubes), and survival—not just complication rates.
- Explicitly inviting patients and families to deliberate over these scenarios and relate them to their own goals and tolerances.

After using this tool, surgeons' OPTION-5 scores increased significantly and qualitative analysis showed a shift from problem-focused, risk-enumeration conversations to decision-focused deliberation that integrated patient values [18,20,31]. This makes tradeoffs more concrete and invites patients to consider whether the potential "best" is worth the possible "worst."

Better Conversations [19] is a conversation framework also developed by Schwarze and colleagues that builds on extensive analysis of recorded consent encounters across surgical specialties. This approach argues that the traditional core of informed consent–understanding, risks, benefits, and alternatives–has inadvertently produced 2 distortions:

1. An overly technical explanation of disease and treatment ("mini-medical school").
2. An overly simplistic narrative that surgery will "fix" the problem, with little discussion of the goals and downsides of surgery as experienced by patients.

Based on this critique, Schwarze and colleagues propose a new core framework to informed consent–"Better Conversations"–with 5 steps:

1. *"Show your cards":* Early in the discussion, the surgeon reveals their initial inclination framed as a professional norm or concern (eg, "We usually do surgery for this," "I'm worried surgery may not help you"). This transparency acknowledges expertise without dictating the decision.
2. *"Clearly describe the goals of surgery":* Surgery can (a) prolong life, (b) improve function or symptoms, (c) prevent disability, and/or (d) establish a diagnosis. The surgeon explicitly states which goal(s) apply and what surgery can *and cannot* accomplish for the particular patient.
3. *"Describe all the downsides of surgery":* Surgeons should reframe risks not just as reportable complications, but rather (a) bad things that happen to everyone (incisions, recovery time, scars, and permanent anatomic changes); (b) bad things that *might* happen (complications and "bumps in the road" that may not be coded as complications, such as urinary retention or chronic diarrhea); (c) the possibility that surgery fails to achieve its goals.
4. *"Deliberate":* Surgeons invite patients to weigh whether the goals are valuable enough to justify the downsides (eg, "Is it worth it to you?" "How do you feel about trading more time in hospital for a chance at...?"). The focus is on reasoning together about tradeoffs, not simply on choosing a checkbox.
5. *"Make an agreement and a plan":* Surgeon and patient arrive at a shared understanding of what they are aiming for and what they are willing to tolerate. This includes acknowledging disagreement when it arises and documenting the rationale.

Better Conversations is not a scripted tool but a conceptual reframing. It meets legal requirements for consent and creates what the authors call a "deliberative space" in which patients can realistically anticipate and prepare for the experience of surgery.

For practicing surgeons, BC/WC and Better Conversations are complementary:

- BC/WC offers structure and visualization for scenario planning
- Better Conversations offers a high-level framework for how to frame goals and downsides and how to use professional judgment ("show your cards") in a way that neither engages in paternalism nor overpowers patients

Question prompt lists and other decision support tools

- *Question prompt lists (QPLs):* In a randomized trial, older adults considering major surgery were given a QPL encouraging them to ask about benefits, risks, recovery, and alternatives; surgeons were cued to invite questions. While deemed feasible, QPLs did not significantly increase patient engagement or satisfaction, although ceiling effects within the study population may have obscured potential benefits [42].
- *Teach-back techniques:* Asking patients to explain in their own words what they understood (eg, "Just so I know I explained things clearly, can you tell me how you'd explain this operation to a family member?") improves comprehension and often reveals surprising misconceptions [2,11].

- *Communication skills training:* Coaching in serious-illness communication, goals-of-care conversations, and SDM can be adapted from critical care and oncology to surgery and may serve as important adjuncts to the informed decision-making process [3,27].

Vulnerable populations

Emergency surgery and trauma

Most consent research focuses on elective or semiurgent cases. Emergency surgery and trauma–where time is severely constrained and patients may lack capacity–pose distinct challenges. Adapting frameworks like BC/WC and Better Conversations for surrogate decision-makers in these contexts is an active area of work but evidence is limited [43].

Patients with cognitive impairment

Many older surgical candidates have dementia, mild cognitive impairment, or delirium. Their capacity may fluctuate, and survey data demonstrate that surrogate decision-makers may struggle to make decisions that are concordant with the patient's wishes, with higher degrees of discordance in patients with dementia despite advance care planning [44,45]. Tailored approaches that incorporate prior documented preferences, supported decision-making, and careful surrogate counseling are needed. These approaches and tools should promote clear, value-concordant recommendations to surrogates that acknowledge the added complexity of substituted judgment without placing the burden of complex surgical decision-making on surrogates alone.

Limited English proficiency and disadvantaged populations

Patients with limited English proficiency, lower socioeconomic status, and marginalized racial or ethnic identities may be more likely to report gaps in understanding and to experience discordant care [2,11,28]. Few interventions are designed to specifically address these additional complexities; future research is needed ensuring optimal integration of high-quality interpreters and other strategies to address social determinants of health in preoperative communication and decision-making.

Measurement and implementation barriers

Despite having reasonable tools to measure SDM and aspects of informed consent, some barriers persist: (1) they are rarely embedded in routine perioperative workflows; (2) there is no consensus surgery-specific PROM for decision quality; and (3) many interventional studies emphasize knowledge and satisfaction but do not assess goal-concordant care, decisional regret, or downstream utilization (ie, ICU days in the last month of life). Furthermore, implementation of existing tools and strategies may be limited by workflow constraints and variable training resources, underscoring the need for future research to leverage implementation science to embed these processes and related training into existing surgical workflows.

Digital and artificial intelligence-enabled tools

Emerging technologies may serve to augment preoperative decision processes, including

- Personalized risk calculators that integrate electronic health record data and machine learning [46].
- Interactive decision aids that tailor content to individual risk and preferences [47].
- Artificial intelligence (AI)-driven summaries of educational content and other AI adjuncts to streamline informed decision-making. However, AI tools require validation for accuracy, bias, readability, and effect on comprehension/decisional conflict before clinical deployment [48,49].

These tools may enhance consistency and personalization but do raise concerns about transparency, information overload, and the potential to widen bias and disparities if not carefully designed and evaluated.

SUMMARY

Data from surveys, observational studies, and interviews demonstrate that substantial numbers of patients lack clear understanding of the major risks, therapeutic alternatives, and postoperative trajectories of surgery–even if they recall signing a consent form. Audio-recordings of real-world encounters reveal that surgeons often emphasize technical explanations and list complication without giving sufficient attention to patient goals and values, functional outcomes, and nonoperative options. The traditional informed-consent framework of "understanding, risks, benefits, and alternatives"–within the time-pressured contexts of clinic visits and inpatient settings–is insufficient to prepare patients for informed decisions about surgical care.

At the same time, research demonstrates that communication is modifiable. Decision aids, risk visualization tools, scenario-based frameworks such as BC/WC, and conceptual innovations like Better Conversations can meaningfully shift conversations toward deliberation and value-alignment. These interventions improve patient knowledge, calibrate expectations, and increase observed SDM behaviors without excessive time burden. Implementing these changes does not need to mean uniformly lengthy encounters for every preoperative conversation; rather, surgeons should recognize that small, structured changes can have meaningful impact.

Finally, there are important knowledge gaps in how to meet the needs of vulnerable surgical patients: emergency settings, cognitively impaired patients, and minoritized populations remain understudied. Addressing these gaps will require ongoing collaboration between surgeons, patients, and health systems.

CLINICS CARE POINTS

- *Ask patients how they want to make decisions.* Avoid assuming one size fits all. Encourage patients to include key family members or caregivers who will help them during recovery.

- *Show your cards early.* Briefly state your professional inclination ("I think surgery is likely to help" or "I'm worried it may not help enough to be worth it") to reduce guesswork and ground the discussion in your expertise.
- *Clarify the goals of surgery in plain language.* Is the primary aim to help them live longer, feel better, prevent disability, or obtain a diagnosis? Spell this out and point out what surgery *cannot* do. Reflect explicitly on whether surgery can reasonably be expected to achieve the patient-specific goal.
- *Describe the full spectrum of downsides, not just complications.* Include expected recovery time, pain, need for rehabilitation or nursing facility, permanent lifestyle changes, and the possibility that surgery will *not* achieve its goals. Tailor these discussions to patients' and families' goals and values.
- *Separate explanation from deliberation.* First ensure the patient understands the problem and options; then explicitly shift to, "Now let's talk about what makes the most sense for *you*."
- *Use scenario planning frameworks for high-stakes decisions.* For frail or seriously ill patients, consider BC/WC: draw simple trajectories for each option and discuss best, worst, and most likely outcomes in terms of function, place of care, and survival.
- *Invite and normalize questions.* Use prompts like, "Many people in your situation ask about..." Consider providing QPLs when possible, and pause after key points.
- *Employ teach-back routinely.* Ask patients to explain the plan and main risks in their own words; address misunderstandings.
- *Use visual aids and decision tools when available.* Risk charts, icon arrays, and online decision aids often improve comprehension and engagement more effectively than verbal descriptions alone.
- *Document the reasoning, not just the signature.* Chart the goals discussed, the options considered (including nonoperative care), and the patient's stated preferences; this helps continuity and supports goal-concordant care.
- *Seek feedback and measure your practice.* Periodically use simple SDM measures (ie, collaboRATE or SDM-Q-9) or patient surveys to identify areas for improvement and track change over time.

Disclosure

The authors report no relevant conflicts of interest.

References

[1] Lloyd A, Hayes P, Bell PR, et al. The role of risk and benefit perception in informed consent for surgery. Med Decis Mak 2001;21(2):141–9.

[2] Glaser J, Nouri S, Fernandez A, et al. Interventions to improve patient comprehension in informed consent for medical and surgical procedures: an updated systematic review. Med Decis Mak 2020;40(2):119–43.

[3] Weiss Y, Zarour S, Neuman MD, et al. Shared decision-making for older adults in the perioperative setting: a narrative review. Eur J Anaesthesiol 2025;42(9):767.

[4] Childress JF, Childress MD. What does the evolution from informed consent to shared decision making teach us about authority in health care? AMA Journal of Ethics 2020;22(5): 423–9.

[5] Braddock CH, Edwards KA, Hasenberg NM, et al. Informed decision making in outpatient practice: time to get back to basics. JAMA 1999;282(24):2313–20.
[6] Brock DW. The ideal of shared decision making between physicians and patients. Kennedy Inst Ethics J 1991;1(1):28–47.
[7] Ochieng J, Buwembo W, Munabi I, et al. Informed consent in clinical practice: patients' experiences and perspectives following surgery. BMC Res Notes 2015;8:765.
[8] Basukala S, Shrestha O, Thapa N, et al. How informed is informed consent?—Evaluating the quality of informed consent among surgical patients in a tertiary care hospital in Nepal. PLoS One 2023;18(7):e0288074.
[9] McKeague M, Windsor J. Patients' perception of the adequacy of informed consent: a pilot study of elective general surgical patients in Auckland. N Z Med J 2003;116 (1170):U355.
[10] Mihiretu MM, Bekele E, Ayele K, et al. Patient knowledge of surgical informed consent and shared decision-making process among surgical patients in Ethiopia: a systematic review and meta-analysis. Patient Saf Surg 2024;18:2.
[11] Schenker Y, Fernandez A, Sudore R, et al. Interventions to improve patient comprehension in informed consent for medical and surgical procedures: a systematic review. Med Decis Mak 2011;31(1):151–73.
[12] Sherman KA, Kilby CJ, Pehlivan M, et al. Adequacy of measures of informed consent in medical practice: a systematic review. PLoS One 2021;16(5):e0251485.
[13] Zaza SI, Arnold RM, Schwarze ML. Innovations in surgical communication 4—Present the downsides of surgery, not just risks. JAMA Surg 2023;158(10):998–1000.
[14] Wilson A, Ronnekleiv-Kelly SM, Pawlik TM. Regret in surgical decision making: a systematic review of patient and physician perspectives. World J Surg 2017;41(6):1454–65.
[15] Kruser JM, Pecanac KE, Brasel KJ, et al. "And I think that we can fix it": mental models used in high-risk surgical decision making. Ann Surg 2015;261(4):678–84.
[16] Elwyn G, Frosch D, Thomson R, et al. Shared decision making: a model for clinical practice. J Gen Intern Med 2012;27(10):1361–7.
[17] Paasche-Orlow MK, Taylor HA, Brancati FL. Readability standards for informed-consent forms as compared with actual readability. N Engl J Med 2003;348(8):721–6.
[18] Stalter LN, Baggett ND, Hanlon BM, et al. Identifying patterns in preoperative communication about high-risk surgical intervention: a secondary analysis of a randomized clinical trial. Med Decis Mak 2023;43(4):487–97.
[19] Schwarze ML, Arnold RM, Clapp JT, et al. Better conversations for better informed consent. Hastings Cent Rep 2024;54(3):11–4.
[20] Taylor LJ, Nabozny MJ, Steffens NM, et al. A framework to improve surgeon communication in high-stakes surgical decisions: best case/worst case. JAMA Surg 2017;152(6): 531–8.
[21] Braddock C, Hudak PL, Feldman JJ, et al. "Surgery is certainly one good option": quality and time-efficiency of informed decision-making in surgery. J Bone Joint Surg Am 2008;90(9):1830–8.
[22] Nabozny MJ, Kruser JM, Steffens NM, et al. Patient-reported limitations to surgical buy-in: a qualitative study of patients facing high-risk surgery. Ann Surg 2017;265(1):97.
[23] Neuman MD, Bosk CL. What we talk about when we talk about risk: refining surgery's hazards in medical thought. Milbank Q 2012;90(1):135–59.
[24] Gillett G. A history and theory of informed consent. J Med Ethics 1987;13(4):219–20.
[25] Kannan S, Seo J, Riggs KR, et al. Surgeons' views on shared decision-making. J Patient Cent Res Rev 2020;7(1):8–18.
[26] Skowron KB, Angelos P. Surgical informed consent revisited: time to revise the routine? World J Surg 2017;41(1):1–4.
[27] Cooper Z, Koritsanszky LA, Cauley CE, et al. Recommendations for best communication practices to facilitate goal-concordant care for seriously ill older patients with emergency surgical conditions. Ann Surg 2016;263(1):1–6.

[28] Karliner LS, Jacobs EA, Chen AH, et al. Do professional interpreters improve clinical care for patients with limited English proficiency? A systematic review of the literature. Health Serv Res 2007;42(2):727–54.
[29] Elwyn G, Frosch D, Volandes AE, et al. Investing in deliberation: a definition and classification of decision support interventions for people facing difficult health decisions. Med Decis Mak 2010;30(6):701–11.
[30] Sebastian A, Wyld L, Morgan J. Examining the variation in consent in general surgery. Ann R Coll Surg Engl 2024;106(2):140–9.
[31] Kruser JM, Nabozny MJ, Steffens NM, et al. "Best case/worst case": qualitative evaluation of a novel communication tool for difficult in-the-moment surgical decisions. J Am Geriatr Soc 2015;63(9):1805–11.
[32] Mylod D, Lee TH. Giving hope as a high reliability function of health care. J Patient Exp 2023;10:23743735221147765.
[33] Mack JW, Smith TJ. Reasons why physicians do not have discussions about poor prognosis, why it matters, and what can be improved. J Clin Orthod 2012;30(22):2715–7.
[34] Stuart B. Managing the hopes of seriously ill patients. Harv Bus Rev 2019. Available at: https://hbr.org/2019/05/managing-the-hopes-of-seriously-ill-patients. Accessed February 23, 2026.
[35] Kriston L, Scholl I, Hölzel L, et al. The 9-item shared decision making questionnaire (SDM-Q-9). Development and psychometric properties in a primary care sample. Patient Educ Counsel 2010;80(1):94–9.
[36] Calderon C, Ferrando PJ, Carmona-Bayonas A, et al. Validation of SDM-Q-Doc questionnaire to measure shared decision-making physician's perspective in oncology practice. Clin Transl Oncol 2017;19(11):1312–9.
[37] Elwyn G, Barr PJ, Grande SW, et al. Developing CollaboRATE: a fast and frugal patient-reported measure of shared decision making in clinical encounters. Patient Educ Counsel 2013;93(1):102–7.
[38] Elwyn G, Hutchings H, Edwards A, et al. The OPTION scale: measuring the extent that clinicians involve patients in decision-making tasks. Health Expect 2005;8(1):34–42.
[39] Stacey D, Lewis KB, Smith M, et al. Decision aids for people facing health treatment or screening decisions. Cochrane Database Syst Rev 2024;1(1):CD001431.
[40] Bilimoria KY, Liu Y, Paruch JL, et al. Development and evaluation of the universal ACS NSQIP surgical risk calculator: a decision aid and informed consent tool for patients and surgeons. J Am Coll Surg 2013;217(5):833–42.e1-3.
[41] Gisladottir U, Nakikj D, Jhunjhunwala R, et al. Effective communication of personalized risks and patient preferences during surgical informed consent using data visualization: qualitative semistructured interview study with patients after surgery. JMIR Hum Factors 2022;9(2): e29118.
[42] Schwarze ML, Buffington A, Tucholka JL, et al. Effectiveness of a question prompt list intervention for older patients considering major surgery: a multisite randomized clinical trial. JAMA Surg 2020;155(1):6–13.
[43] Stalter L, Hanlon BM, Bushaw KJ, et al. Best case/worst Case-ICU: protocol for a multisite, stepped-wedge, randomised clinical trial of scenario planning to improve communication in the ICU in US trauma centres for older adults with serious injury. BMJ Open 2024;14(8): e083603.
[44] Ayalon L, Bachner YG, Dwolatzky T, et al. Preferences for end-of-life treatment: concordance between older adults with dementia or mild cognitive impairment and their spouses. Int Psychogeriatr 2012;24(11):1798–804.
[45] Nicholas LH, Langa KM, Halpern SD, et al. How do surrogates make treatment decisions for patients with dementia: an Experimental Survey Study. Health Econ 2024;33(6):1211–28.
[46] Mahajan A, Esper S, Oo TH, et al. Development and validation of a machine learning model to identify patients before surgery at high risk for postoperative adverse events. JAMA Netw Open 2023;6(7):e2322285.

[47] Coylewright M, Otero D, Lindman BR, et al. An interactive, online decision aid assessing patient goals and preferences for treatment of aortic stenosis to support physician-led shared decision-making: early feasibility pilot study. PLoS One 2024;19(5):e0302378.
[48] Goldschmitt M, Gleim P, Mandelartz S, et al. Digitalizing informed consent in healthcare: a scoping review. BMC Health Serv Res 2025;25(1):893.
[49] Rudra P, Balke WT, Kacprowski T, et al. Large language models for surgical informed consent: an ethical perspective on simulated empathy. J Med Ethics 2025; https://doi.org/10.1136/jme-2024-110652 jme-2024-110652.

Advances in Surgery 60 (2026) 251–257

ADVANCES IN SURGERY

Management of Serous Cystadenoma

Jon M. Harrison, MD[a], Carlos Fernandez-del Castillo, MD[b,*]

[a]Section of Hepatobiliary and Pancreatic Surgery, Division of Surgical Oncology, Department of General Surgery, Massachusetts General Hospital, Boston, USA; [b]Pancreas and Biliary Surgery Program, Division of Surgical Oncology, Department of General Surgery, Massachusetts General Hospital, Harvard Medical School, Boston, USA

Keywords

• Serous cystadenoma • Cystic pancreatic lesion • Endoscopic ultrasonography • Operative management

Key points

- Serous cystadenoma (SCA) is a non-malignant entity commonly found in elderly women.
- Many SCAs have predictable clinical and radiographic findings.
- SCAs lacking these features can be mistaken for other pancreatic cystic lesions.
- Resection is reserved for symptomatic patients or those with rapidly growing cysts and impending symptoms.
- Improved diagnostic accuracy will reduce the number of unnecessary resections.

INTRODUCTION

Serous cystadenoma (SCA) is an unusual but benign cystic pancreatic neoplasm with a propensity to slowly grow and encroach upon the surrounding viscera [1,2]. While resection is *curative*, patients must accept the risk associated with pancreatectomy, which can be significant for a noncancerous pathology. Balancing these aspects leads to complex medical decision-making, which is also influenced by preoperative diagnostic certainty—a unique challenge in this particular entity. This article addresses how such clinical aspects can best inform management of pancreatic serous cystadenomas.

*Corresponding author. Gastrointestinal and Oncologic Surgery, WAC-495, 15 Parkman Street, Boston, MA 02114. *E-mail address:* cfernandez@mgh.harvard.edu

https://doi.org/10.1016/j.yasu.2026.03.010

Abbreviations

CEA	carcinoembryonic antigen
PAS	periodic acid-schiff
SCA	serous cystadenoma
VEGFa	vascular endothelial growth factor A
VHL1	von Hippel Lindau

CLINICAL BACKGROUND AND DIAGNOSTIC FEATURES

Serous cystadenoma can arise throughout the pancreas, however, tend to cause symptoms when originating in the pancreatic head and neck [3]. There is a genetic association with von Hippel Lindau (*VHL1*) disease, characterized by the constellation of renal and pancreatic cysts as well as neurologic findings. Most SCAs, however, are sporadic (Fig. 1A) [4]. Additionally, the genetic profile of SCAs is notable for vascular endothelial growth factor A (*VEGFa*) transcription, which can have diagnostic utility in addition to important operative implications [5]. SCAs importantly show a female predominance (65%–74%), and patients tend to be older or elderly (58–62 year old), owing to the cyst's indolent biology [6,7]. Though debated, malignant transformation has been described in SCAs with a mucinous component though cases of widespread metastatic disease are virtually nonexistent [8]. In addition, no cystadenocarcinomas were reported in any of the 3 recently published large retrospective SCA series [6,7,9].

Histologically, SCAs exhibit broad vacuoles lined with periodic acid-schiff (PAS)-positive, glycogen rich cells (Fig. 1B). Radiographically, SCAs appear as cystic lesions with characteristic internal septa (Fig. 1C) [10]. The presence of a central scar (32%) or speckled calcifications (24%) are other key radiographic clues suggestive of serous cyst adenoma (Fig. 1D and E) [11]. Microcystic and macrocystic variants (44%–58% and 11%–16%, respectively) are also well-known, and while rarer, men tend to have a macrocystic morphology rather than a typical *honeycomb* or *bosselated* appearance (see Fig. 1D) [6,7]. Finally, solid (1%–3%) and unilocular (5%) phenotypes can occur and pose a diagnostic dilemma given their similar appearance to other pancreatic cysts such as mucinous cystic neoplasm or cystic pancreatic neuroendocrine tumor (Fig. 1F) [6,7].

Both pancreas-protocol computed tomography (CT) and magnetic resonance imaging (MRI) axial imaging studies are appropriate for either initial diagnostic modalities or surveillance. Endoscopic ultrasound is a useful adjunct as cyst fluid analysis can discern the etiology of cysts with an equivocal radiographic appearance [12]. In the absence of convincing radiographic findings, only cyst size greater than 4 cm (odds ratio [OR] 8.6, confidence interval [CI]: 2.67–31.2, $P < .001$) has been shown to be predictive of SCA suggesting that many smaller lesions are incorrectly triaged into either surveillance or resection pathways based on additional radiographic features [6].

As there is no pancreatic duct communication or mucin production, amylase and carcinoembryonic antigen (CEA) levels are normal, though false-positives

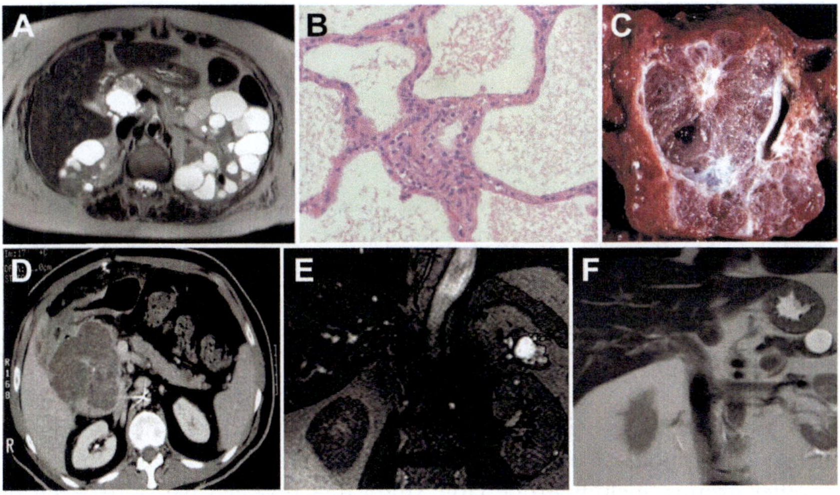

Fig. 1. Histologic and radiographic appearances of serous cystadenomas. (*A*) von Hippel Lindau patient with a large, bosselated SCA of the pancreatic head and innumerable renal cysts, (*B*) 40x magnification of resected SCA showing PAS-positive cells surrounding fluid-filled vacuoles, (*C*) Internal septations and central scar in a resected SCA, (*D*) Radiographic appearance of an SCA with classic central scar, (*E*) Small SCA in the pancreatic tail again with lobular appearance and calcifications, (*F*) Unilocular morphology of an SCA in a male.

are not infrequent (13%) [6,13]. Since these cysts are often intra-parenchymal (62%), pancreatic duct dilation and gland atrophy can be seen in the setting of a growing SCA [6]. Across studies, improved diagnostic accuracy for equivocal pancreatic cysts is attributed to cyst fluid analysis that reveal a normal CEA level (OR = 4.06, CI: 1.32–13.5, $P<.017$), a *VHL* mutation, or *VEGFa* [5,6]. Specifically, a combination of normal CEA levels and elevated *VEGFa* levels had sensitivity and specificity of 96% and 100% in one series of nearly 150 patients with sufficient cytologic analysis [5]. Unfortunately, these assays are commercially unavailable, and in the majority of patients, a VHL mutation is absent. Consequently, additional biochemical testing evaluating for elevated glucose levels can be used [14]. While sensitive for nonmucinous cysts such as SCA, an elevated level (>50 mg/dl) has poor specificity for differentiating between nonmucin producing cystic entities.

DIAGNOSTIC CHALLENGES

Despite some *classic* clinical and radiographic findings, serous cystadenomas can elude even skilled diagnosticians and convincingly masquerade as other pancreatic cyst types. An important study authored by Roldan and colleagues found that from over 30 years of high-volume pancreatic cyst surgery, roughly 25% of the preoperative misdiagnoses were attributable to SCAs [9]. Furthermore, Assawasirsin and colleagues showed that in 172 consecutive SCA resections, the pre-operative diagnosis of SCA occurred in only 33% of cases, with

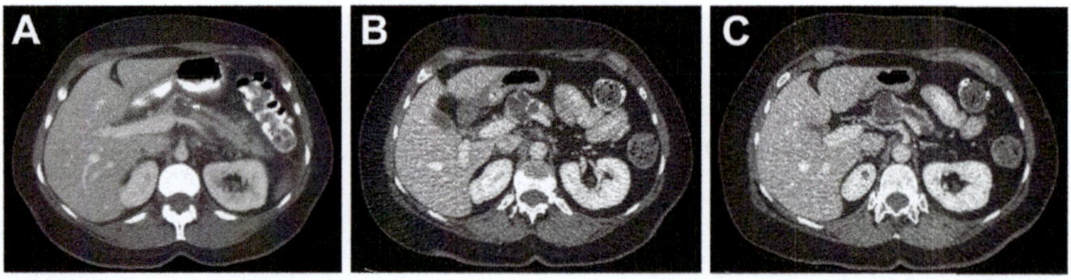

Fig. 2. Evolution of a presumed intraductal papillary mucinous neoplasm that returned as SCA on final pathologic review. (*A*) Lobulated cystic lesion in the pancreatic body with dilation of the upstream main pancreatic duct, (*B*) Interval CT of the lesion 13 years later showing cyst growth with (*C*) increase in pancreatic duct dilation and subsequent and gland atrophy.

an incorrect diagnosis being driven by the presence of a mural nodule (35%) or thickened septation (27%) [6]. Similar rates of misdiagnosis have been reported by other groups, including one large study that revealed parity between preoperative suspicion and pathologic confirmation (19.4% vs 15.7%, *P*=.491) [7]. Again, clinical decision-making guided by the presence of worrisome features or high-risk stigmata such as thickened internal septa (7%), jaundice (6%), or mural nodule/solid component (3%) for a presumed mucinous cyst accounted for the misdiagnoses (Fig. 2A and B) [7,15].

MANAGEMENT CONSIDERATIONS

Serous cystadenoma management highlights the importance of diagnostic certainty. For a benign disease process, resection is generally reserved for fit, symptomatic patients, however, young patients with a progressively enlarging lesion may also be considered for surgery to avoid a more extensive resection at a suboptimal future timepoint. For example, a healthy, middle-aged patient with a modest size SCA may benefit from elective surgery rather than watchful

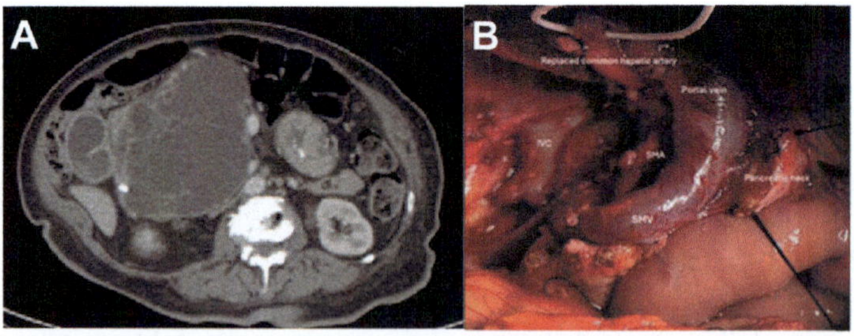

Fig. 3. Serous cystadenoma causing painless jaundice. (*A*) Large SCA compressing the common bile duct and causing displacement of the superior mesenteric vein. Note biliary stent traversing through the mass, (*B*) Whipple resection for this SCA required peeling the mass off a replaced right hepatic artery and superior mesenteric vein to avoid a vascular reconstruction.

Box 1: Indications for serous cystadenoma resection

- Clinical symptoms
- Growth with impending symptoms
- Main pancreatic duct obstruction with significant gland atrophy

waiting in the face of significant cyst growth to the point of needing a more extensive resection at an older age. Again, Assawasirsin and colleagues described *cross over* from surveillance to resection in patients with an enlarging cyst (29%) or new symptoms (14%), and overall growth rate did translate into longer surveillance periods (73 vs 37 months, $P<.001$) [6]. Other studies have shown that larger, growing cysts tend to grow at an accelerated pace compared to stable SCAs. Specifically, Tseng and colleagues showed that cysts greater than 4 cm grew at a rate 4-times faster than cysts < 4 cm, and a subset of SCAs did appear to be *fast growing* and outpace expected growth rates in another large series [7,16,17].

Regarding symptomology, bulky or pancreatic head tumors can cause pain and fullness leading to weight loss and/or biliary or gastric outlet obstructions (Fig. 3A) [18,19]. Unfortunately, a common scenario is an older patient presenting with advanced findings that requires either an extensive or palliative procedure (Fig. 3B). In addition, smaller tumors with parenchymal in-growth can obstruct the main pancreatic duct leading to pancreatic atrophy (Fig. 2C) [6]. Established indications for surgical intervention are outlined in Box 1.

SURGICAL INTERVENTION

Anatomic site guides the decision of resection extent, and SCAs in the uncinate process and pancreatic head are treated with pancreaticoduodenectomy whereas a subtotal or distal pancreatectomy is appropriate for lesions in the body and tail. In suitable cases, neck and proximal body lesions may be treated with central pancreatectomy, however, the surgeon must have sufficient experience to offer this approach (Fig. 4). Enucleation or unroofing is

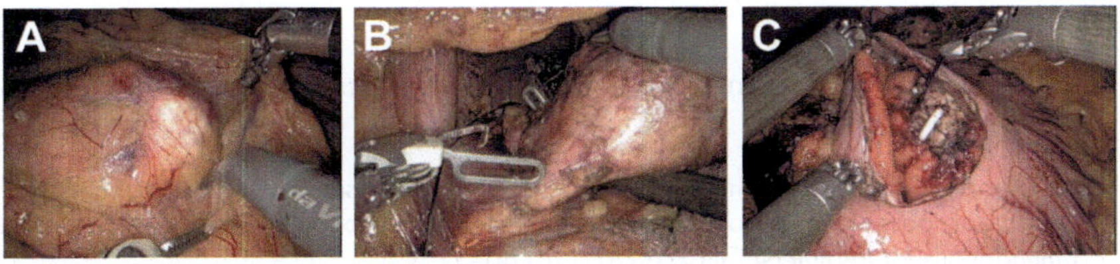

Fig. 4. Robotic resection of a presumed pancreatic body SCA. (*A*) Lobulated texture of the cyst after exposure of the lesser sac through pars flaccida, (*B*) Development of the posterior retroperitoneal plane elevating the cyst anteriorly for proximal transection, (*C*) Creation of a pancreaticogastrostomy through an anterior gastrotomy.

not recommended as these tumors are usually embedded in the pancreatic parenchyma. For appropriate cases without vascular involvement, a minimally invasive, either laparoscopic or robotic approach, can be offered, again, based on the surgeon's experience with these techniques. Note that these lesions can be locally infiltrative given *VEGFa* production and may require vascular resection and reconstruction.

SUMMARY

Serous cyst adenoma management is heavily influenced by symptomology and diagnostic certainty at the time of detection. A common pitfall is ascribing a framework for mucinous cysts to equivocal pancreatic cysts, which leads to long-term surveillance in search of accumulating worrisome features. Unindicated surgery in the face of misdiagnosis is unfortunately common and reinforces the need for improved diagnostics. Still, resection is warranted in the setting of symptoms or anticipated symptoms for growing cysts in appropriate surgical candidates. The extent of resection is dictated by anatomic location, and minimally invasive approaches can be considered at experienced centers. As such, a multidisciplinary approach involving dedicated pancreatobiliary radiologists, interventional gastroenterologists, and pancreatic surgeons is requisite for achieving an accurate diagnosis and steering clinical decision-making away from unwarranted resections.

CLINICS CARE POINTS

- Serous cystadenoma can be found in men and may have a different morphology than those clasically seen in women.
- Sugeons must maintain an appropriate index of suspicion to not misdiagnose a serous cystadenoma as a mucinous cyst as this can lead to unnecessary surveillance or surgery.
- Resection can be challenging as large serous cystadenomas can obliterate normal tissue planes, distort normal anatomy, and tether onto nearby venous structures.

Disclosure

The authors have no financial disclosures or conflicts of interest to disclose.

References

[1] Malleo G, Bassi C, Rossini R, et al. Growth pattern of serous cystic neoplasms of the pancreas: observational study with long-term magnetic resonance surveillance and recommendations for treatment. Gut 2012;61(5):746–51.
[2] Bassi C, Salvia R, Molinari E, et al. Management of 100 consecutive cases of pancreatic serous cystadenoma: wait for symptoms and see at imaging or vice versa? World J Surg 2003;27(3):319–23.
[3] Khashab MA, Shin EJ, Amateau S, et al. Tumor size and location correlate with behavior of pancreatic serous cystic neoplasms. Am J Gastroenterol 2011;106(8):1521–6.

[4] Matsubayashi H, Uesaka K, Kanemoto H, et al. Multiple Endocrine Neoplasms and Serous Cysts of the Pancreas in a Patient with von Hippel-Lindau Disease. J Gastrointest Cancer 2010;41(3):197–202.
[5] Carr RA, Yip-Schneider MT, Dolejs S, et al. Pancreatic cyst fluid vascular endothelial growth factor A and carcinoembryonic antigen: a highly accurate test for the diagnosis of serous cystic neoplasm. J Am Coll Surg 2017;225(1):93–100.
[6] Assawasirisin C, Qadan M, Aimprasittichai S, et al. Pancreatic serous cystadenoma: a continuing diagnostic challenge. Ann Surg 2025;281(3):501–7.
[7] Marchegiani G, Caravati A, Andrianello S, et al. Serous cystic neoplasms of the pancreas management in the real-world: still operating on a benign entity. Ann Surg 2022;276(6): e868–75.
[8] Reid MD, Choi HJ, Memis B, et al. Serous neoplasms of the pancreas: a clinicopathologic analysis of 193 cases and literature review with new insights on macrocystic and solid variants and critical reappraisal of So-called "Serous Cystadenocarcinoma.". Am J Surg Pathol 2015;39(12):1597–610.
[9] Roldán J, Harrison JM, Qadan M, et al. Evolving trends in pancreatic cystic tumors: a 3-Decade single-center experience with 1290 resections. Ann Surg 2023;277(3):491–7.
[10] Choi JY, Kim MJ, Lee JY, et al. Typical and atypical manifestations of serous cystadenoma of the pancreas: imaging findings with pathologic correlation. AJR Am J Roentgenol 2009;193 (1):136–42.
[11] Kimura W, Moriya T, Hirai I, et al. Multicenter study of serous cystic neoplasm of the Japan pancreas society. Pancreas 2012;41(3):380–7.
[12] van der Waaij LA, van Dullemen HM, Porte RJ. Cyst fluid analysis in the differential diagnosis of pancreatic cystic lesions: a pooled analysis. Gastrointest Endosc 2005;62(3): 383–9.
[13] Park WGU, Mascarenhas R, Palaez-Luna M, et al. Diagnostic performance of cyst fluid carcinoembryonic antigen and amylase in histologically confirmed pancreatic cysts. Pancreas 2011;40(1):42–5.
[14] Zikos T, Pham K, Bowen R, et al. Cyst fluid glucose is rapidly feasible and accurate in diagnosing mucinous pancreatic cysts. Am J Gastroenterol 2015;110(6):909–14.
[15] Ohtsuka T, Fernandez-del Castillo C, Furukawa T, et al. International evidence-based Kyoto guidelines for the management of intraductal papillary mucinous neoplasm of the pancreas. Pancreatology 2024;24(2):255–70.
[16] Tseng JF, Warshaw AL, Sahani DV, et al. Serous cystadenoma of the pancreas: tumor growth rates and recommendations for treatment. Ann Surg 2005;242(3):413–9 [discussion: 419–421].
[17] El-Hayek KM, Brown N, O'Rourke C, et al. Rate of growth of pancreatic serous cystadenoma as an indication for resection. Surgery 2013;154(4):794–800 [discussion: 800–802].
[18] Medina DC, Osorno R, Boutros CN. Biliary and gastric drainage in advanced pancreatic serous cystadenoma and portal hypertension in Von Hippel-Lindau syndrome. J Gastrointest Oncol 2014;5(2):E50–3.
[19] Jais B, Rebours V, Malleo G, et al. Serous cystic neoplasm of the pancreas: a multinational study of 2622 patients under the auspices of the International Association of Pancreatology and European Pancreatic Club (European Study Group on Cystic Tumors of the Pancreas). Gut 2016;65(2):305–12.

Advances in Surgery 60 (2026) 259–270

ADVANCES IN SURGERY

Management of Anastomotic Leaks

Endoscopic, Interventional, and Surgical Strategies

Uzma Rahman, MD[a], Stephen C. Yang, MD, MAMSE[b,*]

[a]Division of Cardiothoracic Surgery, The Johns Hopkins Hospital, Baltimore, MD, USA; [b]Division of Thoracic Surgery, Department of Surgery, The Johns Hopkins Medical Institutions, Baltimore, MD, USA

Keywords

• Anastomotic leaks (ALs) • Endoscopic interventions • Conservative management • Surgical interventions • Source control

Key points

- Anastomotic leaks are associated with increased morbidity, mortality, length of stay, cost, and poor quality of life.
- With advances in medical technology, most anastomotic leaks can be managed with nonoperative interventions.
- Surgical intervention may be required depending on the patient's clinical status, or leaks that fail to resolve with nonoperative interventions.

INTRODUCTION

Anastomotic leaks (ALs) after gastrointestinal (GI) surgery remain a major cause of morbidity, mortality, and increased costs for patients and health care system. A lack of consensus on the definition of AL after GI surgery makes it difficult to study the true incidence of this complication and compare outcomes [1,2]. Various definitions have been proposed, the United Kingdom Surgical Infection Study Group's (UKSISG) definition being one of the first. UKSISG differentiated an AL from a subclinical leak. AL was defined as a leak of luminal contents from a surgical joint between two hollow viscera, whereas a subclinical leak was defined as the escape of luminal contents

*Corresponding author. The Johns Hopkins Medical Institutions, Division of Thoracic Surgery, 600 N. Wolfe Street, Blalock 240, Baltimore, MD 21287. *E-mail address:* syang7@jhmi.edu

https://doi.org/10.1016/j.yasu.2026.03.017
0065-3411/26/

Abbreviations

AL	anastomotic leak
EVAC	endoscopic vacuum-assisted closure
FC-SEMS	fully covered self-expanding metal stents
GI	gastrointestinal
ISREC	International Study Group of Rectal Cancer
IV	intravenous
NGT	nasogastric tube
NPO	*nil per os*
PC-SEMS	partially covered self-expanding metal stents
SEMS	self-expanding metal stents
UKSISG	United Kingdom Surgical Infection Study Group

from the site of the anastomosis into an adjacent localized area, detected by imaging, in the absence of clinical symptoms.

Further specifications in these definitions were developed since the clinical sequelae and management of a proximal AL is different from that of a distal AL. For example, according to the Esophagectomy Complications Consensus Group, an AL is defined as a full-thickness GI defect involving esophagus, anastomosis, staple line, or conduit irrespective of presentation or method of identification. The International Study Group of Rectal Cancer (ISREC) deemed that rectal AL are treated differently compared to proximal GI AL; therefore, a specific definition and grading system was developed for rectal AL. ISREC defined an AL as a defect of the intestinal wall at the anastomotic site (including suture and staple lines of neorectal reservoirs) leading to a communication between the intraluminal and extraluminal compartments. [3] According to the ISREC grading system, grade A AL does not require a change in management, grade B requires a therapeutic intervention, whereas grade C requires reoperation. Although historically AL after GI surgery was often managed with reoperation, advances in interventional and endoscopic procedures have enabled us to treat AL with nonoperative measures in a majority of cases. However, surgical intervention remains the cornerstone for patients who are septic, peritonitic or have failed nonoperative management [4].

The diagnosis of AL should always be suspected, whenever there is fever, leukocytosis, or an acute change in hemodynamic status. If drains are left behind around the anastomosis, the amount, color, and chemistries (amylase and bile) should be examined. Radiologic studies, including upper GI series using gastrograffin, and/or computerized tomography (CT) scans with oral contrast, should be performed. Endoscopic approaches should be used judiciously especially with a fresh anastomosis, and should be not only diagnostic but also therapeutic, as will be discussed.

DISCUSSION

AL remains one of the most feared complications after GI surgery. AL can be diagnosed clinically, using biochemical assay, imaging studies, or endoscopy.

In general, treatment is aimed at source control with drainage of fluid collections, intravenous (IV) antibiotics, closure or coverage of leak, salvaging the conduit in esophagectomy patients, and optimizing nutrition. While there are various treatment modalities to manage AL, the optimal method depends on the patient's clinical status, size and location of the defect, severity of symptoms, and time after surgery [5].

Conservative measures

This approach is for clinically stable patients with minimal symptoms and a radiographically proven contained or small leak. Conservative measures for AL consist of keeping the patient *nil per os* (NPO), decompression with a nasogastric tube (NGT), IV antibiotics, and parenteral nutrition or distal alimentary feeding with a jejunostomy tube when feasible. Decompressing the GI tract with an NGT minimizes distention and leakage of fluid through the anastomotic defect, thereby allowing the defect to heal gradually with time. Studies have also reported the use of a double elementary tube placed transnasally, which has two lumens: a proximal lumen to suction and decompress the conduit, and a distal lumen to feed the alimentary tract [6,7]. Current recommendations for the duration of IV antibiotics state that four days of IV antibiotics after adequate source control are sufficient in most patients [8]. The decision to initiate or withhold parenteral nutrition depends on the expected duration for which the patient remains NPO. Fluid collections less than 3cm in size, in a stable patient, usually do not require percutaneous drainage and can be managed as mentioned above. Patient's clinical course and repeat imaging can be used to evaluate whether conservative management is effective. Studies and anecdotal data have shown reassuring results with conservative measures when used for the appropriate patient cohort [9,10].

Nonsurgical interventions

Nonsurgical interventions play a significant role in the management of AL after GI surgery. This is usually the next approach for patients who have failed conservative management of AL. In the past decade, various advances in endoscopic techniques and image-guided procedures have allowed resolution of AL without the need for surgery for many patients. Different endoscopic and percutaneous procedures are often used in conjunction to optimize management of these patients.

Endoscopic interventions

Endoscopic stents. Endoscopic stents are commonly used in the management of AL after GI surgery.

Stents can be placed under endoscopic visualization to cover the area of defect. This controls extraluminal leakage of fluid and allows time for the tissue to heal. The time from stent placement to closure of defect ranges anywhere from 2 to 8 weeks [5,6]. Various stent options are available, such as plastic stents, fully covered self-expanding metal stents (FC-SEMS), or partially covered SEMS (PC-SEMS), each with their own advantages and disadvantages. Studies have failed to show a significant difference in the success rates between different types of stents. However, PC-SEMS have a higher risk of tissue ingrowth, plastic stents have a higher risk of migration, and FC-SEMS are difficult to anchor in place. Although there is no consensus on the maximum defect size that can be managed with an endoscopic stent, they are typically used for defects that involve less than 30% of the luminal surface or staple line.

In general, endoscopic stents are best used for midthoracic and foregut leaks. Stents in the cervical region are difficult to anchor and are associated with globus sensation. If placed too close to the esophageal sphincter (<2 cm between the upper esophageal sphincter and upper edge of the stent) they can increase the risk of airway compromise and aspiration pneumonia. Currently, custom-designed stents for upper esophageal leaks are being developed. Similarly, for colorectal AL, the distal end of the stent must lie 5 cm above the anal verge, to prevent rectal pain and foreign body sensation. Stents are often too narrow for the average colorectal anastomosis and may require securing with endoclips to lower the risk of stent migration [11].

Although endoscopic stents have greater than 85% success rate with SEMS used for leak closure, they can have complications [12]. For example, stent migration can occur in about 25% of patients, they often require reintervention, and in about 15% of cases stents can cause intestinal obstruction. In some cases, stents can also erode through the lumen or form a fistula, and thus care should be taken not to oversize the stent. Similarly, stents should not be used to cover a perforated site of cancer (eg, after dilation), as it will not heal; definitive/palliative resection should be performed. Stenting can also delay the time to definitive surgery should endoscopic treatment fail [13]. Some of these potential complications are overcome by using biodegradable stents made of woven polydioxanone monofilament [5]. These stents gradually degrade by random hydrolysis in a low ambient pH. Therefore, they have been used for AL after esophagectomy and gastric resections. However, these biodegradable stents are expensive and associated with globus sensation.

Endoscopic vacuum-assisted closure. This technique has gained popularity in the past decade and has shown promising results for GI AL's [5,6]. For foregut AL, an NGT with an open-pored polyurethane sponge sutured to its tip is endoscopically placed into or overlying the defect and connected to a low vacuum negative pressure system (about 100 mm of Hg). There are commercially available premade endoscopic vacuum-assisted closures (EVACs) (EsoSPONGE, Braun B. Melsungen, Germany, Fig. 1). This negative pressure not only facilitates drainage of the wound bed but also promotes tissue granulation and angiogenesis. Patients usually need 5 to 6 sponge changes for complete granulation of defect, and the mean healing time is 12 to 36 days. A rendezvous technique using EVAC has also been described where the NGT with the sponge is passed into the esophagus through an existing chest tube drain [14].

EVAC has a success rate of up to 85% in gastric and colorectal AL. For colorectal AL, the sponge is placed transanally, under endoscopic guidance,

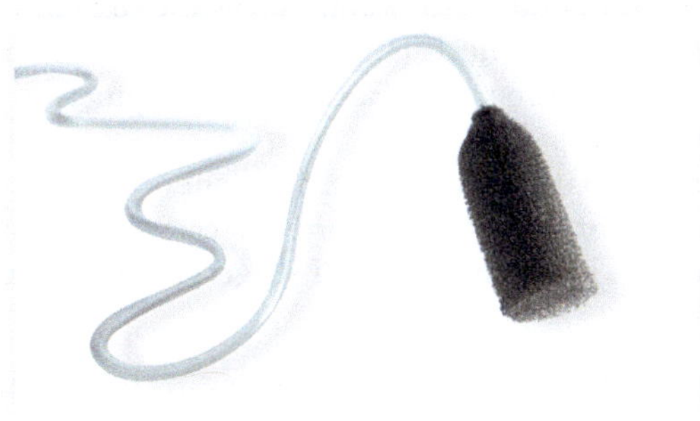

Fig. 1. Endoscopic VAC sponges. (Image provided courtesy of Boston Scientific. © 2026 Boston Scientific Corporation or its affiliates. All rights reserved.)

through the anastomotic defect into the presacral space. The sponge is changed every 2 to 3 days and removed once the cavity is less than 1 cm in size. The presence of a visible vessel in the presacral space is a contraindication to this intervention. EVAC for colorectal AL is more successful when used in conjunction with proximal diversion. Although EVAC has been widely adopted for upper GI AL, its use for colorectal AL has only been reported in case series and case reports [3,15].

Endoscopic stent over sponge. Many centers, also use a combination of SEMS and EVAC or the stent-over-sponge technique [5,6]. The stent secures the sponge in place and optimizes suction. Selected studies have showed encouraging results with this approach, both as a first-line treatment for simple ALs, and for complex leaks that failed EVAC [16–18]. Combined vacuum-assisted closure (*VAC*) stents (see Fig. 1) are now commercially available (MICRO-TECH Europe GmbH, Fig. 2), which consist of a suction catheter attached to a fully covered stent with a polyurethane sponge on its outer surface.

Endoscopic sealants. For defects that are less than 15 mm or residual small defects after the use of EVAC, sealants such as fibrin glues or cyanoacrylates can be used. Fibrin glue consists of fibrinogen, aprotinin, dried thrombin, and calcium chloride. The glue firmly adheres to the wound and rapidly forms a rubber-like adhesive mass. It gains tensile strength gradually, although 70% of this strength

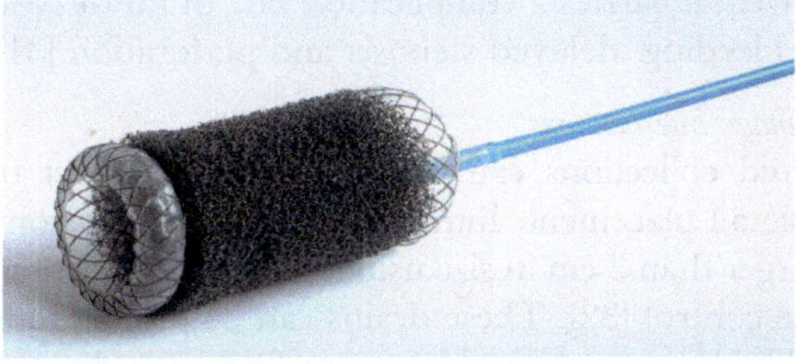

Fig. 2. Combined VAC stent. (Copyright (c) VAC Stent GmbH.)

is achieved within 10 minutes. Aprotinin delays the dissolution process of this adhesive mass as the wound heals [19]. Although data are limited on their use and success rate in this setting, they can be useful adjuncts to other endoscopic interventions for AL [20].

Endosealants are also useful in the management of small fistulae that form as a sequela of AL [21]. Studies have reported successful treatment of small AL and prevention of AL in bariatric and GI surgery, although evidence is inconclusive [19,22].

Endoscopic clips and suturing. Endoscopic suturing technique uses a disposable suturing device mounted on the tip of a double channel endoscope [5,6]. It can place full thickness or mucosal sutures, continuous or intermittent, to close an anastomotic defect. Endosuturing can be used to manage <2 cm AL as well as to close fistula tracts [23,24]. Endoscopic snares are also available, where multiple endoclips are placed along the border of the defect to create pseudopolyps, and then cinched together with a snare in a purse-string [25].

Endoscopic clips are made with nitinol, a biocompatible elastic alloy. These clips are deployed such that they reapproximate the edges of the defect and compress the tissue together. They allow the tissue to remain approximated while healing and usually self-detach within a few weeks. They are typically used for defects smaller than 15 mm and only when the surrounding mucosa is healthy [25].

Although endoscopic clips and suturing are not at the forefront of endoscopic management of AL's, studies are currently evaluating their efficacy and show encouraging results [26,27]. These are more commonly used for staple line leaks after sleeve gastrectomy or mucosal defects after endoscopic submucosal dissections [28,29]. Endoclips are also suitable for small colorectal AL with defects less than 1.5 cm, without a pelvic fluid collection, and ideally in a nonradiated pelvis [3,30].

Endoscopic internal drainage. This technique can be used for bariatric surgical leaks that involve a tract connecting an organized fluid collection to the lumen. A double pigtail stent is placed, under endosonographic guidance, across the defect to facilitate transmural drainage. Although this technique has a reported success rate of greater than 80% for bariatric surgery AL and patients tolerate this procedure well, it carries a complication rate of up to 10%, with complications including bleeding, delayed stenosis and perforation [31].

Percutaneous drainage interventions

Intrathoracic fluid collections can be managed with chest tube drainage or image-guided pigtail placement. Intra-abdominal para-anastomotic fluid collections that are larger than 3 cm in size usually require percutaneous drainage for adequate source control [32]. These drains can be placed under ultrasound or CT guidance. Fluid cultures should be sent from this drainage to guide antibiotic therapy. Although this technique has greater than 85% success rate, repeat imaging is usually obtained to assess for resolution of the abscess cavity [32]. Interloop abscesses or abscesses that are not amenable to percutaneous drainage, may be managed initially with conservative management in stable patients. However, patients who fail to progress clinically should be considered for surgical washout and drainage. For colorectal AL, pelvic fluid collections may require transgluteal, transvaginal, or transanal drain placement by interventional radiology. A surgical intervention will likely be needed if the drain has stool or if extravasation of enteral contrast is noted on imaging [33].

Surgical interventions

With advances in endoscopic and percutaneous interventions, a majority of AL can be managed nonoperatively. However, surgery may be required for early postoperative leaks (within 72 hours), septic patients, and leaks refractory to conservative and procedural interventions [3]. Additionally, multiple studies have supported early surgical intervention (<24 hours since surgery) for bariatric surgery patients solely based on clinical symptoms. AL should be suspected in postoperative bariatric surgery patients who have persistent tachycardia, greater than 120 beats/minute, even if other vitals, physical examination and laboratory values are unremarkable [34–36]. Patients should be resuscitated adequately, started on IV antibiotics, and decompressed with NGT if needed, in preparation for surgery.

Among esophagectomy patients, AL management depends on the location of the anastomosis, extent of contamination, viability of the conduit, and the patient's hemodynamic status. For cervical anastomoses, washout and wide drainage may be adequate if the defect is small and contamination is confined to the neck region. However, patients with infection extending into the mediastinum require prompt surgical washout and wide drainage via open or thoracoscopic approach. For intrathoracic AL in a stable patient with a viable conduit, reinforcing the anastomotic dehiscence site with sutures or debriding necrotic tissue and redoing the anastomosis, are both reasonable options. When revising or reconstructing the anastomosis, reinforcing it with a pedicled pleural, pericardial or intercostal muscle flap when possible, and wide drainage is recommended.

In patients who are septic, hemodynamically unstable, have a necrotic conduit, or tissue is too friable for any repair, an esophageal diversion and exclusion is recommended [37]. The esophagus is resected proximally and distally to remove the necrotic tissue, and the proximal end is delivered through the left neck region as an end esophagostomy. The thoracic cavity is washed out and widely drained. A decompressing gastrostomy tube and a feeding jejunostomy tube should be placed. Once the patient recovers and is optimized, an alternative conduit, such as the colon or jejunum can be used for reconstruction. Although there is no consensus regarding the ideal timing for reconstruction, most patients require at least a few months until they are deemed ready from a nutrition and functional standpoint [38].

An alternative approach is a double-barreled cervical esophagogastric stoma which is feasible when an adequate length of the gastric conduit is available

[39]. The necrotic anastomosis is resected, the distal end (stomach) and the proximal end (esophagus) are both delivered as a stoma in the left neck, and the posterior wall of the anastomosis is created at this time. The advantage of this approach is that once the patient has recovered, completion of the anastomosis only requires closing of the stoma and avoids further dissection in the mediastinum. The stoma can also be used to evaluate the viability of the gastric conduit endoscopically before completing the anastomosis. Studies have also mentioned the use of a T-drain, in combination with wide drainage, under thoracoscopic visualization to manage small AL after esophagectomy [40,41]. A T-drain is inserted through the defect, across the anastomosis, and brought out externally to divert all secretions while creating a low output well-defined fistula. Gradually, over 3 to 4 weeks once the defect has healed, the T-portion of the drain can be cut endoscopically and removed, while the thoracic portion of the tube is slowly retracted out.

Defects in gastric or small bowel anastomoses can be reinforced with sutures or resected and revised. For small defects, debridement and primary repair of the anastomosis can be performed if feasible. However, if the tissue is too friable, edematous, or inflamed, the anastomosis should be resected and reconstructed [42]. When feasible, a pedicled omental flap can be used to reinforce the anastomosis. After reoperation, patients remain on bowel rest, decompression with NGT, and parenteral nutrition if needed. However, patients who are too unstable may need an anastomotic resection for source control and temporary abdominal closure. Once they are resuscitated and stabilized, the anastomosis can be reconstructed.

For colorectal AL, surgical approach depends on the patient's hemodynamic status, location of the AL, and intraoperative findings. Based on these factors, one can revise the anastomosis and divert proximally, or resect the anastomosis and create an end ostomy, with or without a mucus fistula [43]. For septic patients on vasopressor support and with extensive intra-abdominal contamination, it is safest to resect the anastomosis and create an end ostomy. The distal end can be externalized as a mucous fistula, or oversewn and widely drained with multiple surgical drains. In a severely inflamed field, if it is not safe to resect the anastomosis, this area should be irrigated, thoroughly drained, and proximal fecal diversion should be performed. Although this requires another surgery to re-establish GI continuity, the priority in these scenarios is source control and stabilizing the patient.

Patients who are stable with limited intra-abdominal spillage, viable tissue, and anastomotic defect <1 cm, are candidates for revision of the anastomosis, in combination with proximal fecal diversion [44]. If the AL has walled-off, a proximal diversion and drainage may be sufficient to allow healing of the anastomosis without any revision. For larger anastomotic defects or friable tissue, resecting and redoing the anastomosis is recommended, along with proximal diversion. When feasible, a loop ileostomy is preferred to a loop colostomy for diversion, given the ease of reversal in the future and lower rate of parastomal hernia and stoma prolapse associated with loop ileostomies [45]. However, a loop ileostomy does have higher output, therefore, carries a higher risk of dehydration and electrolyte abnormalities.

FUTURE DEVELOPMENTS

Advances in endoscopic equipment and graft material have opened the stage for novel techniques in the management of AL. Case reports have demonstrated the use of human acellular dermis sutured onto the defect area and reinforced with a stent, to heal the anastomotic defect. Another technique using chimera stents, which are a combination of 2 different sized stents proximally and distally, has been used to maximize adherence to gastric conduit defects after esophagectomy [46].

Various animal model studies are investigating minimally invasive ways to treat or prevent AL. For example, the role of bio-artificial esophageal tissue as a scaffold to repair esophageal defects, and the use of stems cells to repair AL is currently in progress [47,48]. Other studies are currently investigating the role of microbiome and animal-derived proteins in preventing and treating AL after GI surgery. One such study drew its inspiration from adhesive proteins in mussels and barnacle cement proteins, to create an adhesive hydrogel [49]. This injectable hydrogel is biodegradable and adheres to the colonic AL site, much like marine animals adhere to wet tissue. Another study is targeting intestinal bacterial production of collagenase as the cause of AL. In mice models, this study was able to reduce the colonization of collagenase producing bacteria, thereby reducing the rate of AL [31]. Although results are encouraging in animal models, more research is needed to assess their applicability in humans.

SUMMARY

ALs are a significant source of morbidity and mortality. Every step should be implemented to prevent AL, including careful patient selection, optimizing patient's clinical and nutritional status, and ensuring proper technique. The appropriate management of an AL depends on several factors, such as the patient's clinical status, type of surgery, location of the AL, and the resources available. Surgeons should be familiar with the armamentarium of treatment modalities available to manage AL and use a patient-tailored approach when selecting the most appropriate treatment.

CLINICS CARE POINTS

Pearls:

- Anastomotic leaks (ALs) are associated with significant increase in morbidity, mortality, and worsened quality of life.
- Although with the advent of medical technology, various nonsurgical options are available for the management of AL, the treatment of AL should be tailored to each patient.

Pitfalls:

- A high index of suspicion, with prompt and appropriate treatment, is imperative to minimize further complications after an AL.

Disclosure

The authors have nothing to disclose.

References

[1] Peel AL, Taylor EW. Proposed definitions for the audit of postoperative infection: a discussion paper. Surgical infection study group. Ann R Coll Surg Engl 1991;73(6):385–8.
[2] Ellis CT, Maykel JA. Defining anastomotic leak and the clinical relevance of leaks. Clin Colon Rectal Surg 2021;34(6):359–65.
[3] Rahbari NN, Weitz J, Hohenberger W, et al. Definition and grading of anastomotic leakage following anterior resection of the rectum: a proposal by the international study group of rectal cancer. Surgery 2010;147(3):339–51.
[4] Turrentine FE, Denlinger CE, Simpson VB, et al. Morbidity, mortality, cost, and survival estimates of gastrointestinal anastomotic leaks. J Am Coll Surg 2015;220(2):195–206.
[5] Fabbi M, Hagens ERC, van Berge Henegouwen MI, et al. Anastomotic leakage after esophagectomy for esophageal cancer: definitions, diagnostics, and treatment. Dis Esophagus 2021;34(1):doaa039.
[6] Famiglietti A, Lazar JF, Henderson H, et al. Management of anastomotic leaks after esophagectomy and gastric pull-up. J Thorac Dis 2020;12(3):1022–30.
[7] Wada T, Takeuchi H, Yoshikawa T, et al. Successful management of anastomotic leakage and lung fistula after esophagectomy. Ann Thorac Surg 2014;97(3):1071–3.
[8] Sawyer RG, Claridge JA, Nathens AB, et al. Trial of short-course antimicrobial therapy for intraabdominal infection. N Engl J Med 2015;372(21):1996–2005.
[9] Manghelli JL, Ceppa DP, Greenberg JW, et al. Management of anastomotic leaks following esophagectomy: when to intervene? J Thorac Dis 2019;11(1):131–7.
[10] Korst RJ, Port JL, Lee PC, et al. Intrathoracic manifestations of cervical anastomotic leaks after transthoracic esophagectomy for carcinoma. Ann Thorac Surg 2005;80(4):1185–90.
[11] Lamazza A, Fiori E, Schillaci A, et al. Treatment of anastomotic stenosis and leakage after colorectal resection for cancer with self-expandable metal stents. Am J Surg 2014;208(3):465–9.
[12] Puli SR, Spofford IS, Thompson CC. Use of self-expandable stents in the treatment of bariatric surgery leaks: a systematic review and meta-analysis. Gastrointest Endosc 2012;75(2):287–93.
[13] Williams RN, Hall AW, Sutton CD, et al. Management of esophageal perforation and anastomotic leak by transluminal drainage. J Gastrointest Surg 2011;15(5):777–81.
[14] Pines G, Bar I, Elami A, et al. Modified endoscopic vacuum therapy for nonhealing esophageal anastomotic leak: technique description and review of literature. J Laparoendosc Adv Surg Tech 2018;28(1):33–40.
[15] Shalaby M, Emile S, Elfeki H, et al. Systematic review of endoluminal vacuum-assisted therapy as salvage treatment for rectal anastomotic leakage. BJS Open 2019;3(2):153–60.
[16] Gubler C, Schneider PM, Bauerfeind P. Complex anastomotic leaks following esophageal resections: the new stent over sponge (SOS) approach. Dis Esophagus 2013;26(6):598–602.
[17] Bludau M, Hölscher AH, Herbold T, et al. Management of upper intestinal leaks using an endoscopic vacuum-assisted closure system (E-VAC). Surg Endosc 2014;28(3):896–901.
[18] Valli PV, Mertens JC, Kröger A, et al. Stent-over-sponge (SOS): a novel technique complementing endosponge therapy for foregut leaks and perforations. Endoscopy 2018;50(2):148–53.

[19] Fang AH, Chao W, Ecker M. Review of colonic anastomotic leakage and prevention methods. J Clin Med 2020;9(12):4061.
[20] Lippert E, Klebl FH, Schweller F, et al. Fibrin glue in the endoscopic treatment of fistulae and anastomotic leakages of the gastrointestinal tract. Int J Colorectal Dis 2011;26(3):303–11.
[21] Rábago LR, Ventosa N, Castro JL, et al. Endoscopic treatment of postoperative fistulas resistant to conservative management using biological fibrin glue. Endoscopy 2002;34(8):632–8.
[22] Clifford RE, Fowler H, Govindarajah N, et al. Early anastomotic complications in colorectal surgery: a systematic review of techniques for endoscopic salvage. Surg Endosc 2019;33(4):1049–65.
[23] Albert JG, Friedrich-Rust M, Woeste G, et al. Benefit of a clipping device in use in intestinal bleeding and intestinal leakage. Gastrointest Endosc 2011;74(2):389–97.
[24] Kirschniak A, Subotova N, Zieker D, et al. The over-the-scope clip (OTSC) for the treatment of gastrointestinal bleeding, perforations, and fistulas. Surg Endosc 2011;25(9):2901–5.
[25] Firkins SA, Simons-Linares R. Management of leakage and fistulas after bariatric surgery. Best Pract Res Clin Gastroenterol 2024;70:101926.
[26] Endoluminal therapies for esophageal perforations and leaks-reference-cited by-同舟云学术. Available at: http://globalauthorid.com/WebPortal/ArticleView?wd=4C5A8D0827-CA78F78E4944691FD734068697282ACE19368953ADED1AF5783E4C. Accessed August 16, 2025.
[27] Haito-Chavez Y, Law JK, Kratt T, et al. International multicenter experience with an over-the-scope clipping device for endoscopic management of GI defects (with video). Gastrointest Endosc 2014;80(4):610–22.
[28] Cai JX, Khashab MA, Okolo PI, et al. Full-thickness endoscopic suturing of staple-line leaks following laparoscopic sleeve gastrectomy. Endoscopy 2014;46(Suppl 1 UCTN):E623–4.
[29] Kantsevoy SV, Bitner M, Mitrakov AA, et al. Endoscopic suturing closure of large mucosal defects after endoscopic submucosal dissection is technically feasible, fast, and eliminates the need for hospitalization (with videos). Gastrointest Endosc 2014;79(3):503–7.
[30] Brunner W, Rossetti A, Vines LC, et al. Anastomotic leakage after laparoscopic single-port sigmoid resection: combined transanal and transabdominal minimal invasive management. Surg Endosc 2015;29(12):3803–5.
[31] Hyoju SK, Klabbers RE, Aaron M, et al. Oral polyphosphate suppresses bacterial collagenase production and prevents anastomotic leak due to Serratia marcescens and Pseudomonas aeruginosa. Ann Surg 2018;267(6):1112–8.
[32] Okita Y, Mohri Y, Kobayashi M, et al. Factors influencing the outcome of image-guided percutaneous drainage of intra-abdominal abscess after gastrointestinal surgery. Surg Today 2013;43(10):1095–102.
[33] Hedrick TL, Kane W. Management of acute anastomotic leaks. Clin Colon Rectal Surg 2021;34(6):400–5.
[34] Jacobsen HJ, Nergard BJ, Leifsson BG, et al. Management of suspected anastomotic leak after bariatric laparoscopic Roux-en-y gastric bypass. Br J Surg 2014;101(4):417–23.
[35] Bellorin O, Abdemur A, Sucandy I, et al. Understanding the significance, reasons and patterns of abnormal vital signs after gastric bypass for morbid obesity. Obes Surg 2011;21(6):707–13.
[36] Sayida S, Obeid A, Jubran L, et al. The relationship between tachycardia after laparoscopic sleeve gastrectomy and the development of postoperative complications. Obes Surg 2022;32(5):1479–85.
[37] Rohatgi A, Papanikitas J, Sutcliffe R, et al. The role of oesophageal diversion and exclusion in the management of oesophageal perforations. Int J Surg 2009;7(2):142–4.
[38] Ubels S, Verstegen MHP, Rosman C, et al. Anastomotic leakage after esophagectomy for esophageal cancer: risk factors and operative treatment. Annals of Esophagus 2021;4(0); https://doi.org/10.21037/aoe-2020-18.

[39] Page RD, Shackcloth MJ, Russell GN, et al. Surgical treatment of anastomotic leaks after oesophagectomy. Eur J Cardio Thorac Surg 2005;27(2):337–43.
[40] Tomita M, Matsuzaki Y, Shimizu T, et al. Retrograde tube drainage for esophageal anastomotic leaks and perforation. Dis Esophagus 2007;20(3):247–50.
[41] Tsuji T, Saito H, Hayashi K, et al. T-drain esophagostomy under thoracoscopy for intrathoracic esophagogastric anastomotic leakage following esophagectomy for esophagogastric junction cancer: a case report. Int J Surg Case Rep 2020;73:79–83.
[42] Jeong SH, Lee JK, Seo KW, et al. Treatment and prevention of postoperative leakage after gastrectomy for gastric cancer. J Clin Med 2023;12(12):3880.
[43] Stafford C, Francone TD, Marcello PW, et al. Is diversion with ileostomy non-inferior to hartmann resection for left-sided colorectal anastomotic leak? J Gastrointest Surg 2018;22(3): 503–7.
[44] Phitayakorn R, Delaney CP, Reynolds HL, et al. Standardized algorithms for management of anastomotic leaks and related abdominal and pelvic abscesses after colorectal surgery. World J Surg 2008;32(6):1147–56.
[45] Krarup PM, Jorgensen LN, Harling H, Danish Colorectal Cancer Group. Management of anastomotic leakage in a nationwide cohort of colonic cancer patients. J Am Coll Surg 2014;218(5):940–9.
[46] Mutignani M, Dioscoridi L, Manta R, et al. "Chimera" fully covered self-expandable metal stent for refractory esophageal anastomotic leak. Endoscopy 2015;47(Suppl 1 UCTN): E376–7.
[47] Haghdel M, Imanieh MH, Hosseinpour H, et al. Development of bio-artificial esophageal tissue engineering utilization for circumferential lesion transplantation: a narrative review. Iran J Basic Med Sci 2022;47(5):406–21.
[48] Xue X, Yan Y, Ma Y, et al. Stem-cell therapy for esophageal anastomotic leakage by autografting stromal cells in fibrin scaffold. Stem Cells Transl Med 2019;8(6):548–56.
[49] Huang J, Jiang Y, Liu Y, et al. Marine-inspired molecular mimicry generates a drug-free, but immunogenic hydrogel adhesive protecting surgical anastomosis. Bioact Mater 2021;6(3): 770–82.

Advances in Surgery 60 (2026) 271–284

ADVANCES IN SURGERY

Watch and Wait in Patients with Clinical Complete Response After Neoadjuvant Therapy with Rectal Cancer: Is it Safe?

Bryan Szeglin, MD[a], John Migaly, MD[b,*]

[a]Department of Surgery, The Johns Hopkins Hospital, 1800 Orleans Street, Baltimore, MD 21287, USA; [b]Colon and Rectal Surgery, Department of Surgery, The Johns Hopkins Hospital, 1800 Orleans Street, Baltimore, MD 21287, USA

Keywords

• Rectal cancer • Watch and wait • Nonoperative management
• Total neoadjuvant therapy

Key points

- Total neoadjuvant therapy allows for nearly 25% to 40% of patients with locally advanced rectal cancer to achieve a pathologic complete response.
- About 50% of patients with a clinical complete response to neoadjuvant therapy who undergo nonoperative management with watch-and-wait can achieve organ preservation.
- Most watch-and-wait patients who develop local regrowth can be salvaged with total mesorectal excision with similar overall survival but higher rates of metastatic recurrence.
- Watch-and-wait is a safe option for select patients in a protocolized environment that can achieve recommended surveillance benchmarks.

INTRODUCTION

The previous article–*Total Neoadjuvant Therapy for The Treatment of Locally Advanced Rectal Cancer* –reviews the evolution of locally advanced rectal cancer (LARC) treatment from a time when 95% of patients recurred after surgery alone to a point when 30% of patients have a complete response with total neoadjuvant therapy (TNT). It naturally follows to consider avoiding surgery

*Corresponding author. *E-mail address:* jmigaly1@jhmi.edu

https://doi.org/10.1016/j.yasu.2026.03.012

Abbreviations

cCR	clinical complete response
CNCT	consolidation chemotherapy
CTX	chemotherapy
DFS	disease-free survival
dMMR	Mismatch repair deficient
DR	distant recurrence
DRE	digital rectal exam
iCR	incomplete response
INCT	induction chemotherapy
IWWD	International Watch and Wait Database
LARC	locally advanced rectal cancer
LRG	local regrowth
MSKCC	Memorial Sloan Kettering Cancer Center
NCCN	National Comprehensive Cancer Network
nCR	near complete response
NPV	negative predictive value
OP	organ preservation
OPRA	Organ Preservation in Patients with Rectal Adenocarcinoma
OS	overall survival
pCR	pathologic complete response
PPV	positive predictive value
RCT	randomized controlled trial
s-cCR	sustained cCR
SCRT	short course radiation therapy
TME	total mesorectal excision
TNT	total neoadjuvant therapy
WW	watch-and-wait

altogether in these patients. This article will focus on a shift to this watch-and-wait (WW) approach. We will discuss early WW experience by Dr. Angelita Habr-Gama that paved the way for key trials that have refined WW in the era of TNT. We will then discuss important aspects of a WW protocol, which ensure its safety. Finally, we will review caveats when implementing WW outside of a clinical trial environment and unique populations who may benefit from organ preservation (OP) approaches.

DEFINITIONS

For this discussion, it is important to define several terms clearly [1]. In the context of WW for LARC, patients first undergo TNT and are then restaged to evaluate the clinical response which will determine eligibility for WW. For patients who undergo surgical resection, pathologic complete response (pCR) refers to complete eradication of the tumor on surgical pathology and represents ypT0N0 disease. For patients being considered for WW, pathologic specimens are not available and so our stage assessment after TNT is referred to as the clinical response. Details of how we determine the clinical response will be discussed later in this article. Patients believed to have a pCR are referred to as having a clinical complete response (cCR). Patients who continue to have evidence of a cCR beyond the first 2 years from initial restaging are referred to as having a sustained cCR (s-cCR). Patients with a dramatic response to treatment, but with subtle abnormalities on their restaging examination are referred to as having a near complete response (nCR). Patients with clearly residual tumor are referred to as having an incomplete response (iCR).

Patients managed with WW may develop new signs of disease at the prior tumor site, which is referred to as a local regrowth (LRG). This occurs most commonly within the rectal wall but may also present in the mesorectal tissue or lateral pelvic nodes (internal iliac or obturator) [1]. LRG must be distinguished from a local recurrence (LR) which represents recurrent disease after surgical resection, or in the case of nonoperative management would indicate new disease in the pelvis outside the mesorectum or lateral pelvic nodes. Patients who develop LRG undergo salvage surgery, which refers to surgical resection of the tumor in the fashion initially considered at the time of restaging before selection of WW and implies an R0 resection. Patients who have not developed LRG and continue to have an s-cCR may be referred to as having achieved OP. Both the rate of LRG and OP are key outcomes in WW studies.

EARLY EXPERIENCE

The first experience with WW is universally credited to surgeon Angelita Habr-Gama. In 2004, she published a prospective series of 265 patients initially treated with neoadjuvant chemoradiation (CRT) followed by restaging 8 weeks later [2]. 71 patients (26.8%) achieved cCR and were managed with WW while the remaining went to surgical resection, of which 22 were found to have pCR. In the WW group compared to the resection group with pCR, the 5-year overall survival (OS) was 100% versus 88% and the 10-year distant recurrence (DR) rate was 4.2% versus 13.6%, respectively. The 10-year LRG rate for WW patients was 2.8%. LRG occurred at a median of 52 months. These early results indicated that a subset of patients could be effectively managed nonoperatively with excellent long-term oncologic outcomes.

A follow-up report from Habr-Gama 2 years later of 122 patients showed comparable results and other groups began to report similar findings [3]. An early retrospective review from Memorial Sloan Kettering Cancer Center (MSKCC) of 32 patients treated with WW showed an LRG rate of 18.8% presenting at a median of 11 months from completing CRT; all LRG patients successfully underwent salvage surgery with no difference in 2-year disease-free survival (DFS) or OS [4]. Series from Maastricht University and The Royal Devon & Exeter Hospital in the United Kingdom incorporated MRI in the restaging and surveillance protocol and showed similar results [5,6]. Over the years, several other institutional series, databases, and meta-analyses including thousands of patients together reported LRG rate of 15% to 35% and 3-year OS over 95% with no difference when compared to patients managed surgically after CRT [7–13]. It is important to remember that patients in these reports were overwhelmingly treated with CRT alone before the era of TNT which confers even greater rates of pCR and improved DFS and OS.

While most studies supported that WW was a safe alternative, there is one notable exception with significant follow up. The MSKCC group published 5-year data on a series of 113 patients treated with WW with a more contemporary TNT regimen [14]. In this series, 70% of WW patients received either induction chemotherapy (INCT) or consolidation chemotherapy (CNCT) in addition to CRT while 61% of patients received CRT without chemotherapy (CTX) in the pCR group. 19.4% of WW patients developed LRG and all underwent salvage surgery. When compared to a group of patients not managed with WW who were found to have pCR at surgery, 5-year OS was significantly worse in the WW group (73% vs 94%), although DFS and disease-specific survival were similar. Furthermore, WW patients with LRG had higher rates of distant metastasis compared to WW patients who did not have LRG (36% vs 1%). There was no association between treatment regimen and OS. It is unclear why these outcomes differ from prior work. Wide variability exists across studies in eligibility for WW, definitions of cCR and nCR, and neoadjuvant therapy regimens. WW patients with LRG also likely represent a manifestation of worse disease biology and it may be unreasonable to compare them to pCR patients as a control group. Nevertheless, this study provides a warning for overstating the early results of WW series.

WATCH AND WAIT IN THE ERA OF TOTAL NEOADJUVANT THERAPY

Given the practice variability with respect to TNT, restaging, and surveillance, a randomized controlled trial (RCT) evaluating WW was critically needed. This first came with the Organ Preservation in Patients with Rectal Adenocarcinoma (OPRA) Trial [15]. 324 LARC patients were randomized to either INCT followed by CRT (INCT-CRT) or CRT followed by CNCT (CRT-CNCT). Patients in both groups were then restaged and those with a cCR were assigned to WW. There was no difference in 3-year DFS or metastasis-free survival. 71% of patients in the INCT-CRT group and 76% in the CRT-CNCT underwent WW and the LRG rate was 40% and 27%, respectively. At 5 years, the total mesorectal excision (TME)-free survival was 39% in the INCT-CRT group and 54% in the CRT-CNCT group [16]. For patients with LRG who underwent salvage therapy, DFS was similar to those who had surgery initially. Nearly 50% of all patients achieved OP with this WW approach.

The data from retrospective studies, prospective studies, and an RCT collectively show that a significant proportion of LARC patients who are treated with neoadjuvant therapy and achieve cCR can be managed nonoperatively largely without affecting oncologic outcomes. With respect to quality-of-life outcomes, few studies have reported long-term results. While several studies using various quality of life measures show improvement with OP compared to TME, there are still effects from neoadjuvant therapy alone such as bowel dysfunction and sexual dysfunction in both males and females, although each at lower rates than after TME [17–19].

IMPORTANT CONSIDERATIONS FOR SAFELY OFFERING WATCH AND WAIT

The data presented thus far support that WW for LARC patients who achieve cCR is safe and achieves comparable oncologic outcomes to traditional TNT with TME. The specific details of TNT, patient selection, surveillance, and ability to manage LRG are believed to be critical to achieving these outcomes. We will discuss this treatment timeline in detail (Fig. 1).

Total neoadjuvant therapy regimens

After diagnosis and staging of LARC, patients should undergo TNT. Patients should receive neoadjuvant RT with either INCT or CNCT. While there is growing evidence that a CRT-CNCT approach has higher rates of cCR, there is no literature consensus [15,20]. With respect to CTX agent, 5-fluorouracil-based therapy is standard of care and often combined with oxaliplatin in a doublet fashion. Several trials are considering the necessity of oxaliplatin to reduce toxicity, and investigating the addition of irinotecan or bevacizumab, but at present there is insufficient evidence for their routine use in TNT [21–23]. For neoadjuvant RT, most literature uses a CRT approach. While there are reports of similar outcomes with short course radiation therapy (SCRT), most studies show higher cCR rates with CRT and ongoing clinical trials seek to resolve this debate [24–27].

Restaging

After completion of TNT, patients require restaging to assess clinical response. Timing of restaging is important to allow for tumor regression. While most trials restage 6 to 12 weeks after completion of CRT, it can take up to 16 weeks to achieve cCR and data suggest that it is safe to wait this time for restaging in

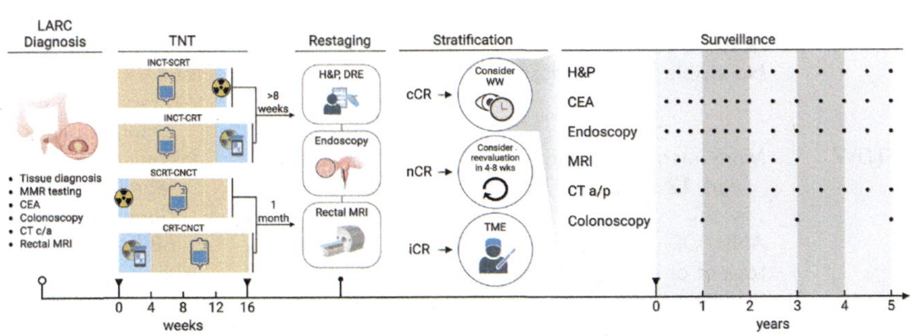

Fig. 1. Timeline of LARC treatment in the context of WW. Patients undergo standard-of-care workup and those with LARC are treated with TNT through 1 of 4 accepted TNT protocols. After a period of waiting, patients are restaged and those with a cCR are eligible for WW. Patients with a nCR can be considered for a reevaluation to allow for progression to cCR. Patients with an iCR undergo TME. WW patients enter a multimodal surveillance protocol with more frequent examinations within the first 2 to 3 years. Treatment and surveillance protocols in this figure are consistent with NCCN 4.2025 guidelines. (Created in BioRender. Szeglin, B. (2025) https://BioRender.com/l2safgr.)

patients with a nCR [25,28–31]. In practice, most institutions restage at 8 weeks. A multimodal restaging assessment should include physical examination with digital rectal exam (DRE), endoscopy, and rectal MRI. Table 1 displays the Memorial Sloan Kettering Regression Schema, which was used in the OPRA trial and largely adopted in the latest National Comprehensive Cancer Network (NCCN) rectal cancer guidelines [32,33]. DRE should be performed for all patients, but has low sensitivity for identifying either cCR or LR/LRG [34]. Endoscopic evaluation should show a flat white scar with telangiectasias in the setting of cCR, while an irregular mucosa with erythema, superficial ulceration, or nodularity is indicative of a nCR [35]. Grossly visible tumor would be characterized as an iCR. With respect to rectal MRI, a radiologist experienced in reading rectal MRI should assess both T2 and diffusion weighted images to assess both the rectal wall and regional lymph nodes with close

Table 1
Memorial Sloan Kettering regression schema from the organ preservation in patients with rectal adenocarcinoma trial protocol

	Complete response	Near complete response	Incomplete response
Endoscopy	Flat, white scar Telangiectasia No ulcer No nodularity	Irregular mucosa Small mucosal nodules or minor mucosal abnormality Superficial ulceration Mild persisting erythema of the scar	Visible tumor
DRE	Normal	Smooth induration or minor mucosal abnormalities	Palpable tumor nodules
MRI-T2W	Only dark T2 signal, no intermediate T2 signal AND No visible lymph nodes	Mostly dark T2 signal, some remaining intermediate signal AND/OR Partial regression of lymph nodes	More intermediate than dark T2 signal, no T2 scar AND/OR No regression of lymph nodes
MRI-DW	More intermediate than dark T2 signal, no T2 scar AND/OR Lack of or low signal on apparent diffusion coefficient (ADC) map Uniform, linear signal in wall above tumor is ok	Significant regression of signal on B800-B1000 AND/OR Minimal or low residual signal on ADC map	Insignificant regression of signal on B800-B1000 AND/OR Obvious low signal on ADC map

Source Rectal Cancer Consortium, Smith JJ, Chow OS, et al. Organ Preservation in Rectal Adenocarcinoma: a phase II randomized controlled trial evaluating 3-year disease-free survival in patients with locally advanced rectal cancer treated with chemoradiation plus induction or consolidation chemotherapy, and total mesorectal excision or nonoperative management. *BMC Cancer.* 2015;15(1):767. https://doi.org/10.1186/s12885-015-1632-z [32].

comparison to baseline imaging [36]. It is important to note that pelvic CT has poor accuracy at identifying cCR [37].

The performance of these restaging assessments are highly variable, although endoscopy is generally accepted to have the highest accuracy for identifying cCR with an estimated positive predictive value (PPV) of 73% to 100% and a negative predictive value (NPV) of 50% to 94% [38]. This is followed by MRI with an estimated PPV of 30% to 100% and NPV of 85% to 96%. The wide range of reported test performance particularly with MRI is reflective of the interuser variability with these modalities and supports the consultation of a radiologist with significant experience with rectal MRI. With these caveats, combination assessment of both endoscopic and radiographic data should be employed [39].

The near-complete response

Patients determined to have cCR on their restaging examination can be offered WW, but the management of nCR is less clear. Most nCR cases in the historical WW literature were treated as iCR and managed with TME. A notable exception is the OPRA trial, which allowed nCR patients to enter the WW arm, and while a higher LRG rate was observed when compared to cCR, nearly 40% of nCR patients could achieve OP at 3 years [15,40]. Similarly, a cohort study from MSKCC compared patients with cCR and nCR with 89% and 43% managed with WW, respectively [41]. More than 50% of nCR patients undergoing WW achieved OP at 5 years compared to 73% in the cCR group. nCR patients did have a higher 3-year LRG rate (40% vs 24%) and slightly lower DFS compared to cCR patients (73% vs 82%), but no difference in 5-year OS. Supporting these findings is also a study from the International Watch and Wait Database (IWWD) comparing cCR which was identified on the first assessment (a more traditional cCR definition) to cCR identified on the second assessment (indicating nCR on the first assessment with conversion to cCR) [42]. There was no difference in 2-year OP rate, metastasis-free survival, or OS. These data suggest that a more dramatic clinical response to TNT is associated with improved oncologic outcomes, but a significant proportion of nCR patients can still be managed successfully with WW. Further prospective studies should be completed before WW is routinely recommended for patients who achieve nCR, but it is reasonable to consider additional observation time to assess downstaging to cCR.

Several studies have examined the role of local excision of residual disease in the case of either nCR or iCR, but patient selection is variable, it is often only offered in node negative disease, long-term follow-up is limited, and most studies are not done in the context of WW [43–47]. There is also concern that local excision may affect the ability to undergo successful salvage surgery for patients who develop LRG and that patients have worse functional outcomes after local excision compared to WW [47,48]. The ongoing STAR-TREC trial is randomizing stage cT3b or lower N0M0 patients to TME or an OP approach with either SCRT or CRT [49]. For the OP arm, patients with cCR are treated with WW and iCR patients are offered local excision with transanal endoscopic microsurgery or other transanal techniques. Results of this study may more clearly define a role for local excision in WW, but there is insufficient evidence to recommend its routine use at this time.

Surveillance

After the decision to proceed with WW is made, patients enter a surveillance protocol consisting of regular re-examinations with the goal of identifying LRG quickly to enable expeditious TME. Surveillance frequency is greatest during the first 2 years when the far majority of LRG presents. The guidelines to follow are recommended in the NCCN Rectal Cancer Clinical Practice Guidelines Version 4.2025 and were largely adapted from OPRA trial protocol [15,33]. Endoscopic assessment should be completed every 3 to 4 months for 2 years, and then every 6 months for 5 years. This should be accompanied by a history and physical examination and carcinoembryonic antigen every 3 to 6 months for 2 years, followed by every 6 months for 5 years. Radiographically, rectal MRI should be completed every 6 months for 3 years, and computed tomography of the chest and abdomen should be completed every 6 to 12 months for 5 years. Circulating tumor DNA has been considered as an adjunct to surveillance, but assays in their present form lack adequate sensitivity [50].

Management of local regrowth

Up to 40% of patients managed with WW will develop LRG and should undergo prompt salvage surgery with TME. Over 95% of LRG is found in the rectal wall and more than 90% of patients can be salvaged [7,51,52]. However, developing an LRG is an independent risk factor for distant metastasis in several studies with reported incidence of metastasis as high as 36% [14,53]. With respect to survival, patients with LRG have been shown to have worse DFS than patients who achieve s-cCR [14]. However, these patients seem to behave more similarly to patients who were found to have iCR and underwent initial TME than those with s-cCR. In the OPRA trial, for example, both the DFS and the rate of R0 resection after TME was the same in these groups. It is important to consider that LRG represents a unique disease state from s-cCR and comparisons of oncologic outcomes between these groups may not fairly assess WW.

CAVEATS AND UNIQUE POPULATIONS

Real-world experience with watch and wait

The far majority of literature evidence supporting WW is derived from large academic centers and often in the context of a protocolized, resource-rich environment. The use of WW in a more real-world implementation, even in a high-resource environment, has yet to be studied at scale. Reports at present show low adherence to surveillance protocols often less than 50% over the first 2 years [54,55]. Given that nearly 40% of patients are expected to develop LRG within this time, poor adherence to surveillance raises questions as to whether WW should be offered outside of an environment that can deliver the benchmarks which ensure its safety. This exists at the hospital level to ensure adequate resources are available to offer timely assessments, and also at the patient level to ensure that patients can adhere to strict multi-year protocols, which are time-intensive.

Center-specific variability in WW outcomes has also been observed, even in the context of clinical trials. In the NORWAIT trial, a WW protocol was implemented across 7 hospitals but was terminated early for protocol violations particularly at one center where only 2 out of 31 patients managed with WW had a documented cCR [56]. About 77% of these patients developed LRG and mortality was 23%. Patients treated at the other 6 hospitals had outcomes comparable to the broader literature.

It is also important to consider that patients may opt for surgery over a WW strategy. Patient preference for WW over surgery varies with some studies reporting 80% of patients opting for a WW approach, while others show preference for surgery depending on the specific options presented in the neoadjuvant setting and the reported effect that WW could have on recurrence or survival [57–59]. Furthermore, there is limited evidence in the WW literature about patient opinions regarding surveillance anxiety, which is unfortunately common in patients with cancer and may be more prevalent with a WW approach, particularly during the first 2 years [60].

Mismatch repair deficient rectal cancer

Mismatch repair deficient (dMMR) rectal cancer represents another potential opportunity for WW. These tumors are exquisitely sensitive to checkpoint blockade in nearly all patients [61]. A recent phase 2 trial treated stage I–III dMMR patients with rectal cancer with the PD-1 antagonist dostarlimab followed by restaging up to 8 weeks after completion of treatment. Almost 100% of patients developed an initial cCR, all proceeded with WW, and at 1 year 75% continued to have a cCR without CTX or RT [62]. Whether LRG salvage would be in the form of TME or restarting checkpoint blockade is unclear and warrants further research.

Young onset rectal cancer

While the overall incidence of rectal cancer has been declining over the past 30 years, there is an alarming increase among patients younger than 50 year old at diagnosis and the etiology of this trend is poorly understood [63]. While these tumors often present at more advanced stage, survival is similar in this generally healthier population who is more resilient to aggressive therapy [64]. Furthermore, with the known long-term complications of TME, this is a unique population for which OP could confer significant benefit for the remainder of the lifespan. A series of young-onset patients from the IWWD managed with WW showed similar rates of 3-year LRG (24% vs 26%), 3-year disease-specific survival (98% vs 97%), and metastasis (10% in both groups) compared to older patients [65]. Further study in this area is unfortunately lacking. At present, WW should be considered for young-onset LARC patients only after clear and transparent discussions with patients about the possible risks and benefits.

SUMMARY

The treatment of LARC has evolved significantly over the past century. With the adoption of TNT, a significant proportion of patients develop pCR at time of TME. With careful patient selection and protocolized surveillance, a select group can avoid surgery altogether in a WW paradigm. While large, prospective, long-term follow-up of WW in the TNT era is limited, initial reports are promising and the historical refinement of neoadjuvant therapy supports the safety of this method. Salvage surgery remains an option for patients who develop LRG with little negative effect on oncologic outcomes. In a protocolized environment with careful patient selection that involves shared decision-making, WW is a reasonable option for many patients.

CLINICS CARE POINTS

- WW is a reasonable approach for patients with clinical complete response after total neoadjuvant therapy.
- Early evidence suggests that near complete response patients can be managed with watch-and-wait (WW) but have higher rates of local regrowth and distant recurrence.
- Ensuring adherence to strict surveillance protocols is essential to safe implementation of a WW program.
- Shared decision-making is imperative in deciding whether a WW approach is appropriate for a given patient.

Disclosure

The authors have no commercial or financial disclosures.

References

[1] Cerdán-Santacruz C, Vailati BB, São Julião GP, et al. Watch and wait: why, to whom and how. Surg Oncol 2022;43:101774; https://doi.org/10.1016/j.suronc.2022.101774.
[2] Habr-Gama A, Perez RO, Nadalin W, et al. Operative versus nonoperative treatment for stage 0 distal rectal cancer following chemoradiation therapy: long-term results. Ann Surg 2004;240(4):711–7 [discussion: 717–718].
[3] Habr-Gama A, Perez RO, Proscurshim I, et al. Patterns of failure and survival for nonoperative treatment of stage c0 distal rectal cancer following neoadjuvant chemoradiation therapy. J Gastrointest Surg Off J Soc Surg Aliment Tract 2006;10(10):1319–28 [discussion: 1328–1329].
[4] Smith JD, Ruby JA, Goodman KA, et al. Nonoperative management of rectal cancer with complete clinical response after neoadjuvant therapy. Ann Surg 2012;256(6): 965–72.
[5] Maas M, Beets-Tan RGH, Lambregts DMJ, et al. Wait-and-see policy for clinical complete responders after chemoradiation for rectal cancer. J Clin Oncol Off J Am Soc Clin Oncol 2011;29(35):4633–40.

[6] Dalton RSJ, Velineni R, Osborne ME, et al. A single-centre experience of chemoradiotherapy for rectal cancer: is there potential for nonoperative management? Colorectal Dis 2012;14(5):567–71.
[7] van der Valk MJM, Hilling DE, Bastiaannet E, et al. Long-term outcomes of clinical complete responders after neoadjuvant treatment for rectal cancer in the International Watch & Wait Database (IWWD): an international multicentre registry study. Lancet Lond Engl 2018;391(10139):2537–45.
[8] Dattani M, Heald RJ, Goussous G, et al. Oncological and survival outcomes in watch and wait patients with a clinical complete response after neoadjuvant chemoradiotherapy for rectal cancer: a systematic review and pooled analysis. Ann Surg 2018;268(6):955–67.
[9] Sammour T, Price BA, Krause KJ, et al. Nonoperative management or "Watch and Wait" for rectal cancer with complete clinical response after neoadjuvant chemoradiotherapy: a critical appraisal. Ann Surg Oncol 2017;24(7):1904–15.
[10] Habr-Gama A, Gama-Rodrigues J, São Julião GP, et al. Local recurrence after complete clinical response and watch and wait in rectal cancer after neoadjuvant chemoradiation: impact of salvage therapy on local disease control. Int J Radiat Oncol 2014;88(4):822–8.
[11] Martens MH, Maas M, Heijnen LA, et al. Long-term outcome of an organ preservation program after neoadjuvant treatment for rectal cancer. J Natl Cancer Inst 2016;108(12): djw171; https://doi.org/10.1093/jnci/djw171.
[12] Renehan AG, Malcomson L, Emsley R, et al. Watch-and-wait approach versus surgical resection after chemoradiotherapy for patients with rectal cancer (the OnCoRe project): a propensity-score matched cohort analysis. Lancet Oncol 2016;17(2):174–83.
[13] Appelt AL, Pløen J, Harling H, et al. High-dose chemoradiotherapy and watchful waiting for distal rectal cancer: a prospective observational study. Lancet Oncol 2015;16(8):919–27.
[14] Smith JJ, Strombom P, Chow OS, et al. Assessment of a watch-and-wait strategy for rectal cancer in patients with a complete response after neoadjuvant therapy. JAMA Oncol 2019;5(4):e185896; https://doi.org/10.1001/jamaoncol.2018.5896.
[15] Garcia-Aguilar J, Patil S, Gollub MJ, et al. Organ preservation in patients with rectal adenocarcinoma treated with total neoadjuvant therapy. J Clin Oncol Off J Am Soc Clin Oncol 2022;40(23):2546–56.
[16] Verheij FS, Omer DM, Williams H, et al. Long-term results of organ preservation in patients with rectal adenocarcinoma treated with total neoadjuvant therapy: the randomized phase II OPRA trial. J Clin Oncol Off J Am Soc Clin Oncol 2024;42(5):500–6.
[17] Custers PA, van der Sande ME, Grotenhuis BA, et al. Long-term quality of life and functional outcome of patients with rectal cancer following a watch-and-wait approach. JAMA Surg 2023;158(5):e230146; https://doi.org/10.1001/jamasurg.2023.0146.
[18] Hilty Chu BK, Loria A, Dhimal T, et al. Patient-reported outcomes after neoadjuvant therapy and watch-and-wait for rectal cancer: a systematic review and meta-analysis. Ann Surg Open Perspect Surg Hist Educ Clin Approaches 2025;6(3):e602; https://doi.org/10.1097/AS9.0000000000000602.
[19] Quezada-Diaz FF, Smith JJ, Jimenez-Rodriguez RM, et al. Patient-reported bowel function in patients with rectal cancer managed by a watch-and-wait strategy after neoadjuvant therapy: a case-control study. Dis Colon Rectum 2020;63(7):897–902.
[20] Fokas E, Schlenska-Lange A, Polat B, et al. Chemoradiotherapy plus induction or consolidation chemotherapy as total neoadjuvant therapy for patients with locally advanced rectal cancer: long-term results of the CAO/ARO/AIO-12 randomized clinical trial. JAMA Oncol 2022;8(1):e215445; https://doi.org/10.1001/jamaoncol.2021.5445.
[21] Alvarez JA, Shi Q, Dasari A, et al. Alliance A022104/NRG-GI010: the Janus rectal cancer trial: a randomized phase II/III trial testing the efficacy of triplet versus doublet chemotherapy regarding clinical complete response and disease-free survival in patients with locally advanced rectal cancer. BMC Cancer 2024;24(1):901.
[22] Akiyoshi T, Shinozaki E, Taguchi S, et al. Non-operative management after chemoradiotherapy plus consolidation or sandwich (induction with bevacizumab and consolidation)

chemotherapy in patients with locally advanced rectal cancer: a multicentre, randomised phase II trial (NOMINATE trial). BMJ Open 2022;12(3):e055140; https://doi.org/10.1136/bmjopen-2021-055140.
[23] Habr-Gama A, São Julião GP, Ortega CD, et al. A multi-centre randomized controlled trial investigating consolidation chemotherapy with and without oxaliplatin in distal rectal cancer and watch & wait. BMC Cancer 2023;23(1):546.
[24] Reddy AV, Safar B, Jia AY, et al. Nonoperative management following complete response in rectal cancer after short-course radiation therapy and consolidation chemotherapy: clinical outcomes and quality of life measures. Am J Clin Oncol 2022;45(7):298–305.
[25] Liu IC, Gearhart S, Hu C, et al. Sustained organ preservation in patients with rectal cancer after sequential short-course radiation therapy and chemotherapy. Am Surg 2025;91(11): 1913–22.
[26] Wurschi G, Kesselmeier M, Schneider M, et al. Short-course radiotherapy versus long-course chemoradiotherapy in total neoadjuvant therapy of rectal cancer - a multicenter analysis of early outcomes and toxicity. Radiother Oncol J Eur Soc Ther Radiol Oncol 2025;213:111194; https://doi.org/10.1016/j.radonc.2025.111194.
[27] Bercz A, Park BK, Pappou E, et al. Organ preservation after neoadjuvant long-course chemoradiotherapy versus short-course radiotherapy. Ann Oncol Off J Eur Soc Med Oncol 2024;35(11):1003–14.
[28] Garcia-Aguilar J, Chow OS, Smith DD, et al. Effect of adding mFOLFOX6 after neoadjuvant chemoradiation in locally advanced rectal cancer: a multicentre, phase 2 trial. Lancet Oncol 2015;16(8):957–66.
[29] Habr-Gama A, São Julião GP, Fernandez LM, et al. Achieving a complete clinical response after neoadjuvant chemoradiation that does not require surgical resection: it may take longer than you think. Dis Colon Rectum 2019;62(7):802–8.
[30] Sloothaak DaM, Geijsen DE, van Leersum NJ, et al. Optimal time interval between neoadjuvant chemoradiotherapy and surgery for rectal cancer. Br J Surg 2013;100(7):933–9.
[31] Kalady MF, de Campos-Lobato LF, Stocchi L, et al. Predictive factors of pathologic complete response after neoadjuvant chemoradiation for rectal cancer. Ann Surg 2009;250(4): 582–9.
[32] Rectal Cancer Consortium, Smith JJ, Chow OS, et al. Organ preservation in rectal adenocarcinoma: a phase II randomized controlled trial evaluating 3-year disease-free survival in patients with locally advanced rectal cancer treated with chemoradiation plus induction or consolidation chemotherapy, and total mesorectal excision or nonoperative management. BMC Cancer 2015;15(1):767.
[33] NCCN clinical practice guidelines in oncology: Rectal cancer (Version 4.2025). 2025. Available at: nccn.org.
[34] Guillem JG, Chessin DB, Shia J, et al. Clinical examination following preoperative chemoradiation for rectal cancer is not a reliable surrogate end point. J Clin Oncol Off J Am Soc Clin Oncol 2005;23(15):3475–9.
[35] Williams H, Thompson HM, Lin ST, et al. Endoscopic predictors of residual tumor after total neoadjuvant therapy: a post hoc analysis from the organ preservation in rectal adenocarcinoma trial. Dis Colon Rectum 2024;67(3):369–76.
[36] Williams H, Omer DM, Thompson HM, et al. MRI predicts residual disease and outcomes in watch-and-wait patients with rectal cancer. Radiology 2024;312(3):e232748; https://doi.org/10.1148/radiol.232748.
[37] Guillem JG, Ruby JA, Leibold T, et al. Neither FDG-PET nor CT can distinguish between a pathological complete response and an incomplete response after neoadjuvant chemoradiation in locally advanced rectal cancer: a prospective study. Ann Surg 2013;258(2): 289–95.
[38] Munk NE, Bondeven P, Pedersen BG. Diagnostic performance of MRI and endoscopy for assessing complete response in rectal cancer after neoadjuvant chemoradiotherapy: a systematic review of the literature. Acta Radiol Stockh Swed 1987 2023;64(1):20–31.

[39] Maas M, Lambregts DMJ, Nelemans PJ, et al. Assessment of clinical complete response after chemoradiation for rectal cancer with digital rectal examination, endoscopy, and MRI: selection for organ-saving treatment. Ann Surg Oncol 2015;22(12):3873–80.
[40] Thompson HM, Omer DM, Lin S, et al. Organ preservation and survival by clinical response grade in patients with rectal cancer treated with total neoadjuvant therapy: a secondary analysis of the OPRA randomized clinical trial. JAMA Netw Open 2024;7(1):e2350903; https://doi.org/10.1001/jamanetworkopen.2023.50903.
[41] Rosen RY, Bercz AP, Omer DM, et al. Correlation between grade of clinical response to neoadjuvant therapy for rectal cancer and oncologic outcomes in the era of watch-and-wait. Dis Colon Rectum 2025;68(3):300–7.
[42] Temmink SJD, Peeters KCMJ, Bahadoer RR, et al. Watch and wait after neoadjuvant treatment in rectal cancer: comparison of outcomes in patients with and without a complete response at first reassessment in the International watch & Wait Database (IWWD). Br J Surg 2023;110(6):676–84.
[43] Stijns RCH, de Graaf EJR, Punt CJA, et al. Long-term oncological and functional outcomes of chemoradiotherapy followed by organ-sparing transanal endoscopic microsurgery for distal rectal cancer: the CARTS study. JAMA Surg 2019;154(1):47–54.
[44] Verseveld M, de Graaf EJR, Verhoef C, et al. Chemoradiation therapy for rectal cancer in the distal rectum followed by organ-sparing transanal endoscopic microsurgery (CARTS study). Br J Surg 2015;102(7):853–60.
[45] Hupkens BJP, Maas M, Martens MH, et al. Organ preservation in rectal cancer after chemoradiation: should we extend the observation period in patients with a clinical near-complete response? Ann Surg Oncol 2018;25(1):197–203.
[46] Serra-Aracil X, Pericay C, Cidoncha A, et al. Chemoradiotherapy and local excision vs total mesorectal excision in T2-T3ab, N0, M0 rectal cancer: the TAUTEM randomized clinical trial. JAMA Surg 2025;160(7):783–93.
[47] Rullier E, Vendrely V, Asselineau J, et al. Organ preservation with chemoradiotherapy plus local excision for rectal cancer: 5-year results of the GRECCAR 2 randomised trial. Lancet Gastroenterol Hepatol 2020;5(5):465–74.
[48] Habr-Gama A, Lynn PB, Jorge JMN, et al. Impact of organ-preserving strategies on anorectal function in patients with distal rectal cancer following neoadjuvant chemoradiation. Dis Colon Rectum 2016;59(4):264–9.
[49] Rombouts AJM, Al-Najami I, Abbott NL, et al. Can we save the rectum by watchful waiting or TransAnal microsurgery following (chemo) radiotherapy versus total mesorectal excision for early REctal cancer (STAR-TREC study)?: protocol for a multicentre, randomised feasibility study. BMJ Open 2017;7(12):e019474; https://doi.org/10.1136/bmjopen-2017-019474.
[50] Akiyoshi T, Shinozaki E, Maeda Y, et al. Circulating tumor DNA longitudinal analysis during total neoadjuvant therapy and non-operative management for locally advanced rectal cancer: a biomarker study from the NOMINATE trial. Clin Cancer Res Off J Am Assoc Cancer Res 2025; https://doi.org/10.1158/1078-0432.CCR-25-1242.
[51] Habr-Gama A, Gama-Rodrigues J, São Julião GP, et al. Local recurrence after complete clinical response and watch and wait in rectal cancer after neoadjuvant chemoradiation: impact of salvage therapy on local disease control. Int J Radiat Oncol Biol Phys 2014;88(4):822–8.
[52] Fernandez LM, Figueiredo NL, Habr-Gama A, et al. Salvage surgery with organ preservation for patients with local regrowth after watch and wait: is it still possible? Dis Colon Rectum 2020;63(8):1053–62.
[53] Fernandez LM, São Julião GP, Renehan AG, et al. The risk of distant metastases in patients with clinical complete response managed by watch and wait after neoadjuvant therapy for rectal cancer: the influence of local regrowth in the international watch and wait database. Dis Colon Rectum 2023;66(1):41–9.

[54] Hilty Chu BK, Loria A, Dhimal T, et al. Challenges of surveillance in implementing nonoperative management for rectal cancer. JAMA Netw Open 2024;7(12):e2448682; https://doi.org/10.1001/jamanetworkopen.2024.48682.
[55] Rubens M, Oduyale O, Eltahir AA, et al. "Watch-and-Wait" or "Lost to follow-up"? Adherence to nonoperative management of rectal cancer. J Surg Res 2025;311:273–9.
[56] Wasmuth HH, Færden AE. The Norwegian watch and wait study: norwait for rectal cancer. A report from a failed study-a word of caution. Updat Surg 2024;76(5):1635–9.
[57] Kennedy ED, Borowiec AM, Schmocker S, et al. Patient and physician preferences for nonoperative management for low rectal cancer: is it a reasonable treatment option? Dis Colon Rectum 2018;61(11):1281–9.
[58] Gani C, Gani N, Zschaeck S, et al. Organ preservation in rectal cancer: the patients' perspective. Front Oncol 2019;9:318.
[59] Alvarez J, Zambare W, George M, et al. Utilizing patient input in rectal cancer trial design. J Natl Cancer Inst 2025;117(7):1421–8.
[60] Khatri R, Quinn PL, Wells-Di Gregorio S, et al. Surveillance-associated anxiety after curative-intent cancer surgery: a systematic review. Ann Surg Oncol 2025;32(1):47–62.
[61] Cercek A, Lumish M, Sinopoli J, et al. PD-1 blockade in mismatch repair–deficient, locally advanced rectal cancer. N Engl J Med 2022;386(25):2363–76.
[62] Cercek A, Foote MB, Rousseau B, et al. Nonoperative management of mismatch repair–deficient tumors. N Engl J Med 2025;392(23):2297–308.
[63] Sung H, Siegel RL, Laversanne M, et al. Colorectal cancer incidence trends in younger versus older adults: an analysis of population-based cancer registry data. Lancet Oncol 2025;26(1):51–63.
[64] Suresh RS, Garcia LE, Gearhart SL. Young-onset rectal cancer: is it for real? Adv Surg 2024;58(1):275–91.
[65] Bahadoer RR, Peeters KCMJ, Beets GL, et al. Watch and wait after a clinical complete response in rectal cancer patients younger than 50 years. Br J Surg 2021;109(1):114–20.

Advances in Surgery 60 (2026) 285–298

ADVANCES IN SURGERY

Surgery on Patients Taking Glucagon-Like Peptide-1 Receptor Agonists

Claire B. Rosen, MD, MSME*, Denise W. Gee, MD

Division of GI Surgery, Department of Surgery, Massachusetts General Brigham, Boston, MA, USA

Keywords

• GLP-1R agonists • Obesity • Perioperative management • Bariatric surgery • Weight loss

Key points

- GLP-1R agonists are established treatments for type 2 diabetes mellitus and obesity (first approved in 2005; obesity indication in 2014) with about 15 agents.
- Weight loss efficacy varies by agent, and is higher with dual agents (eg tirzepatide with additional gastric inhibitory peptide action).
- Perioperative management: American Society of Anesthesiologists suggests holding daily GLP-1R agonists on day of surgery and weekly agents for one week prior; evaluate gastric fullness if not held; continue standard fasting.
- Safety and risks: common gastrointestinal side effects (nausea, vomiting) and delayed gastric emptying with potential aspiration risk; possible hypoglycemia in insulin-treated patients; gallstones and concerns about pancreatitis; black-box warning for medullary thyroid cancer.
- GLP-1R agonists and bariatric surgery: can be used neoadjuvantly; adjuvant use cna help with weight regain or insufficient weight loss.

OBESITY

Obesity is a major health concern globally and in the United States. Per most recent Centers for Disease Control and Prevention report–data from August 2021 to August 2023–40.3% of US adults are obese (body mass index [BMI] 30.0 kg/m^2 or greater) and 9.4% of US adults are severely obese (BMI

*Corresponding author. Department of Surgery, Massachusetts General Hospital, 55 Fruit Street, Wang 460, Boston, MA 02114. *E-mail address:* cbrosen@mgh.harvard.edu

https://doi.org/10.1016/j.yasu.2026.03.011

Abbreviations

ASA	American Society of Anesthesiologists
BMI	body mass index
FDA	Food and Drug Administration
GLP-1	glucagon-like peptide-1
GLP-1R	glucagon-like peptide-1 receptor
RCT	randomized controlled trial
RYGB	Roux-en-Y gastric bypass
T2DM	type 2 diabetes mellitus

of obesity are far-reaching, including increased risk of multiple chronic comorbidities (diabetes, hypertension, heart disease, lung disease, depression, and cancer) [2–8] and increased risk of perioperative complications among obese surgical patients undergoing elective or emergent surgery [9,10]. As such, efforts to reduce obesity, including lifestyle changes, bariatric surgery, and medical weight management are now a frequent aspect of many surgical patients' care. Understanding the impact of medical weight management, specifically the use of glucagon-like peptide-1 (GLP-1) receptor agonists, on surgical patients is an important aspect of perioperative evaluation, management, and consideration.

HISTORY

GLP-1 receptor agonists are not *new* medications in 2025. Glucagon was first discovered in 1922 by Kimball and Murlin, termed *glucagon* as a *gluc*ose *agon*ist [11]. In the late 1960s, scientists noted glucagon-like immunoreactivity in the intestines of humans and dogs, with greater reactivity in response to intraduodenal (instead of intravenous) glucose administration–the so-called incretin effect [12–15]. However, it wasn't until the 1980s that it was confirmed that intestinal *proglucagon* (a peptide precursor to glucagon) was an entirely distinct entity from pancreatic proglucagon [12]. In 1983, Bell, Santerre, and Mullenbach designated glucagon-like peptides 1 and 2 (GLP-1 and GLP-2) through animal-model preproglucagon sequencing [16]. In 1987, GLP-1 was then identified as a potential incretin hormone [17]. Through further investigation it was determined that GLP-1 is secreted by L-cells throughout the intestines, most notably in the ileum and colon, in response to dietary carbohydrates, glucose, lipids, and protein and secondary to neuroendocrine reflexes involving gastric inhibitory peptide (GIP) and vagal stimulation [12,18,19]. GLP-1 then binds to the GLP-1 receptor (GLP-1R), a G-protein coupled receptor, expressed in many areas, including the pancreas, brain, kidneys, stomach, heart, adipocytes, and skeletal muscle [20–23]. Though the broad glucose-lowering impacts of GLP-1 (to be discussed in the next section) offered enticing pharmacologic prospects, exogenous supplementation of GLP-1 (as with insulin or glucagon) was limited by the very short half-life of endogenous GLP-1, thus shifting focus toward creation of GLP-1R agonists [12,24].

In 2005, the Food and Drug Administration (FDA) approved the first GLP-1R agonist: exenatide (Byetta; AstraZeneca, Cambridge, UK) as a twice daily injection for treating type 2 diabetes mellitus (T2DM) [25]. Later, in 2014, the FDA approved the first GLP-1R agonist for treatment of obesity: liraglutide (Saxenda; Novo Nordisk) [26]. Since then, GLP-1R agonist development, production, FDA approval, and patient use has blossomed, with 15 currently FDA-approved GLP-1R agonists available for treatment of T2DM and/or obesity (Table 1) [27].

EFFECTS OF GLUCAGON-LIKE PEPTIDE-1 AND GLUCAGON-LIKE PEPTIDE-1 RECEPTOR AGONISTS

As mentioned, the GLP-1R is expressed in many areas of the human body, including the pancreas, brain, kidneys, stomach, heart, adipocytes, and skeletal muscle. Accordingly, the impacts of GLP-1 (and thus GLP-1R agonists) on glucose balance, metabolism, health, appetite, and digestion are broad. To start, GLP-1 is an incretin hormone, and enhances glucose-induced insulin secretion [12,17]. GLP-1 binds to GLP-1R on pancreatic β cells to induce insulin secretion, promote insulin synthesis, increase β cell proliferation, and to prevent β cell apoptosis [12,28,29]. Through these effects, GLP-1 is over 100 times more potent than glucagon to stimulate insulin secretion [30]. To further impact glucose balance, GLP-1 also decreases glucagon secretion and inhibits gluconeogenesis in the liver [12,31,32].

There are many benefits of GLP-1 on health and weight loss [33–37]. Regarding energy and health, GLP-1 improves insulin sensitivity in skeletal muscle, increases cardiac output, lowers blood pressure, and improves overall cardiovascular outcomes (independent of associated decreases in body weight) [12,38,39]. GLP-1 has a centrally regulated anorexigenic effect and alters non–hunger-related feeding via central pathways related to reward and addiction [12,40–44]. Through delaying gastric emptying by slowing gastric smooth muscle contraction and inhibiting pyloric relaxation, GLP-1 increases the sensation of fullness and reduces hunger for long periods of time after eating [45,46].

On the downside, through the gastrointestinal and central effects mentioned above, GLP-1R agonists can causes nausea, emesis, and taste avoidance [12,24]. GLP-1R agonists can also contribute to dehydration, decreasing water intake (independent of food) [47], and act directly on the kidneys, stimulating the excretion of urine and sodium, though this decreases with time [48].

INDICATIONS FOR GLUCAGON-LIKE PEPTIDE-1 RECEPTOR AGONIST USE

GLP-1R agonists are currently indicated for management of T2DM and for weight loss in adults (≥18 years old) with BMI ≥ 30 kg/m^2, or those with BMI ≥ 27 kg/m^2 with weight-related comorbidities (including T2DM, hypertension, dyslipidemia, polycystic ovarian syndrome, obstructive sleep apnea, metabolic dysfunction-associated steatohepatitis, and/or cardiovascular disease) [49–52]. There are also indications for weight loss in children ≥ 12 years old with BMI at or above the 95% percentile for age and sex [52,53].

Table 1
Food and Drug Administration–approved glucagon-like peptide-1 receptor agonists (as of 2025) [27]

GLP-1R agonist	Brand Names	Pharmaceutical company	Year of approval	Available formulation
Exenatide	Byetta	Amylin	2009	300 ugm/1.2 mL and 600 ugm/2.4 mL subcutaneous solution
	(generic)	Amneal	2024	300 ugm/1.2 mL and 600 ugm/2.4 mL subcutaneous solution
Liraglutide	Victoza	Novo Nordisk Inc	2010	18 mg/3 mL subcutaneous solution
	Saxenda	Novo	2014 (≥18 y/o) 2020 (≥12 y/o)	18 mg/3 mL subcutaneous solution
	(generic)	Hikma	2024	18 mg/3 mL subcutaneous solution
	(generic)	Lupin LTD	2025	18 mg/3 mL subcutaneous solution
	(generic)	Nanjing King-Friend	2025	18 mg/3 mL subcutaneous solution
Lixisenatide	Adlyxin	Sanofi-Aventis US	2016	0.15 mg/3 mL, 0.3 mg/3 mL subcutaneous solution
Dulaglutide	Trulicity	Eli Lilly and Co	2014	0.75 mg/0.5 mL, 1.5 mg/0.5 mL, 3 mg/0.5 mL, 4.5 mg/0.5 mL injectable injection
Semaglutide	Ozempic	Novo	2017	0.25 mg/0.5 mL, 0.5 mg/0.5 mL, 1 mg/0.5 mL, 1.7 mg/0.75 mL, 2.4 mg/0.75 mL subcutaneous solution
	Wegovy	Novo	2021	0.25 mg/0.5 mL, 0.5 mg/0.5 mL, 1 mg/0.5 mL, 1.7 mg/0.75 mL, 2.4 mg/0.75 mL subcutaneous solution
	Rybelsus	Novo	2019	1.5 mg, 3 mg, 4 mg, 7 mg, 9 mg, 14 mg oral tablet
	Rybelsus	Novo Nordisk Inc	2020	3 mg, 7 mg oral tablet
Tirzepatide (dual GLP-1 and GIP Receptor Agonist)	Mounjaro	Eli Lilly and Co	2022	2.5 mg/0.5 mL, 5 mg/0.5 mL, 7.5 mg/0.5 mL, 10 mg/0.5 mL, 12.5 mg/0.5 mL, 15 mg/0.5 mL subcutaneous solution
	Zepbound	Eli Lilly and Co	2023	2.5 mg/0.5 mL, 5 mg/0.5 mL, 7.5 mg/0.5 mL, 10 mg/0.5 mL, 12.5 mg/0.5 mL, 15 mg/0.5 mL subcutaneous solution

WEIGHT LOSS WITH GLUCAGON-LIKE PEPTIDE-1 RECEPTOR USE

There are several randomized controlled trials (RCTs) providing data on expected weight loss for common GLP-1R agonists. Liraglutide 3.0 mg injected daily, when compared to placebo, led to a mean weight loss of 8.4 ± 7.3 kg of total body weight (5.6 kg more weight loss [95% confidence interval (CI) 5.1–6 kg] than placebo) at 56 weeks [54]. Pi-Sunyer and colleagues also noted that over a third (33.1%) of patients in the liraglutide 3.0 mg daily group lost more than 10% of their body weight (compared to 10.6% of patients in the placebo group, $P<.001$) [54]. Another RCT comparing liraglutide 3.0 mg daily versus 1.8 mg liraglutide daily versus placebo found that at 56 weeks, higher-dose liraglutide was associated with higher rates of greater than 5% or greater than 10% weight loss [55]. Unfortunately, but not surprisingly, patients receiving liraglutide, and especially higher-dose liraglutide, noted higher rates of gastrointestinal disorders compared to placebo [54,55]. Regarding semaglutide, patients receiving 2.4 mg injected weekly were noted to have almost 15% mean weight loss at 16 months (compared to 2.4% with placebo, $P<.001$) [56]. Comparing semaglutide to liraglutide (to placebo), semaglutide is associated with greater weight loss at 5 years: −15.8% weight loss with semaglutide versus 6.4% with liraglutide versus 1.9% with placebo ($P<.001$) [57]. On the other hand, exenatide (currently approved for T2DM but not for weight loss) only led to 2.5 ± 0.7 kg mean weight loss at 16 weeks (compared to 0.43 ± 0.6 kg with placebo) when studied among obese women without diabetes [58].

For potentially improved glycemic control, and greater weight loss, tirzepatide combines GLP-1 receptor agonism with gastric inhibitory peptide (GIP) receptor agonism. In RCT evaluation, this has shown greater weight loss, up to more than 20% weight loss at 72 weeks for patients receiving 15 mg weekly injections (compared to 3.1% loss with placebo, $P<.001$). Further, tirzepatide has shown benefit in maintenance of weight reduction, with patients having 5.5% further weight loss from 36 to 88 weeks (after 20.9% mean weight loss in the initial 36 weeks) compared to 14% weight gain among patients receiving placebo after the initial 36 weeks of treatment ($P<.001$) [59]. In a 2024 meta-analysis of RCTs by Yao and colleagues, including 39,246 patients from 76 trials investigating 15 GLP-1R agonist medications, tirzepatide was noted to have greatest impact on glycemic control and weight loss, compared to singular GLP-1R agonists [60].

Table 2 below lists the most used GLP-1R agonists, along with indication, route, dosage, frequency, and comments on weight loss.

CONCERNS ABOUT GLUCAGON-LIKE PEPTIDE-1 RECEPTOR AGONISTS

Though there are many beneficial impacts of GLP-1R agonists for patient health and weight loss, there are also some side effects and risks to be aware of. Gastrointestinal distress, including nausea, vomiting, diarrhea, delayed

Table 2
Commonly used glucagon-like peptide-1 receptor agonists, indications, route, dosing, frequency, and weight loss comments

GLP-1R agonist	Brand Names	Indication	Route	Dosing	Frequency	Comments on weight loss
Liraglutide	Victoza	Type II diabetes	Subcutaneous injection	*Initial:* 0.6 mg *Max:* 1.8 mg	Daily	Weight loss of 5%–10% total body weight in 1 year
	Saxenda	Weight loss	Subcutaneous injection	*Initial:* 0.6 mg *Max:* 3 mg	Daily	
Dulaglutide	Trulicity	Type II diabetes; cardiovascular risk reduction	Subcutaneous injection	*Initial:* 0.75 mg *Max:* 4.5 mg	Weekly	Weight loss benefits secondary to diabetes management
Semaglutide	Ozempic	Type II diabetes; weight loss	Subcutaneous injection	*Initial:* 0.25 mg *Max:* 2 mg	Weekly	Up to 15% weight loss at 1 year
	Wegovy	Weight loss	Subcutaneous injection	*Initial:* 0.25 mg *Max:* 2.4 mg	Weekly	
	Rybelsus	Type II diabetes	Oral tablet	*Initial:* 3 mg *Max:* 14 mg	Daily	Only oral option
Tirzepatide (dual GLP-1 and GIP Receptor Agonist)	Mounjaro	Type II diabetes	Subcutaneous injection	*Initial:* 2.5 mg *Max:* 15 mg	Weekly	>20% weight loss
	Zepbound	Weight loss	Subcutaneous injection	*Initial:* 2.5 mg *Max:* 15 mg	Weekly	
Lixisenatide	Adylixin	Type II diabetes	Subcutaneous injection	*Initial:* 10 mcg *Max:* 20 mcg	Daily	Less effective for weight loss
Exenatide	Byetta	Type II diabetes	Subcutaneous injection	*Initial:* 5 mcg *Max:* 10 mcg	Twice Daily	Less effective for weight loss

gastric emptying, constipation, and abdominal pain, are commonly noted, and can impact adherence to medications [57,60–63]. Further, delayed gastric emptying, though beneficial for reducing appetite and increasing weight loss, can predispose patients to higher risk of aspiration pneumonia, especially if undergoing sedation or anesthesia. Further serious side effects of GLP-1R agonist use include hypoglycemia (especially among patients with insulin-dependance), gallstones/biliary disease, and concerns regarding loss of lean body mass [64]. As such, especially among patients greater than 65 years old, extra caution should be used, and patients should be encouraged to incorporate healthy eating and exercise into a holistic approach to weight loss and health [49,52,64].

Rooted mostly in data from animal models, there is also concern about increased risk of pancreatitis and pancreas cancer associated with GLP-1R agonist use. In an FDA database study of reported adverse events from 2004 to 2009, exenatide (and sitagliptin, a dipeptidyl peptidase-4 inhibitor also used to treat T2DM) were associated with six times higher odds of reported pancreatitis compared with other control (non–GLP-1R agonist) diabetic medications ($P < .008$) [65]. Another study of FDA adverse event reports found liraglutide to be associated with the greatest risk of upper-abdominal pain and pancreatitis and semaglutide associated with the greatest risk of nausea, diarrhea, vomiting, and constipation [62]. In a retrospective analysis of patients with T2DM, patients taking GLP-1R agonists were found to have 2 times higher odds of hospitalization for pancreatitis when matched (case–control) to non–GLP-1R using diabetic patients [66]. Despite these concerns, a systematic review of RCTs did not find significantly increased risk of pancreatitis or pancreas cancer among GLP-1R agonist users [64]. Further, a systematic review and meta-analysis did not find clear evidence of an increased risk of pancreatitis among patients using GLP-1R agonists and noted that data are too sparse to comment on association with pancreatic cancer [67]. Of note, given that animal studies have indicated an increased risk of medullary thyroid cancer associated with GLP-1R agonist use, there is a black box warning against using GLP-1R agonists among patients with a personal or family history of multiple endocrine neoplasia type II or medullary thyroid cancer [60,61].

PERIOPERATIVE MANAGEMENT OF GLUCAGON-LIKE PEPTIDE-1 RECEPTOR AGONISTS

As noted above, with the delayed gastric emptying effects of GLP-1R agonists, there is concern about increased risk of regurgitation and aspiration of gastric contents during general anesthesia and deep sedation [68–71]. It has been noted that there are higher risks of gastrointestinal side effects among patients newly taking GLP-1R agonists, among those on higher doses, and among those on weekly dosing (compared to daily) [72–74]. Despite these concerns, there is conflicting advice regarding perioperative fasting and GLP-1R agonist protocols.

The American Society of Anesthesiologists (ASA), in a consensus-based guideline, recommend the following regarding perioperative management of GLP-1R agonists [75].

- For patients on daily dosing, hold the day of surgery
- For patients on weekly dosing, hold 1 week before surgery
- If GLP-1R agonist is held for longer than the dosing schedule in a diabetic patient, one should consider endocrinologist recommendations for bridging antidiabetic therapy
- If a patient presents on day of surgery with gastrointestinal symptoms (vomiting, nausea, retching, bloating, pain) despite holding GLP-1R agonist per the above recommendations, then consideration should be given to delaying an elective procedure
- If a patient has held the GLP-1R agonist and is asymptomatic on day of surgery, then one can proceed as usual
- If a patient has not held the GLP-1R agonist, despite a lack of gastrointestinal symptoms, then rapid sequence intubation or ultrasound to evaluate gastric fullness before intubation should be considered
- Regarding fasting, providers should follow current ASA fasting guidelines (as there is inconclusive evidence to do otherwise)

A British group does not advocate holding GLP-1R agonists in the perioperative period, and instead recommends continued dosing (including on day of surgery), as even the medication can remain in a patients system despite withholding a GLP-1R agonist for a week before surgery, and there are risks of hyperglycemia or needing insulin if the GLP-1R agonist is held [76]. Regarding the pharmacokinetics of GLP-1R agonists, 88% clearance would require that the medications be held for 3+ half-lives for weekly agents and 5+ half-lives for daily administered agents–which should prompt endocrinology consult for any diabetic patients for bridging management given risk of hyperglycemia [77].

Despite differences in official guidelines, depending on the country and organization and often in flux as new data emerges, there are a few key points that should be considered when operating on patients taking GLP-1R agonists (at least as of 2025) [75,77–80].

- Discussion of the possible increased risk of aspiration should be included in the informed consent process around surgery and anesthesia in all patients using GLP-1R agonists
- Continue GLP-1R agonists in the perioperative setting for most patients, though consider an individualized approach to aspiration risk, especially in patients at higher risk for gastroparesis (diabetic, bowel dysmotility, Parkinson's disease, patients newly using GLP-1R agonists)
- Consider rapid sequence intubation, endotracheal intubation (instead of sedation or laryngeal mask airway), head-up positioning for induction, and orogastric suctioning before extubation
- Always consider delaying an elective procedure if there is true concern for increased aspiration risk

- Consider the use of imaging (ultrasound vs radiograph) to assess gastric fullness before induction
- Continue general perioperative fasting guidelines, or consider a liquid diet the day before surgery, and only clear liquids for 8 to 12 hours before *nil per os*, as this is a low-risk intervention
- Resume agents as soon as the patient is eating, or on discharge for day surgery patients

COMBINED GLUCAGON-LIKE PEPTIDE-1 RECEPTOR AGONISM AND BARIATRIC SURGERY FOR IMPROVED WEIGHT LOSS

For patients pursuing bariatric surgery, some may be using GLP-1R agonists preoperatively. As such, for these patients, providers should be aware of the potential risks associated with GLP-1R agonist use and general anesthesia and surgery (as discussed above). Furthermore, GLP-1R agonists could be considered a neoadjuvant approach to weight loss before surgery, particularly for patients with extremely high BMI or as part of a *shrink the liver* preoperative protocol [81–83].

For patients undergoing bariatric surgery, there should be consideration as to whether GLP-1R agonists can (or should) be used in the adjuvant setting for continued weight loss. In the immediate postoperative period, it is often recommended that patients hold GLP-1R agonists (if using for weight loss purposes). This is partially due to the endogenously increased levels of GLP-1 after bariatric surgery [84]. That being said, for patients with weight recurrence or insufficient weight loss at least 1 year after bariatric surgery, adjuvant GLP-1R agonist use can add positive effects.

Among patients with prior bariatric surgery, liraglutide 3.0 mg daily has been associated with an average of 6.3 kg of weight loss at 8 months and an average of 8% reduction in body weight, though with frequently noted side effect of nausea [85,86]. In a study comparing adjuvant pharmacotherapy among patients after gastric sleeve versus Roux-en-Y gastric bypass (RYGB), RYGB patients were significantly more likely to lose up to 5% of total body weight [86]. Another study noted, though, that regardless of procedure type, semaglutide was more effective than liraglutide for treating postbariatric surgery weight recurrence [87]. Further, a retrospective observational study found semaglutide to be associated with a loss of 67% of regained weight after bariatric surgery [88].

Taken together, these results should cue providers into a few important concerns. First, just because a patient has had prior bariatric surgery does not mean that they are no longer taking a GLP-1R agonist. Further, patients who have had prior bariatric surgery may be at higher risk for aspiration at the time of surgery (given smaller gastric reservoir), and these effects may be more dramatic in patients taking GLP-1R agonists. Finally, patients with insufficient weight loss after bariatric surgery, or weight recurrence, can consider using GLP-1R agonists for further weight loss. Overall, the combined use of GLP-1R agonists and surgery, in the neoadjuvant or adjuvant setting is still an area of evolving investigation and data.

SUMMARY

Despite increased attention in medical literature and lay press, GLP-1R agonists are not new medications in 2025. Initially developed and produced to help manage the hyperglycemic effects of T2DM, many are now indicated for weight loss in adults (and even in adolescents). GLP-1R agonists act in various ways in the human body to improve health and energy expenditure, increase insulin and lower blood glucose, and to reduce hunger and increase weight loss. It is important to consider the side effect profile of GLP-1R agonists among surgical patients, and to discuss individualized risks with patients before any procedures. GLP-1R agonists can also serve as an adjunct to bariatric surgery, both in the neoadjuvant and adjuvant settings, although further research is still needed to determine best practices.

CLINICS CARE POINTS

- Hospital and National guidelines for perioperative management of surgical patients taking GLP-1R agonists can be variable, though the American Society of Anesthesiologists recommend holding daily agents on day of surgery and weekly agents for one week. Consider rapid sequence intubation or gastric emptying.
- GLP-1R agonists are not new medications, their safety profile has been established over greater than two decades among patients with diabetes.
- GLP-1R agonists can be used in the neoadjuvant and adjuvent settings to treat obestiy, along with bariatric surgery (rather than simply an alternative to surgery).

Disclosure

The authors have no financial disclosures or conflicts of interest to disclose.

References

1 Emmerich SD, Fryar CD, Stierman B, Ogden CL. Obesity and severe obesity prevalence in adults: United States, August 2021-August 2023 key findings data from the national health and nutrition examination survey. 2021. Available at: https://www.cdc.gov/nchs/products/index.htm. Accessed August 27, 2025.

[2] Lega IC, Lipscombe LL. Review: diabetes, obesity, and cancer-pathophysiology and clinical implications. Endocr Rev 2020;41(1):bnz014.

[3] Fletcher GF, Landolfo C, Niebauer J, et al. Promoting physical activity and exercise: JACC health promotion series. J Am Coll Cardiol 2018;72(14):1622–39.

[4] Kohl HW, Craig CL, Lambert EV, et al. The pandemic of physical inactivity: global action for public health. Lancet 2012;380(9838):294–305.

[5] Bauer UE, Briss PA, Goodman RA, et al. Prevention of chronic disease in the 21st century: elimination of the leading preventable causes of premature death and disability in the USA. Lancet 2014;384(9937):45–52.

[6] Ser WCWHOTR, 2000 undefined. Obesity: preventing and managing the global epidemic. iris.who.int. 2000. Available at: https://iris.who.int/bitstream/handle/10665/42330/WHO_TRS_894.pdf. Accessed August 27, 2025.

[7] Silveira EA, Kliemann N, Noll M, et al. Visceral obesity and incident cancer and cardiovascular disease: an integrative review of the epidemiological evidence. Obes Rev 2021;22(1); https://doi.org/10.1111/OBR.13088.
[8] Silveira EA, Mendonça CR, Delpino FM, et al. Sedentary behavior, physical inactivity, abdominal obesity and obesity in adults and older adults: a systematic review and meta-analysis. Clin Nutr ESPEN 2022;50:63–73.
[9] Quante M, Dietrich A, Elkhal A, et al. Obesity-related immune responses and their impact on surgical outcomes. Int J Obes 2015;39(6):877–83.
[10] Bazurro S, Ball L, Pelosi P. Perioperative management of obese patient. Curr Opin Crit Care 2018;24(6):560–7.
[11] Kimball CP, Murlin JR. Aqueous extracts of pancreas. J Biol Chem 1923;58(1):337–46.
[12] Müller TD, Finan B, Bloom SR, et al. Glucagon-like peptide 1 (GLP-1). Mol Metab 2019;30:72.
[13] Drucker DJ. Mechanisms of action and therapeutic application of glucagon-like Peptide-1. Cell Metab 2018;27(4):740–56.
[14] Unger RH, Ohneda A, Valverde I, et al. Characterization of the responses of circulating glucagon-like immunoreactivity to intraduodenal and intravenous administration of glucose. J Clin Investig 1968;47(1):48–65.
[15] Nauck MA, Meier JJ. Incretin hormones: their role in health and disease. Diabetes Obes Metab 2018;20:5–21.
[16] Bell GI, Santerre RF, Mullenbach GT. Hamster preproglucagon contains the sequence of glucagon and two related peptides [20]. Nature 1983;302(5910):716–8.
[17] Kreymann B, Ghatei MA, Williams G, et al. Glucagon-like peptide-1 7-36: a physiological incretin in man. Lancet 1987;330(8571):1300–4.
[18] Bryant MG, Bloom SR, Polak JM, et al. Measurement of gut hormonal peptides in biopsies from human stomach and proximal small intestine. Gut 1983;24(2):114.
[19] Steinert RE, Feinle-Bisset C, Asarian L, et al. Ghrelin, CCK, GLP-1, and PYY(3-36): secretory controls and physiological roles in eating and glycemia in health, obesity, and after RYGB. Physiol Rev 2017;97(1):411–63.
[20] Mayo KE, Miller LJ, Bataille D, et al. International union of pharmacology. XXXV. The glucagon receptor family. Pharmacol Rev 2003;55(1):167–94.
[21] Vendrell J, El Bekay R, Peral B, et al. Study of the potential association of adipose tissue GLP-1 receptor with obesity and insulin resistance. Endocrinology 2011;152(11):4072–9.
[22] Wei Y, Mojsov S. Tissue-specific expression of the human receptor for glucagon-like peptide-I: brain, heart and pancreatic forms have the same deduced amino acid sequences. FEBS Lett 1995;358(3):219–24.
[23] Bullock BP, Heller RS, Habener JF. Tissue distribution of messenger ribonucleic acid encoding the rat glucagon-like peptide-1 receptor. Endocrinology 1996;137(7):2968–78.
[24] Müller TD, Clemmensen C, Finan B, et al. Anti-obesity therapy: from rainbow pills to polyagonists. Pharmacol Rev 2018;70(4):712–46.
[25] Bray GM, Bonk ME. Exenatide. Am J Health Syst Pharm 2006;63(5):411–8.
[26] Manigault KR, Thurston MM. Liraglutide: a glucagon-like peptide-1 agonist for chronic weight management. Consult Pharm 2016;31(12):685–97.
[27] Drugs@FDA: FDA-approved drugs. Available at: https://www.accessdata.fda.gov/scripts/cder/daf/index.cfm. Accessed August 24, 2025.
[28] Drucker DJ, Philippe J, Mojsov S, et al. Glucagon-like peptide I stimulates insulin gene expression and increases cyclic AMP levels in a rat islet cell line. Proc Natl Acad Sci U S A 1987;84(10):3434.
[29] Wang X, Zhou J, Doyle ME, et al. Glucagon-like peptide-1 causes pancreatic duodenal homeobox-1 protein translocation from the cytoplasm to the nucleus of pancreatic β-cells by a cyclic adenosine monophosphate/protein kinase A-dependent mechanism. Endocrinology 2001;142(5):1820–7.
[30] Weir GC, Mojsov S, Hendrick GK, et al. Glucagonlike peptide I (7-37) actions on endocrine pancreas. Diabetes 1989;38(3):338–42.

[31] Hare KJ, Vilsbøll T, Asmar M, et al. The glucagonostatic and insulinotropic effects of glucagon-like peptide 1 contribute equally to its glucose-lowering action. Diabetes 2010;59(7):1765.
[32] Prigeon RL, Quddusi S, Paty B, et al. Suppression of glucose production by GLP-1 independent of islet hormones: a novel extrapancreatic effect. Am J Physiol Endocrinol Metab 2003;285(4 48–4):701–7.
[33] Sandoval DA, D'Alessio DA. Physiology of proglucagon peptides: role ofglucagon and GLP-1 in health and disease. Physiol Rev 2015;95(2):513–48.
[34] Campbell JE, Drucker DJ. Pharmacology, physiology, and mechanisms of incretin hormone action. Cell Metab 2013;17(6):819–37.
[35] Sivertsen J, Rosenmeier J, Holst JJ, et al. The effect of glucagon-like peptide 1 on cardiovascular risk. Nature Reviews Cardiology 2012;9(4):209–22.
[36] Holst JJ. The physiology of glucagon-like peptide 1. Physiol Rev 2007;87(4):1409–39.
[37] Drucker DJ. The biology of incretin hormones. Cell Metab 2006;3(3):153–65.
[38] Marso SP, Daniels GH, Brown-Frandsen K, et al. Liraglutide and cardiovascular outcomes in type 2 diabetes. N Engl J Med 2016;375(4):311.
[39] Sun F, Wu S, Guo S, et al. Impact of GLP-1 receptor agonists on blood pressure, heart rate and hypertension among patients with type 2 diabetes: a systematic review and network meta-analysis. Diabetes Res Clin Pract 2015;110(1):26–37.
[40] van Bloemendaal L, Veltman DJ, Ten Kulve JS, et al. Brain reward-system activation in response to anticipation and consumption of palatable food is altered by glucagon-like peptide-1 receptor activation in humans. Diabetes Obes Metab 2015;17(9):878–86.
[41] De Silva A, Salem V, Long CJ, et al. The gut hormones PYY 3-36 and GLP-1 7-36 amide reduce food intake and modulate brain activity in appetite centers in humans. Cell Metab 2011;14(5):700–6.
[42] Van Bloemendaal L, IJzerman RG, Ten Kulve JS, et al. GLP-1 receptor activation modulates appetite- and reward-related brain areas in humans. Diabetes 2014;63(12):4186–96.
[43] Jelsing J, Vrang N, Hansen G, et al. Liraglutide: short-lived effect on gastric emptying-long lasting effects on body weight. Diabetes Obes Metab 2012;14(6):531–8.
[44] Dickson SL, Shirazi RH, Hansson C, et al. The glucagon-like peptide 1 (GLP-1) analogue, exendin-4, decreases the rewarding value of food: a new role for mesolimbic GLP-1 receptors. J Neurosci 2012;32(14):4812–20.
[45] Willms B, Werner J, Holst JJ, et al. Gastric emptying, glucose responses, and insulin secretion after a liquid test meal: effects of exogenous glucagon-like peptide-1 (GLP-1)-(7-36) amide in type 2 (Noninsulin-dependent) diabetic patients. J Clin Endocrinol Metab 1996;81(1):327–32.
[46] Little TJ, Pilichiewicz AN, Russo A, et al. Effects of intravenous glucagon-like peptide-1 on gastric emptying and intragastric distribution in healthy subjects: relationships with postprandial glycemic and insulinemic responses. J Clin Endocrinol Metab 2006;91(5):1916–23.
[47] Mckay NJ, Kanoski SE, Hayes MR, et al. Glucagon-like peptide-1 receptor agonists suppress water intake independent of effects on food intake. Am J Physiol Regul Integr Comp Physiol 2011;301(6):R1755.
[48] Tonneijck L, Smits MM, Muskiet MHA, et al. Renal effects of DPP-4 inhibitor sitagliptin or GLP-1 receptor agonist liraglutide in overweight patients with type 2 diabetes: a 12-week, randomized, double-blind, placebo-controlled trial. Diabetes Care 2016;39(11):2042–50.
[49] Garvey WT, Mechanick JI, Brett EM, et al. American association of clinical endocrinologists and American college of endocrinology comprehensive clinical practice guidelines for medical care of patients with obesity. Endocr Pract 2016;22:1–203.
[50] Grunvald E, Shah R, Hernaez R, et al. AGA clinical practice guideline on pharmacological interventions for adults with obesity. Gastroenterology 2022;163(5):1198–225.
[51] Apovian CM, Aronne LJ, Bessesen DH, et al. Pharmacological management of obesity: an endocrine society clinical practice guideline. J Clin Endocrinol Metab 2015;100(2):342–62.

[52] Gudzune KA, Kushner RF. Medications for obesity: a review. JAMA 2024;332(7):571–84.
[53] Hampl SE, Hassink SG, Skinner AC, et al. Clinical practice guideline for the evaluation and treatment of children and adolescents with obesity. Pediatrics 2023;151(2):e2022060640.
[54] Pi-Sunyer X, Astrup A, Fujioka K, et al. A randomized, controlled trial of 3.0 mg of liraglutide in weight management. N Engl J Med 2015;373(1):11–22.
[55] Davies MJ, Bergenstal R, Bode B, et al. Efficacy of liraglutide for weight loss among patients with type 2 diabetes: the SCALE diabetes randomized clinical trial. JAMA, J Am Med Assoc 2015;314(7):687–99.
[56] Wilding JPH, Batterham RL, Calanna S, et al. Once-weekly semaglutide in adults with overweight or obesity. N Engl J Med 2021;384(11):989–1002.
[57] Rubino DM, Greenway FL, Khalid U, et al. Effect of weekly subcutaneous semaglutide vs daily liraglutide on body weight in adults with overweight or obesity without diabetes: the STEP 8 randomized clinical trial. JAMA 2022;327(2):138–50.
[58] Dushay J, Gao C, Gopalakrishnan GS, et al. Short-term exenatide treatment leads to significant weight loss in a subset of obese women without diabetes. Diabetes Care 2012;35(1):4–11.
[59] Aronne LJ, Sattar N, Horn DB, et al. Continued treatment with tirzepatide for maintenance of weight reduction in adults with obesity: the SURMOUNT-4 randomized clinical trial. JAMA 2024;331(1):38–48.
[60] Yao H, Zhang A, Li D, et al. Comparative effectiveness of GLP-1 receptor agonists on glycaemic control, body weight, and lipid profile for type 2 diabetes: systematic review and network meta-analysis. The BMJ 2024;384:e076410.
[61] Reiss AB, Gulkarov S, Lau R, et al. Weight reduction with GLP-1 agonists and paths for discontinuation while maintaining weight loss. Biomolecules 2025;15(3):408.
[62] Liu L, Chen J, Wang L, et al. Association between different GLP-1 receptor agonists and gastrointestinal adverse reactions: a real-world disproportionality study based on FDA adverse event reporting system database. Front Endocrinol 2022;13:1043789.
[63] Jastreboff AM, Aronne LJ, Ahmad NN, et al. Tirzepatide once weekly for the treatment of obesity. N Engl J Med 2022;387(3):205–16.
[64] Monami M, Nreu B, Scatena A, et al. Safety issues with glucagon-like peptide-1 receptor agonists (pancreatitis, pancreatic cancer and cholelithiasis): data from randomized controlled trials. Diabetes Obes Metab 2017;19(9):1233–41.
[65] Elashoff M, Matveyenko AV, Gier B, et al. Pancreatitis, pancreatic, and thyroid cancer with Glucagon-like peptide-1based therapies. Gastroenterology 2011;141(1):150–6.
[66] Singh S, Chang HY, Richards TM, et al. Glucagonlike peptide 1–based therapies and risk of hospitalization for acute pancreatitis in type 2 diabetes mellitus: a population-based matched case-control study. JAMA Intern Med 2013;173(7):534–9.
[67] Nreu B, Dicembrini I, Tinti F, et al. Pancreatitis and pancreatic cancer in patients with type 2 diabetes treated with glucagon-like peptide-1 receptor agonists: an updated meta-analysis of randomized controlled trials. Minerva Endocrinology 2023;48(2):206–13.
[68] Mahase E. GLP-1 agonists may raise risk of pulmonary aspiration during surgery, MHRA warns. BMJ 2025;388:r205.
[69] Weber M, Siddarthan I, Mack PF. Clinically significant emesis in a patient taking a long-acting GLP-1 receptor agonist for weight loss. Br J Anaesth 2023;131(2):e37–9.
[70] Klein SR, Hobai IA. Semaglutide, delayed gastric emptying, and intraoperative pulmonary aspiration: a case report. Can J Anesth 2023;70(8):1394–6.
[71] Avraham SA, Hossein J, Somri F, et al. Pulmonary aspiration of gastric contents in two patients taking semaglutide for weight loss. Anaesth Rep 2024;12(1):e12278.
[72] van Zuylen ML, Siegelaar SE, Plummer MP, et al. Perioperative management of long-acting glucagon-like peptide-1 (GLP-1) receptor agonists: concerns for delayed gastric emptying and pulmonary aspiration. Br J Anaesth 2024;132(4):644–8.
[73] Silveira SQ, da Silva LM, de Campos Vieira Abib A, et al. Relationship between perioperative semaglutide use and residual gastric content: a retrospective analysis of patients undergoing elective upper endoscopy. J Clin Anesth 2023;87:111091.

[74] Kindel TL, Wang AY, Wadhwa A, et al. Multisociety clinical practice guidance for the safe use of glucagon-like peptide-1 receptor agonists in the perioperative period. Surg Obes Relat Dis 2024;20(12):1183–6.
[75] American society of anesthesiologists consensus-based guidance on preoperative management of patients (adults and children) on glucagon-like Peptide-1 (GLP-1) receptor agonists I American society of anesthesiologists (ASA). Available at: https://www.asahq.org/about-asa/newsroom/news-releases/2023/06/american-society-of-anesthesiologists-consensus-based-guidance-on-preoperative. Accessed August 25, 2025.
[76] Dhatariya K, Levy N, Russon K, et al. Perioperative use of glucagon-like peptide-1 receptor agonists and sodium-glucose cotransporter 2 inhibitors for diabetes mellitus. Br J Anaesth 2024;132(4):639–43.
[77] Goldenberg RM, Gilbert JD, Houlden RL, et al. Perioperative and periprocedural management of GLP-1 receptor-based agonists and SGLT2 inhibitors: narrative review and the STOP-GAP and STOP DKA-2 algorithms. Curr Med Res Opin 2025;41(3):403–19.
[78] El-Boghdadly K, Dhesi J, Fabb P, et al. Elective peri-operative management of adults taking glucagon-like peptide-1 receptor agonists, glucose-dependent insulinotropic peptide agonists and sodium-glucose cotransporter-2 inhibitors: a multidisciplinary consensus statement: a consensus statement from the association of anaesthetists, association of British clinical diabetologists, British obesity and metabolic surgery society, centre for perioperative care, joint British diabetes societies for inpatient care, royal college of anaestheti. Anaesthesia 2025;80(4):412.
[79] Li XY, Jin Y, Feng XY, et al. Perioperative management of patients on GLP-1 receptor agonists: risks, recommendations, and future directions—A narrative review. J Clin Anesth 2025;104; https://doi.org/10.1016/j.jclinane.2025.111871.
[80] Oprea AD, Ostapenko LJ, Sweitzer BJ, et al. Perioperative management of patients taking glucagon-like peptide 1 receptor agonists: society for perioperative assessment and quality improvement (SPAQI) multidisciplinary consensus statement. Br J Anaesth 2025;135(1):48–78.
[81] Hughes DL, Elmasry M, Wilson I, et al. Evaluating the evidence for a liver shrinkage diet for obese patients prior to laparoscopic cholecystectomy: a systematic review and meta-analysis. J Minim Access Surg 2024;20(1):1–6.
[82] Liao C, Liang X, Zhang X, et al. The effects of GLP-1 receptor agonists on visceral fat and liver ectopic fat in an adult population with or without diabetes and nonalcoholic fatty liver disease: a systematic review and meta-analysis. PLoS One 2023;18(8):e0289616.
[83] Shantaram D, Rima XY, Bradley D, et al. The GLP-1 receptor agonist dulaglutide attenuates hepatic steatosis in obesity via a weight-independent mechanism. Diabetes 2025;74(9):1512–24.
[84] Hindsø M, Hedbäck N, Svane MS, et al. The importance of endogenously secreted GLP-1 and GIP for postprandial glucose tolerance and β-cell function after Roux-en-Y gastric bypass and sleeve gastrectomy surgery. Diabetes 2023;72(3):336–47.
[85] Wharton S, Kuk JL, Luszczynski M, et al. Liraglutide 3.0 mg for the management of insufficient weight loss or excessive weight regain post-bariatric surgery. Clin Obes 2019;9(4):e12323.
[86] Mok J, Adeleke MO, Brown A, et al. Safety and efficacy of liraglutide, 3.0 mg, once daily vs placebo in patients with poor weight loss following metabolic surgery: the BARI-OPTIMISE randomized clinical trial. JAMA Surg 2023;158(10):1003–11.
[87] Murvelashvili N, Xie L, Schellinger JN, et al. Effectiveness of semaglutide versus liraglutide for treating post-metabolic and bariatric surgery weight recurrence. Obesity 2023;31(5):1280–9.
[88] Jensen AB, Renström F, Aczél S, et al. Efficacy of the glucagon-like peptide-1 receptor agonists liraglutide and semaglutide for the treatment of weight regain after bariatric surgery: a retrospective observational study. Obes Surg 2023;33(4):1017–25.

Advances in Surgery 60 (2026) 299–313
ADVANCES IN SURGERY

Total Neoadjuvant Therapy for the Treatment of Locally Advanced Rectal Cancer

Bryan Szeglin, MD[a], John Migaly, MD[b,*]
[a]Department of Surgery, The Johns Hopkins Hospital, 1800 Orleans Street, Baltimore, MD 21287, USA; [b]Colon and Rectal Surgery, Department of Surgery, The Johns Hopkins Hospital, 1800 Orleans Street, Baltimore, MD 21287, USA

Keywords
• Locally advanced rectal cancer • Total neoadjuvant therapy • Chemoradiation
• Induction and consolidation chemotherapy

Key points

- Locally advanced rectal cancer treatment has been transformed from 95% recurrence with surgery before total mesorectal excision adoption, to 40% complete response after neoadjuvant therapy.
- Total neoadjuvant therapy constitutes preoperative chemotherapy and chemoradiation, followed by total mesorectal excision, and is the standard-of-care treatment for locally advanced rectal cancer.
- Neoadjuvant therapy greatly improves chemotherapy compliance compared to adjuvant treatment.

INTRODUCTION

Rectal cancer is a leading cause of global morbidity and mortality, and in the United States an estimated 46,000 new rectal cancers will be diagnosed in 2025 [1,2]. In this article, we will focus on the one-third of patients with locally advanced rectal cancer (LARC). Over the last 100 years, a new treatment approach has transformed outcomes from a time when 95% of patients developed recurrence after surgical excision alone to a point when 40% of patients can achieve sustained complete response to chemotherapy (CTX) and radiation therapy (RT). We will explore the historical evidence that has led to the

*Corresponding author. *E-mail address:* jmigaly1@jhmi.edu

https://doi.org/10.1016/j.yasu.2026.03.013
0065-3411/26/

Abbreviations

5-FU	5-fluorouracil
APR	abdominoperineal resection
CNCT	consolidation chemotherapy
CRT	chemoradiation
CRT-CNCT	chemoradiation followed by consolidation chemotherapy
CTX	chemotherapy
DFS	disease-free survival
DR	distant recurrence
EORTC	European Organization for Research and Treatment of Cancer
GITSG	Gastrointestinal Tumor Study Group
INCT	induction chemotherapy
INCT-CRT	induction chemotherapy followed by chemoradiation
LARC	locally advanced rectal cancer
LCRT	long-course radiation therapy
LR	local recurrence
NSABP	National Surgical Adjuvant Breast and Bowel Project
OS	overall survival
pCR	pathologic complete response
RT	radiation therapy
SCRT	short-course radiation therapy
SCRT-CNCT	chemoradiation followed by consolidation chemotherapy
TME	total mesorectal excision
TNT	total neoadjuvant therapy

adoption of the total mesorectal excision (TME) and total neoadjuvant therapy (TNT) as the standard of care. We will then demonstrate how our stepwise refinement of treatment has led to improved locoregional control and set the stage for nonoperative management which will be further discussed by Bryan Szeglin and John Migaly's article, "Watch and Wait in Patients with Clinical Complete Response After Neoadjuvant Therapy with Rectal Cancer: Is it Safe?," in this issue.

THE TOTAL MESORECTAL EXCISION

Rectal resections with abdominal, perineal, and combined approaches have been described for nearly 200 years, but early experience had near-universal recurrence in even experienced surgical hands [3]. In 1908, Ernest Miles described the first abdominoperineal resection (APR) with special attention to the areas where recurrent disease was believed to develop: "the operation should be carried out as widely as possible so that the lateral and downward zones of spread may be effectively extirpated." [4] He reported a dramatic decrease in recurrence rates from 95% in studies published just a few years before to 16% at 2 years in his series. Several decades later, Claude Dixon would report on the anterior resection to preserve the sphincter complex [5]. With these new techniques, experienced surgeons could achieve local recurrence (LR) rates less than 15%, but rates of 30% to 40% were commonly observed in less specialized centers [6–8].

In the 1970s, the advent of circular stapling devices allowed for lower sphincter-preserving resections, but there was concern that inadequate dissections could result in higher rates of LR [7,8]. In a pathologic analysis of such patients, surgeon Richard J. *Bill* Heald identified foci of adenocarcinoma several centimeters distal to the distal resection margin in patients without nodal disease on pathology [9]. Subsequent studies would show that greater depth of invasion into the mesorectal tissue was associated with worse overall survival (OS) [10]. To address this disease, Heald described the complete removal of the intact mesorectum as the TME in 1982. In his initial series of 115 patients, no patient developed pelvic or staple-line recurrence at initial 2-year follow up and only 3.3% of patients recurred locally at 9 years [11,12].

The importance of removing the intact mesorectum is critical to successful resection for rectal cancer with several studies demonstrating that incomplete excision is associated with higher rates of LR (11%–13% incomplete vs 3%–5% complete) and distant recurrence (DR, 19.2%–27.6% vs 12.2–19.7, respectively) [13–15]. As operative techniques have transitioned to minimally invasive approaches, ensuring TME quality remains imperative. Many studies have examined the difference between laparoscopic and open approaches with mixed results, and 2 large randomized controlled trials (RCTs) failed to meet the criteria for noninferiority for a primary composite outcome of pathologic factors [16,17]. A meta-analysis has also shown higher rates of incomplete mesorectal excision with the laparoscopic approach when compared to open (13.2% vs 10.4%, respectively) [18]. Nearly 50% of TMEs are now performed robotically, which has been shown to be either equivalent to or outperform both open and laparoscopic approaches, particularly for low rectal tumors [19–24]. Transanal TME has achieved similar oncologic results in several studies, although it carries significant perioperative morbidity and requires a high level of training [20,25,26].

RADIATION

Before the widespread adoption of TME, efforts to address LR focused on the adjuvant setting given concerns that preoperative CTX and RT would lead to increased surgical morbidity. RCTs demonstrated variable efficacy with either CTX or RT alone. Most trials showed some benefit to adjuvant RT at sufficiently high doses over 25 Gy, but combination CTX and RT generally demonstrated decreased rates of LR from 30% to 55% with surgery alone to 12% to 33% with combination, even if DR was often unchanged [27–34]. Concurrent CTX and long-course RT (LCRT)–termed chemoradiation (CRT)–was developed to increase the efficacy of RT and demonstrated improved relapse-free survival and OS [35,36]. A summary of the major RCTs that we will discuss is presented in Table 1.

A major shift in LARC treatment occurred as evidence began to build that neoadjuvant RT could have oncologic benefit with minimal effect on surgical morbidity [37–46]. This early work led to several large RCTs which

Table 1
Major randomized controlled trials supporting the use of total neoadjuvant therapy

Study	Years of accrual	N	Experimental arms	Control arm	Experimental arm LR rate	Main conclusions
GITSG GI-7175 [61]	1975–1980	227	3 adj arms: CTX, RT, or RT and CTX	No adj therapy	10.8% in RT and CTX arm at 5 y	Improved oncologic outcomes with adjuvant CTX and RT
NSABP R-01 [62]	1977–1986	555	2 adj arms: CTX or LCRT	No adj therapy	16.3% in RT arm, 21.4% in CTX arm at 6.7 y	Either adjuvant CTX or LCRT had improved DFS and OS.
Stockholm I [47]	1980–1987	849	SCRT + surgery	Surgery alone	14% at 8.9 y	Neoadjuvant SCRT has improved locoregional control compared to surgery alone but may lead to worse perioperative outcomes in the elderly.
Rich et al [35].	1986–1990	660	Adj extended infusion 5-FU with concurrent CTX	Adj intermittent bolus 5-FU with concurrent CTX	LR 37% at 5 y	Extended infusion 5-FU given concurrently with radiation has improved oncologic outcomes.
Swedish Trial [50]	1987–1990	1168	Neoadj SCRT + surgery	Surgery alone	9% at 13 y	SCRT with surgery has improved locoregional control and OS benefit without effecting postoperative outcomes beyond 6 mo.

Stockholm II [48]	1987–1993	557	Neoadj SCRT + surgery	Surgery alone	12% at 8.8 y	SCRT with surgery has improved locoregional control compared without effect on postoperative outcomes after 6 mo.
EORTC 22921 [64]	1993–2003	1011	3 arms: neoadj CRT; neoadj RT + adj CTX; neoadj CRT + adj CTX	Neoadj RT	LR 7.6%–9.6% at 5 y	Receiving any CTX in addition to RT improves locoregional control.
Dutch TME [52,53]	1996–1999	1861	Neoadj SCRT + TME	Surgery alone	LR 5% at 10 y	SCRT with TME has improved locoregional control.
CAO/ARO/AIO-94 German Trial [56]	1995–2002	402	Neoadj CRT + surgery + adj CTX	Surgery + adj CRT + CTX	LR 7.1% at 10 y	Preoperative CRT has improved LR compared to postoperative CRT.
Grupo Cáncer de Recto 3 [65]	2006–2007	108	INCT-CRT + TME	CRT + TME + adjuvant CTX	NA	No difference in pCR if CTX is delivered in the neoadjuvant setting with greatly improved compliance.
TIMING [66]	2004–2012	292	3 arms: neoadj CRT followed by either 2, 4, or 6 cycles of mFOLFOX6 + TME	Neoadj CRT + TME	NA	Improved pCR with increasing dose of neoadjuvant CTX.
RAPIDO [71]	2011–2016	920	SCRT-CNCT + TME	Neoadj CRT + TME ± adj CTX	LR 10% at 5.6 y	Similar rates of pCR can be achieved with SCRT-CNCT compared to traditional CRT with adjuvant CTX, but with higher rates of LR.

(*continued on next page*)

Table 1
(*continued*)

Study	Years of accrual	N	Experimental arms	Control arm	Experimental arm LR rate	Main conclusions
CAO/ARO/AIO-12 German Trial	2015–2018	311	INCT-CRT + TME	CRT-CNCT + TME	LR 5% and 6% at 3 y	CRT-CNCT has higher rates of pCR compared to INCT-CRT.
PRODIGE 23 [72]	2012–2017	461	INCT-CRT + TME + adj CTX	CRT + TME + adj CTX	LR 4.3% at 3.9 y	A TNT approach has improved pCR, 3-y DFS, and OS compared to CRT with adjuvant CTX.

Abbreviations: adj, adjuvant; neoadj, neoadjuvant.

simultaneously accrued patients in the 1980s and 1990s. The Stockholm I trial compared short-course RT (SCRT) followed by rectal resection to surgery alone and found a near 50% decrease in LR with SCRT and no effect on DR or OS [47]. However, significant perioperative morbidity and mortality in the SCRT group was observed, particularly in elderly patients. The follow up Stockholm II Trial had a similar design as Stockholm I but excluded patients greater than 80 years and limited radiation volume in an attempt to decrease toxicity [48]. Similar effect on LR, DR, and OS were observed with no difference in immediate perioperative morbidity, although the authors noted a small increase in cardiovascular death within the first 6 months in the SCRT group.

Similarly, the Swedish Rectal Cancer Trial compared SCRT followed by rectal resection to surgery alone and demonstrated not only improved LR but improved OS in the SCRT group with durable benefit at 13-year follow up [49,50]. While SCRT patients were at increased risk for admission in the first 6 months with the most severe indication being bowel obstruction, no difference in morbidity was observed after 6 months [51]. Together, these 3 trials showed an improvement in LR from 25% to 28% with surgery alone to 11% to 14% with SCRT and surgery.

The Stockholm I and II Trials and the Swedish Trial each accrued before widespread adoption of TME and so even though the benefit of SCRT was significant, it was unclear how this benefit would change in combination with TME. The Dutch TME Trial sought to answer this question [52]. Patients were randomized to SCRT followed by TME or TME alone. At 12-year follow up, LR was 5% in the SCRT with TME group and 11% in the TME-alone group with no difference in 10-year OS [53]. Stage III patients with a negative resection margin were noted to have an improved 10-year OS of 50% in the SCRT group compared to 40% in the TME group. With respect to surgical complications, patients in the SCRT group had marginal increase in intraoperative blood loss and more perineal complications with APR, but no difference in perioperative mortality [54].

CHEMORADIATION

To further compare if RT should be delivered before or after surgery, and to capitalize on the proven benefits of concurrent CTX with RT in a CRT fashion, the CAO/ARO/AIO-94 German Trial randomized LARC patients to receive either preoperative or postoperative CRT administered as a 120-hour extended infusion of 5-fluorouracil (5-FU) in the first and fifth week of 50.4 Gy LCRT [55]. Both groups received 4 cycles of adjuvant 5-FU. The 5- and 10-year cumulative incidence of LR was 5.0% and 7.1% in the preoperative group and 9.7% and 10.1% in the postoperative group, respectively [56]. Similarly to other RT studies with the exception of the Swedish Trial, there was no difference in 5- or 10-year OS. Furthermore, short- and long-term toxicity were significantly less common in the preoperative group. These data collectively support the use of neoadjuvant CRT.

ADJUVANT CHEMOTHERAPY

Given that most RT and CRT trials have failed to show any improvement in DR or mortality, investigators turned to adjuvant CTX. Most of the early trials supporting the use of adjuvant CTX for rectal cancer that ultimately contributed to its inclusion in consensus guidelines in 1990 were drawn from studies with predominantly colon cancer patients [57–59]. Two pivotal rectal cancer-specific trials that supported this recommendation were the Gastrointestinal Tumor Study Group (GITSG) GI-7175 Trial and the National Surgical Adjuvant Breast and Bowel Project (NSABP) R-01 Trial. The GITSG GI-7175 Trial randomized LARC patients to 4 groups: no adjuvant therapy, adjuvant LCRT, adjuvant CTX, or adjuvant CTX and LCRT [60,61]. A benefit in LR, DR, and OS was observed in all groups compared to no adjuvant therapy, but combined CTX and LCRT had the greatest effect. The NSABP R-01 Trial randomized patients to no adjuvant therapy, adjuvant CTX, or adjuvant LCRT and found a benefit in disease-free survival (DFS) and OS in both treatment groups compared to control [62]. Support for adjuvant CTX in the context of neoadjuvant RT would come nearly 2 decades later when the European Organization for Research and Treatment of Cancer (EORTC) Radiotherapy Group Trial 22921 randomized patients to receive preoperative LCRT or preoperative CRT each with or without adjuvant CTX [63]. Receiving any CTX improved locoregional control, but there was no benefit to 5- or 10-year OS when added to LCRT [64].

THE ERA OF TOTAL NEOADJUVANT THERAPY

Compliance with adjuvant CTX is unfortunately low. In the GITSG GI-7175 Trial, 81% of patients in the postoperative CTX group received at least 1 year of therapy and with the addition of LCRT in the combination group only 65% of patients received the full dose. In the NSABP R-01 Trial CTX group, only 47% of patients received the full dose. Patients in both arms of the CAO/ARO/AIO-94 German Trial were assigned adjuvant CTX in addition to either preoperative or postoperative CRT and while 89% of patients in the preoperative CRT group received the full CTX dose, full compliance was only 50% in the postoperative group. And finally, in the EORTC 22921 Trial, while over 95% of patients received RT as prescribed and 85% of patients received the full dose of concurrent CTX as a part of CRT, less than 50% of patients received the full dose of adjuvant CTX.

Given this poor compliance to adjuvant CTX despite a clear benefit that was observed even with intention-to-treat analyses, it became reasonable to consider offering CTX in the neoadjuvant setting. Fig. 1 outlines the major TNT sequences that we will discuss. The Grupo Cáncer de Recto 3 Study randomized LARC patients to receive either neoadjuvant capecitabine and oxaliplatin-based (CAPOX) CRT followed by TME and adjuvant CAPOX, or CAPOX first (termed *induction chemotherapy* [INCT]) followed by CAPOX-based CRT followed by TME (abbreviated INCT-CRT) [65]. Greatly improved CTX compliance was observed with 94% of patients in the INCT-CRT group compared to

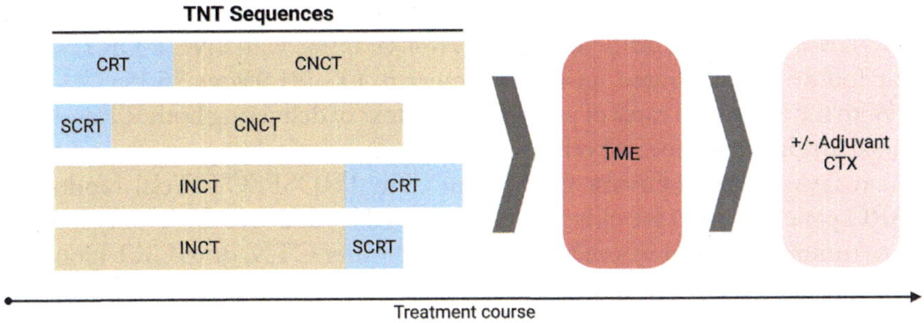

Fig. 1. TNT treatment sequences. CNCT, consolidation chemotherapy; CRT, chemoradiation therapy; INCT, induction chemotherapy; SCRT, short-course radiation therapy; TNT, total neoadjuvant therapy. (*Created in* BioRender. Szeglin, B. (2025) https://BioRender.com/77zqn5r.)

57% of patients in the adjuvant group receiving the prescribed dose. Similar rates of pathologic complete response (pCR) were observed in each group.

The TIMING Trial further refined this approach by randomizing patients to receive CRT followed by either 0, 2, 4, or 6 cycles of neoadjuvant mFOLFOX6 CTX (termed *consolidation chemotherapy* [CNCT]) before TME (abbreviated CRT-CNCT) [66]. They demonstrated a dose-dependent rate of pCR with increasing neoadjuvant CTX cycles: 18%, 25%, 30%, and 38% in the 0, 2, 4, and 6 cycle groups, respectively. It is important to note that patients with more CTX cycles have a greater time delay from the end of CRT to surgery and that pCR rates are known to increase over time, making it likely that these impressive pCR rates represent the combined effect of both neoadjuvant CRT and a greater time to allow for pCR.

THE MODERN ERA OF TOTAL NEOADJUVANT THERAPY AND UNANSWERED QUESTIONS

Further refinement of a neoadjuvant approach to LARC was investigated in several subsequent trials.

To compare INCT and CNCT, the CAO/ARO/AIO-12 German Trial randomized patients to either INCT-CRT or CRT-CNCT [67]. The rate of pCR was 17% in the INCT-CRT group and 25% in the CRT-CNCT group with no difference in 3- or 5-year LR, DFS, or OS [68,69]. While this and other data that we will discuss show improved oncologic outcomes with CRT-CNCT over INCT-CRT, it remains controversial.

The RAPIDO Trial investigated the role of SCRT in neoadjuvant therapy for LARC. Patients were randomized to either SCRT without concomitant CTX followed by CNCT (SCRT-CNCT) or standard neoadjuvant CRT in a long-course fashion with adjuvant CTX. While they demonstrated higher rates of pCR in the SCRT-CNCT group, a higher 5-year LR was also observed in these patients [70,71]. It remains unclear if SCRT is an appropriate alternative for CRT in the context of neoadjuvant therapy.

And finally, the PRODIGE 23 Trial compared INCT-CRT followed by TME to CRT followed by TME, with both groups receiving adjuvant CTX

[72]. At the initial report, there was a significant improvement in the rate of pCR (28% vs 12%) and 3-year DFS (76% vs 69%) with INCT-CRT, and 7-year follow demonstrated an improvement in OS (81.9% vs 76.1%).

With the improved rates of pCR in the context of delivering both RT and CTX before surgical resection, it became reasonable to ask if select patients could avoid RT in favor of neoadjuvant CTX alone. The PROSPECT Trial randomized LARC patients to receive either INCT followed by selective CRT only if the primary tumor decreased in size by less than 20% after CTX, or to CRT alone [73]. 89.6% of patients in the selective CRT group avoided RT, and with respect to DFS, neoadjuvant CTX was noninferior to CRT, supporting that there may be a group of patients with excellent response who could avoid RT. Long-term follow up of these patients has yet to be reported.

This novel neoadjuvant approach to LARC is referred to as TNT where patients receive both CTX and CRT before TME. Twenty-five percent to 40% of patients can achieve a pCR with TNT compared to 15% treated with CRT and adjuvant CTX. The greatest evidence to date supports the use of CRT with an LCRT protocol followed by CNCT, although INCT and SCRT regimens remain common with some studies showing similar outcomes [66,74,75]. With a significant percentage of patients achieving pCR, investigators have begun to ask if a select group of patients could avoid surgery altogether. We will explore this nonoperative management approach in Bryan Szeglin and John Migaly's article, "Watch and Wait in Patients with Clinical Complete Response After Neoadjuvant Therapy with Rectal Cancer: Is it Safe?," in this issue.

SUMMARY

We have traced the evolution of LARC treatment from the development of the TME as the standard-of-care surgical resection, to the widespread adoption of TNT. Growing evidence supports a CRT-CNCT approach; however, the roles of INCT and SCRT remain controversial. Given the success of TNT achieving pCR rates of 25% to 40% in many studies, the role of surgery altogether has been brought into question.

CLINICS CARE POINTS

- Rich mesorectal excision (TME) is the standard-of-care rectal resection technique for locally advanced rectal cancer and leads to superior oncologic outcomes compared to non-TME resections.
- Compliance for neoadjuvant therapy is significantly improved compared to adjuvant treatment.
- Chemoradiation and chemotherapy should be given in the neoadjuvant setting as total neoadjuvant therapy (TNT) and lead to improved locoregional control.
- A subset of patients with complete response to TNT may be able to avoid surgery altogether.

Disclosure

The authors have no commercial or financial disclosures.

References

[1] Bray F, Laversanne M, Sung H, et al. Global cancer statistics 2022: GLOBOCAN estimates of incidence and mortality worldwide for 36 cancers in 185 countries. CA Cancer J Clin 2024;74(3):229–63.
[2] Siegel RL, Kratzer TB, Giaquinto AN, et al. Cancer statistics. CA Cancer J Clin 2025;75(1): 10–45.
[3] Ernest Miles W. A method of performing abdomino-perineal excision for carcinoma of the rectum and of the terminal portion of the pelvic colon. Lancet 1908;172(4451):1812–3.
[4] Miles WE. The treatment of carcinoma of the rectum and pelvic Colon. Glasg Med J 1912;77(2):81–104.
[5] Dixon CF. Anterior resection for malignant lesions of the upper part of the rectum and lower part of the sigmoid. Ann Surg 1948;128(3):425–42.
[6] Cullen KP, Mayo CW. A further evaluation of the one-stage low-anterior resection. Dis Colon Rectum 1963;6(6):415–21.
[7] Lasson AL, Ekelund GR, Lindström CG. Recurrence risk after stapled anastomosis for rectal carcinoma. Acta Chir Scand 1984;150(1):85–9.
[8] Hurst PA, Prout WG, Kelly JM, et al. Local recurrence after low anterior resection using the staple Gun. J Br Surg 1982;69(5):275–6.
[9] Heald RJ, Husband EM, Ryall RDH. The mesorectum in rectal cancer Surgery—The clue to pelvic recurrence? J Br Surg 1982;69(10):613–6.
[10] Cawthorn SJ, Caffarey SM, Broughton CIM, et al. Extent of mesorectal spread and involvement of lateral resection margin as prognostic factors after surgery for rectal cancer. Lancet 1990;335(8697):1055–9.
[11] Heald RJ, Ryall RDH. Recurrence and survival after total mesorectal excision for rectal cancer. Lancet 1986;327(8496):1479–82.
[12] Heald RJ. The 'Holy Plane' of rectal surgery. J R Soc Med 1988;81(9):503–8.
[13] Kitz J, Fokas E, Beissbarth T, et al. Association of plane of total mesorectal excision with prognosis of rectal cancer: secondary analysis of the CAO/ARO/AIO-04 phase 3 randomized clinical trial. JAMA Surg 2018;153(8):e181607; https://doi.org/10.1001/jamasurg.2018.1607.
[14] Quirke P, Steele R, Monson J, et al. Effect of the plane of surgery achieved on local recurrence in patients with operable rectal cancer: a prospective study using data from the MRC CR07 and NCIC-CTG CO16 randomised clinical trial. Lancet 2009;373(9666): 821–8.
[15] Nagtegaal ID, Van De Velde CJH, Van Der Worp E, et al. Macroscopic evaluation of rectal cancer resection specimen: clinical significance of the pathologist in quality control. J Clin Oncol 2002;20(7):1729–34.
[16] Fleshman J, Branda M, Sargent DJ, et al. Effect of laparoscopic-assisted resection vs open resection of stage II or III rectal cancer on pathologic outcomes: the ACOSOG Z6051 randomized clinical trial. JAMA 2015;314(13):1346–55.
[17] Stevenson ARL, Solomon MJ, Lumley JW, et al. Effect of laparoscopic-assisted resection vs open resection on pathological outcomes in rectal cancer: the ALaCaRT randomized clinical trial. JAMA 2015;314(13):1356–63.
[18] Martínez-Pérez A, Carra MC, Brunetti F, et al. Pathologic outcomes of laparoscopic vs open mesorectal excision for rectal cancer: a systematic review and meta-analysis. JAMA Surg 2017;152(4):e165665; https://doi.org/10.1001/jamasurg.2016.5665.
[19] Feng Q, Yuan W, Li T, et al. Robotic vs laparoscopic surgery for middle and low rectal cancer: the REAL randomized clinical trial. JAMA 2025;334(2):136–48.
[20] Rouanet P, Guerrieri M, Lemercier P, et al. A prospective European trial comparing laparotomy, laparoscopy, robotic-assisted, and transanal total mesorectal excision procedures in

high-risk patients with rectal cancer: the RESET trial. Ann Surg 2024; https://doi.org/10.1097/SLA.0000000000006534.
[21] Duhoky R, Rutgers MLW, Burghgraef TA, et al. Long-term outcomes of robotic versus laparoscopic total mesorectal excisions: a propensity-score matched cohort study of 5-year survival outcomes. Ann Surg Open Perspect Surg Hist Educ Clin Approaches 2024;5(2):e404; https://doi.org/10.1097/AS9.0000000000000404.
[22] Liu C, Wu Y, Liu H, et al. Robotic versus laparoscopic total mesorectal excision for mid-low rectal cancer after neoadjuvant chemoradiotherapy: a systematic review and meta-analysis of oncological, perioperative, and survival-related outcomes. J Robot Surg 2025;19(1):570.
[23] Cardelli S, Stocchi L, Merchea A, et al. Comparative outcomes of robotic versus open proctectomy for rectal cancer at high risk of positive circumferential resection margin. Dis Colon Rectum 2024;67(11):1475–84.
[24] Simon EF, Westfall KM, Erozkan K, et al. The rise of robotics: surgical approaches for rectal cancer over time. Surg Endosc 2025;39(10):6702–18.
[25] Zeng Z, Luo S, Zhang H, et al. Transanal vs laparoscopic total mesorectal excision and 3-Year disease-free survival in rectal cancer: the TaLaR randomized clinical trial. JAMA 2025;333(9):774.
[26] Chen GY, Liao CK, You JF, et al. Comparison of short- and long-term outcomes among laparoscopic, robotic-assisted, and transanal total mesorectal excision procedures in patients with rectal cancer: a propensity score-matching analysis. Tech Coloproctol 2025;29(1):163.
[27] Fountzilas G, Zisiadis A, Dafni U, et al. Postoperative radiation and concomitant bolus fluorouracil with or without additional chemotherapy with fluorouracil and high-dose leucovorin in patients with high-risk rectal cancer: a randomized phase III study conducted by the Hellenic cooperative oncology group. Ann Oncol Off J Eur Soc Med Oncol 1999;10(6):671–6.
[28] Tveit KM, Guldvog I, Hagen S, et al. Randomized controlled trial of postoperative radiotherapy and short-term time-scheduled 5-fluorouracil against surgery alone in the treatment of Dukes B and C rectal cancer. Norwegian Adjuvant Rectal Cancer Project Group. Br J Surg 1997;84(8):1130–5.
[29] Treurniet-Donker AD, van Putten WL, Wereldsma JC, et al. Postoperative radiation therapy for rectal cancer. An interim analysis of a prospective, randomized multicenter trial in the Netherlands. Cancer 1991;67(8):2042–8.
[30] Krook JE, Moertel CG, Gunderson LL, et al. Effective surgical adjuvant therapy for high-risk rectal carcinoma. N Engl J Med 1991;324(11):709–15.
[31] Mameghan H, Gray BN, de Zwart J, et al. Adjuvant post-operative radiotherapy in rectal cancer: results from the ANZ bowel cancer trial (protocol 8202). Australas Radiol 1991;35(1):61–5.
[32] Hafström L, Domellöf L, Rudenstam CM, et al. Adjuvant chemotherapy with 5-fluorouracil, vincristine and CCNU for patients with Dukes' C colorectal cancer. The Swedish Gastrointestinal Tumour Adjuvant Therapy Group. Br J Surg 1990;77(12):1345–8.
[33] Balslev I, Pedersen M, Teglbjaerg PS, et al. Postoperative radiotherapy in rectosigmoid cancer Dukes' B and C: interim report from a randomized multicentre study. Br J Cancer 1982;46(4):551–6.
[34] Balslev I, Pedersen M, Teglbjaerg PS, et al. Postoperative radiotherapy in Dukes' B and C carcinoma of the rectum and rectosigmoid. A randomized multicenter study. Cancer 1986;58(1):22–8.
[35] Rich TA, Lokich JJ, Chaffey JT. A pilot study of protracted venous infusion of 5-fluorouracil and concomitant radiation therapy. J Clin Oncol Off J Am Soc Clin Oncol 1985;3(3):402–6.
[36] O'Connell MJ, Martenson JA, Wieand HS, et al. Improving adjuvant therapy for rectal cancer by combining protracted-infusion fluorouracil with radiation therapy after curative surgery. N Engl J Med 1994;331(8):502–7.

[37] Stearns MW, Deddish MR, Quan SH. Preoperative roentgen therapy for cancer of the rectum. Surg Gynecol Obstet 1959;109(2):225–9.

[38] Cafiero F, Gipponi M, Di Somma C, et al. Adjuvant post-operative radiotherapy vs radiotherapy plus 5-FU and levamisole in patients with TNM stage II-III resectable rectal cancer. A phase III randomized clinical trial. P.A.R. Cooperative Study Group. Eur J Surg Oncol 1995;21(4):391–2.

[39] Goldberg PA, Nicholls RJ, Porter NH, et al. Long-term results of a randomised trial of short-course low-dose adjuvant pre-operative radiotherapy for rectal cancer: reduction in local treatment failure. Eur J Cancer Oxf Engl 1990 1994;30A(11):1602–6.

[40] Dahl O, Horn A, Morild I, et al. Low-dose preoperative radiation postpones recurrences in operable rectal cancer. Results of a randomized multicenter trial in western Norway. Cancer 1990;66(11):2286–94.

[41] Horn A, Halvorsen JF, Dahl O. Preoperative radiotherapy in operable rectal cancer. Dis Colon Rectum 1990;33(10):823–8.

[42] Reis Neto JA, Quilici FA, Reis JA. A comparison of nonoperative vs. preoperative radiotherapy in rectal carcinoma. A 10-year randomized trial. Dis Colon Rectum 1989;32(8): 702–10.

[43] Higgins GA, Humphrey EW, Dwight RW, et al. Preoperative radiation and surgery for cancer of the rectum. Veterans Administration Surgical Oncology Group Trial II. Cancer 1986;58(2):352–9.

[44] Gérard A, Buyse M, Nordlinger B, et al. Preoperative radiotherapy as adjuvant treatment in rectal cancer. Final results of a randomized study of the European Organization for Research and Treatment of Cancer (EORTC). Ann Surg 1988;208(5):606–14.

[45] Roswit B, Higgins GA, Keehn RJ. Preoperative irradiation for carcinoma of the rectum and rectosigmoid colon: reportof a National Veterans Administration randomized study. Cancer 1975;35(6):1597–602.

[46] Higgins GA, Conn JH, Jordan PH, et al. Preoperative radiotherapy for colorectal cancer. Ann Surg 1975;181(5):624–31.

[47] Cedermark B, Johansson H, Rutqvist LE, et al. The Stockholm I trial of preoperative short term radiotherapy in operable rectal carcinoma. A prospective randomized trial. Stockholm Colorectal Cancer Study Group. Cancer 1995;75(9):2269–75.

[48] Martling A, Holm T, Johansson H, et al, Stockholm Colorectal Cancer Study Group. The Stockholm II trial on preoperative radiotherapy in rectal carcinoma: long-term follow-up of a population-based study. Cancer 2001;92(4):896–902.

[49] Cedermark B, Dahlberg M, Glimelius B, et al, Swedish Rectal Cancer Trial. Improved survival with preoperative radiotherapy in resectable rectal cancer. N Engl J Med 1997;336(14):980–7.

[50] Folkesson J, Birgisson H, Pahlman L, et al. Swedish Rectal Cancer Trial: long lasting benefits from radiotherapy on survival and local recurrence rate. J Clin Oncol Off J Am Soc Clin Oncol 2005;23(24):5644–50.

[51] Birgisson H, Påhlman L, Gunnarsson U, et al, Swedish Rectal Cancer Trial Group. Adverse effects of preoperative radiation therapy for rectal cancer: long-term follow-up of the Swedish Rectal Cancer Trial. J Clin Oncol Off J Am Soc Clin Oncol 2005;23(34):8697–705.

[52] Kapiteijn E, Marijnen CA, Nagtegaal ID, et al. Preoperative radiotherapy combined with total mesorectal excision for resectable rectal cancer. N Engl J Med 2001;345(9): 638–46.

[53] van Gijn W, Marijnen CAM, Nagtegaal ID, et al. Preoperative radiotherapy combined with total mesorectal excision for resectable rectal cancer: 12-year follow-up of the multicentre, randomised controlled TME trial. Lancet Oncol 2011;12(6):575–82.

[54] Marijnen CaM, Kapiteijn E, van de Velde CJH, et al. Acute side effects and complications after short-term preoperative radiotherapy combined with total mesorectal excision in primary rectal cancer: report of a multicenter randomized trial. J Clin Oncol Off J Am Soc Clin Oncol 2002;20(3):817–25.

[55] Sauer R, Becker H, Hohenberger W, et al. Preoperative versus postoperative chemoradiotherapy for rectal cancer. N Engl J Med 2004;351(17):1731–40.
[56] Sauer R, Liersch T, Merkel S, et al. Preoperative versus postoperative chemoradiotherapy for locally advanced rectal cancer: results of the German CAO/ARO/AIO-94 randomized phase III trial after a median follow-up of 11 years. J Clin Oncol Off J Am Soc Clin Oncol 2012;30(16):1926–33.
[57] Heriot AG, Kumar D. Adjuvant therapy for resectable rectal and colonic cancer. Br J Surg 1998;85(3):300–9.
[58] Buyse M, Zeleniuch-Jacquotte A, Chalmers TC. Adjuvant therapy of colorectal cancer. Why we still don't know. JAMA 1988;259(24):3571–8.
[59] NIH consensus conference. Adjuvant therapy for patients with colon and rectal cancer. JAMA 1990;264(11):1444–50.
[60] Thomas PR, Lindblad AS. Adjuvant postoperative radiotherapy and chemotherapy in rectal carcinoma: a review of the Gastrointestinal tumor study group experience. Radiother Oncol J Eur Soc Ther Radiol Oncol 1988;13(4):245–52.
[61] Gastrointestinal Tumor Study Group. Prolongation of the disease-free interval in surgically treated rectal carcinoma. N Engl J Med 1985;312(23):1465–72; https://doi.org/10.1056/NEJM198506063122301.
[62] Fisher B, Wolmark N, Rockette H, et al. Postoperative adjuvant chemotherapy or radiation therapy for rectal cancer: results from NSABP protocol R-01. J Natl Cancer Inst 1988;80(1):21–9.
[63] Bosset JF, Collette L, Calais G, et al. Chemotherapy with preoperative radiotherapy in rectal cancer. N Engl J Med 2006;355(11):1114–23.
[64] Bosset JF, Calais G, Mineur L, et al. Fluorouracil-based adjuvant chemotherapy after preoperative chemoradiotherapy in rectal cancer: long-term results of the EORTC 22921 randomised study. Lancet Oncol 2014;15(2):184–90.
[65] Fernández-Martos C, Pericay C, Aparicio J, et al. Phase II, randomized study of concomitant chemoradiotherapy followed by surgery and adjuvant capecitabine plus oxaliplatin (CAPOX) compared with induction CAPOX followed by concomitant chemoradiotherapy and surgery in magnetic resonance imaging-defined, locally advanced rectal cancer: grupo cancer de recto 3 study. J Clin Oncol Off J Am Soc Clin Oncol 2010;28(5):859–65.
[66] Garcia-Aguilar J, Chow OS, Smith DD, et al. Effect of adding mFOLFOX6 after neoadjuvant chemoradiation in locally advanced rectal cancer: a multicentre, phase 2 trial. Lancet Oncol 2015;16(8):957–66.
[67] Fokas E, Allgäuer M, Polat B, et al. Randomized phase II trial of chemoradiotherapy plus induction or consolidation chemotherapy as total neoadjuvant therapy for locally advanced rectal cancer: CAO/ARO/AIO-12. J Clin Oncol Off J Am Soc Clin Oncol 2019;37(34):3212–22.
[68] Fokas E, Schlenska-Lange A, Polat B, et al. Chemoradiotherapy plus induction or consolidation chemotherapy as total neoadjuvant therapy for patients with locally advanced rectal cancer: long-term results of the CAO/ARO/AIO-12 randomized clinical trial. JAMA Oncol 2022;8(1):e215445; https://doi.org/10.1001/jamaoncol.2021.5445.
[69] Diefenhardt M, Kosmala R, Fleischmann M, et al. Chemotherapy before or after preoperative chemoradiotherapy and surgery for locally advanced rectal cancer: 5-year results of the CAO/ARO/AIO-12 trial - a general pairwise comparison. ESMO Open 2025;10(3):104483; https://doi.org/10.1016/j.esmoop.2025.104483.
[70] Bahadoer RR, Dijkstra EA, van Etten B, et al. Short-course radiotherapy followed by chemotherapy before total mesorectal excision (TME) versus preoperative chemoradiotherapy, TME, and optional adjuvant chemotherapy in locally advanced rectal cancer (RAPIDO): a randomised, open-label, phase 3 trial. Lancet Oncol 2021;22(1):29–42.
[71] Dijkstra EA, Nilsson PJ, Hospers GAP, et al. Locoregional failure during and after short-course radiotherapy followed by chemotherapy and surgery compared with long-course

chemoradiotherapy and surgery: a 5-Year Follow-up of the RAPIDO trial. Ann Surg 2023;278(4):e766–72.
[72] Conroy T, Bosset JF, Etienne PL, et al. Neoadjuvant chemotherapy with FOLFIRINOX and preoperative chemoradiotherapy for patients with locally advanced rectal cancer (UNI-CANCER-PRODIGE 23): a multicentre, randomised, open-label, phase 3 trial. Lancet Oncol 2021;22(5):702–15.
[73] Schrag D, Shi Q, Weiser MR, et al. Preoperative treatment of locally advanced rectal cancer. N Engl J Med 2023;389(4):322–34.
[74] Kasi A, Abbasi S, Handa S, et al. Total neoadjuvant therapy vs standard therapy in locally advanced rectal cancer: a systematic review and meta-analysis. JAMA Netw Open 2020;3(12):e2030097; https://doi.org/10.1001/jamanetworkopen.2020.30097.
[75] Turri G, Ostuzzi G, Vita G, et al. Treatment of locally advanced rectal cancer in the era of total neoadjuvant therapy: a systematic review and network meta-analysis. JAMA Netw Open 2024;7(6):e2414702; https://doi.org/10.1001/jamanetworkopen.2024.14702.

9780443472268